A Mental Healthcare Model for Mass Trauma Survivors

Control-Focused Behavioral Treatment of Earthquake, War, and Torture Trauma

A Mental Healthcare Model for Mass Trauma Survivors

Control-Focused Behavioral Treatment of Earthquake, War, and Torture Trauma

Metin Başoğlu and Ebru Şalcıoğlu

Trauma Studies, Department of Psychological Medicine, Institute of Psychiatry, King's College London & Istanbul Center for Behavior Research and Therapy

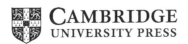

CAMBRIDGE
UNIVERSITY PRESS

CAMBRIDGE
UNIVERSITY PRESS

University Printing House, Cambridge CB2 8BS, United Kingdom

One Liberty Plaza, 20th Floor, New York, NY 10006, USA

477 Williamstown Road, Port Melbourne, VIC 3207, Australia

314-321, 3rd Floor, Plot 3, Splendor Forum, Jasola District Centre, New Delhi - 110025, India

79 Anson Road, #06-04/06, Singapore 079906

Cambridge University Press is part of the University of Cambridge.

It furthers the University's mission by disseminating knowledge in the pursuit of education, learning and research at the highest international levels of excellence.

www.cambridge.org
Information on this title: www.cambridge.org/9780521880008

First published 2011

A catalogue record for this publication is available from the British Library

ISBN 978-0-521-88000-8 Hardback

mesele esir düşmekte değil,
teslim olmamakta bütün mesele!

falling captive is not the problem,
the problem is not to surrender!

İşte Böyle Laz İsmail, Nazım Hikmet Ran, Yatar Bursa Kalesinde,
Yapı Kredi Yayınları, 2002, p. 170.

(Translated by Metin Başoğlu)

Contents

Preface

Despite significant advances in treatment of psychological trauma in the last two decades, current knowledge in this field falls short of addressing the care needs of millions of mass trauma survivors around the world, particularly in developing countries. Such a challenging task requires brief and effective treatments that can be cost-effectively disseminated to survivors through all possible means, including health professionals, lay therapists, self-help tools, and even mass media. None of the current trauma treatments are suitable for this purpose. Drawing on 20 years of research aimed at development of brief and effective interventions and cost-effective treatment dissemination methods, this book represents a visionary approach to this problem with recourse to sound theory and evidence.

With its broad scope, this book will be of interest to a wide readership. A learning theory formulation of earthquake, war, and torture trauma in Part 1 might be useful for researchers as well as care providers in understanding mechanisms of traumatic stress common to different types of trauma events. A sound theory-based understanding of mechanisms of traumatic stress is essential in choice of interventions likely to be useful in helping trauma survivors. In view of the fact that the evidence base of learning theory originated largely from experimental work with animals, evidence pertaining to human behavior in support of this theoretical model might be of interest to students of learning theory. Such evidence in relation to torture trauma might also be of interest to human rights workers and legal professionals because of its relevance to definitional issues surrounding torture and the controversy regarding the distinction between torture and cruel, inhuman, and degrading treatment.

In view of the urgent need for evidence-based interventions for mass trauma survivors, Part 2 provides a step-by-step description of brief assessment and behavioral treatment strategies for earthquake, war, and torture survivors developed in the course of our work. Part 3 provides a mental healthcare model for earthquake survivors based on brief and largely self-help interventions together with the tools needed for implementation of the model in earthquake-prone countries. These tools include various screening and assessment instruments and two manuals designed for cost-effective dissemination of treatment knowledge to professional and lay therapists as well as to survivors. As such, the book might be of interest to individual care providers, disaster relief organizations, psychosocial aid groups, as well as governments of countries at risk of earthquakes. Also presented is a critical review of various issues in care of mass trauma survivors in the light of evidence in support of a learning theory formulation of trauma.

The mental healthcare approach described in this book aims at empowerment of mass trauma survivors. Although the importance of empowerment in recovery from trauma is widely recognized among care providers, the rather broad, elusive, and ill-defined nature of the concept has somewhat limited its usefulness in clinical or fieldwork with mass trauma survivors. A learning theory approach to trauma sheds light on the nature of psychosocial interventions that are conducive to empowerment of survivors. As such, the interventions described in the book are likely to be of interest to all care providers who believe empowerment is the way forward in effective care of survivors.

Acknowledgments

Ebru Şalcıoğlu and I dedicate this book, a product of nearly 20 years of research, to our good friend Marianne Gerschel, President of Spunk Fund, Inc. and Spunk Foundation International. She has had the insight and vision to recognize the importance of scientific research for the human rights cause and effective care of mass trauma survivors. She started supporting our research on mental health effects of torture trauma in the early 1990s at a time when torture was widely perceived in the Western world as an esoteric issue confined to remote dictatorships and when few funders were cognizant of the importance of scientific research in this area. Ms. Gerschel's support also made possible the large multi-site research project on cognitive effects of war and torture trauma in former Yugoslavia. When the 1999 earthquake in Turkey occurred, she was again there to help us launch a research program that led to the development of brief treatments for earthquake survivors. We were fortunate to have her with us at every stage of our work, taking part in shaping research ideas and providing us with moral support in dealing with the trials and tribulations of running large projects. Although she is too modest to acknowledge it, the work reviewed in this book would not have been possible without her loyal support over the years.

We are also indebted to the Bromley Trust for their regular support for our work since the early 1990s. The late Mr. Keith Bromley's faith in the value of our work for the human rights cause has always been a source of inspiration for us. Together with Spunk Fund, Inc. and Spunk Foundation International, the Bromley Trust made possible much of our work, including this book.

We also appreciate Teresa Elwes' kind efforts to promote our work.

Part of our work with earthquake survivors between 2000 and 2003 was supported by CORDAID from the Netherlands. We are indebted to more than 60 colleagues internationally, who contributed to our work over the years. Special thanks are due to Maria Livanou, who made significant contributions to all aspects of our work. Her scientific and executive input as the International Projects Coordinator, together with the diligent work of our colleagues Cvetana Crnobarić, Tanja Frančišković, Enra Suljić, and Dijana Đurić as regional project coordinators and their hard-working teams made high-quality research possible in the difficult post-war circumstances of former Yugoslavia. Thanks are also due to Deniz Kalender and Gönül Acar for their part in running treatment studies with earthquake survivors in difficult post-disaster circumstances and Tamer Aker who contributed to our work with torture and earthquake survivors in Turkey. Special thanks are due to Susan Mineka for her major contribution to the 1992 book on torture regarding the parallels between the experimental models of anxiety/depression and human experience under torture. She provided us with valuable insights into learning theory, which inspired the work in this book. The first author also learned a great deal from Metin Özek and Isaac Marks during many years of work with them. Finally, we are grateful to all survivors of war, torture, and earthquake who participated in our studies and shared their experiences with us.

Introduction

Mass trauma events, such as wars, armed conflicts, acts of terror, political violence, torture, and natural disasters affect millions of people around the world. The 'New World Order' following the collapse of the Soviet Union has seen an escalation in political violence of all kinds around the globe and a 'war on terror' leading to the invasion of Iraq and Afghanistan by the United States and its allies. According to the Office of the United Nations High Commissioner for Refugees (UNHCR, 2009) figures, the number of forcibly displaced people in the world was 42 million at the end of 2008, including 15.2 million refugees, 827 000 asylum-seekers, and 26 million internally displaced people, 20% of whom were in industrialized countries. According to World Health Organization estimates (Van Ommeren et al., 2005), 20% of people exposed to mass trauma events develop post-traumatic stress disorder (PTSD). This suggests that 8.4 million war survivors worldwide (about 1.7 million in industrialized countries and 6.7 million in developing countries) are likely to need mental healthcare. These figures do not include non-displaced civilians exposed to various war events, political violence, or torture. Although reliable estimates of the prevalence of torture are not available, it is known to be systematically practiced in at least 81 countries (Amnesty International, 2009). Torture is known to be associated with long-term mental health consequences (Başoğlu et al., 2001; Campbell, 2007; Johnson & Thompson, 2008; Steel et al., 2009).

Among natural disasters earthquakes are a major contributor to the public health problem posed by mass trauma events. Over the 30 years between 1974 and 2003 a total of 660 earthquakes occurred worldwide which resulted in the death of 559 608 people and affected more than 82 million people (Guha-Sapir et al., 2004). Earthquakes make a disproportionate impact in developing countries (Guha-Sapir et al., 2004). Indeed, of all people killed by earthquakes worldwide in the last decade, more than 72% were in Asia (Guha-Sapir et al., 2004). Evidence (e.g. Armenian et al., 2000; Başoğlu et al., 2004b; Durkin, 1993; Lai et al., 2004; Önder et al., 2006; Wang et al., 2000) suggests that exposure to earthquakes is associated with increased psychiatric morbidity.

Currently there is no mental healthcare model that is capable of addressing the needs of millions of mass trauma survivors around the world, particularly the dispossessed populations of developing countries that often bear the brunt of these trauma events. Effective dealing with this problem requires interventions that are (1) *theoretically sound*, (2) *proven to be effective*, (3) *brief*, (4) *easy to train therapists in their delivery*, (5) *practicable in different cultures*, and (6) *suitable for dissemination through media other than professional therapists, such as lay people, self-help tools, and mass media*. Current treatments commonly used with trauma survivors do not meet more than two or three of these requirements. The last requirement is particularly important, as even the most effective treatment is of limited use if it cannot be widely disseminated to millions of people who may be in need of help.

Evolution of control-focused behavioral treatment

This book essentially tells the story of a nearly 20-year-long odyssey in search of a mental healthcare approach that satisfies the above requirements. Such a model requires a sound theoretical framework. In a previous book (Başoğlu, 1992) on *Torture and Its Consequences: Current Treatment Approaches*, we had examined the parallels between animal and human responses to unpredictable and uncontrollable stressors and presented a learning theory formulation of torture trauma (Başoğlu & Mineka, 1992) drawing on the work of Martin E. P. Seligman, Steve Maier, Bruce Overmier, Susan Mineka, and many other prominent learning theorists and anxiety researchers. As much of the evidence in support of this formulation had originated from experimental work with animals, its relevance to human experience was not entirely clear. Accordingly, we set out on a long journey to explore the parallels between animal and human experience under extreme duress and gather evidence pointing to the relevance of this formulation to humans. First, we conducted a series of three studies in Turkey between 1993 and 1999 to examine the role of unpredictable and uncontrollable stressors in psychological responses to torture. After the cessation of hostilities in former Yugoslavia countries we launched a 5-year multi-site research program in Bosnia-Herzegovina, Croatia, and Serbia to examine the same issue in 1358 survivors of war trauma, including combat, internal displacement, refugee experience, aerial bombardment, and torture. These studies provided ample evidence in support of a learning theory model of traumatic stress. Such evidence implied that traumatic stress can be reversed by interventions that enhance sense of control over (or resilience against) traumatic stressors. This hypothesis ultimately led to the development of Control-Focused Behavioral Treatment (CFBT).

The important role of sense of control in treatment of anxiety disorders is well known to anxiety researchers. Indeed, Barlow (2002) provided an excellent review of the work on this issue in his book on *Anxiety and its Disorders*. There have been few attempts, however, to develop a behavioral intervention specifically designed to enhance sense of control over or resilience against anxiety cues or traumatic stressors. Such an intervention needs to aim for anxiety tolerance and control rather than anxiety reduction. Indeed, in a recent review of the processes of change in exposure treatment, Craske et al. (2008) found no conclusive evidence to suggest an association between treatment outcome and the extent of fear reduction during and between sessions. Craske and Mystkowski (2006) suggested that "... *it is time to shift away from an emphasis on fear reduction during exposure therapy as an index of learning at the process level toward a model of exposure therapy that emphasizes ... weakening of avoidance and strengthening tolerance of aversive internal states and fear*" (pp. 233).

This is indeed what we have done in the 1990s in the light of findings from our studies pointing to the important role of sense of control in the development (Başoğlu et al., 1997) as well as treatment (Başoğlu et al., 1994a; Başoğlu et al., 1994b) of anxiety disorders. We shifted treatment focus from habituation to

enhancement of sense of control over anxiety cues and anxiety tolerance. For reasons detailed in Chapter 6, we thought such a paradigm change might enhance the efficacy of behavioral treatment. This not only led to important procedural changes in the application of exposure treatment but also a broader treatment focus including but not limited to avoidance behaviors. Hence, CFBT came into existence.

In 1999 a 7.4 magnitude earthquake struck the Marmara region of Turkey, killing more than 17 000 people and exposing millions of people to severe trauma. Until then much of our experience with behavioral treatment was limited to patients with anxiety disorders in clinical settings. Our knowledge on the development and course of traumatic stress reactions in naturalistic settings was rather limited. This disaster turned out to be a major milestone for our work in providing not only an opportunity to test CFBT more extensively but also valuable insights into natural processes of recovery from trauma. We learned a great deal by simply observing how people recover from traumatic stress without any help from a therapist. Having experienced the earthquake and the aftershocks ourselves, we also learned a great deal from our own experience.

In 1999 we established a research-driven treatment delivery project and conducted fieldwork with more than 10 000 survivors in 6 years. When we set out to test CFBT in the early days of the disaster, inundated by demands for help from thousands of survivors, we quickly realized that CFBT delivered in 8 to 10 sessions was too long for post-disaster circumstances. Furthermore, due to demographic mobility in the disaster region and day-to-day survival problems, many survivors were not able to attend treatment for more than one session. Therefore, we had no choice but to deliver treatment in a single session and hope for the best. Given that not much can be squeezed into a 60-minute session, treatment was limited to instructions for self-exposure to fear-evoking trauma cues presented with a treatment rationale designed to enhance sense of control over fear. Although we knew from previous experience that much of the improvement in anxiety disorders with exposure treatment occurs within the first few weeks after a few exposure sessions (Marks et al., 1988; Marks et al., 1993), we were not certain whether the survivors would comply with self-exposure instructions in a post-disaster setting without regular monitoring of progress. In the meantime we conducted research to examine treatment outcome.

To our own surprise, an open trial (Başoğlu et al., 2003b) showed that 80% of the cases improved after a single treatment session, which was confirmed by later randomized controlled studies (Başoğlu et al., 2005b; Başoğlu et al., 2007b). Thus, single-session CFBT came into being, proving once again that necessity is the mother of invention!

We then embarked on a search for an explanation for this somewhat serendipitous discovery. Examining how survivors coped with debilitating fear of earthquakes, we discovered that many survivors, without any instructions or guidance from a mental health professional, used self-exposure in their natural environment to overcome their fear of earthquakes. This discovery was an eye opener for us in several ways. Most importantly, it suggested that self-help is not only a viable approach in survivor care but also one that carries great potential. This may not be surprising from an evolutionary point of view, considering that trauma is as old as human history and our survival could not have been possible without the secret key to trauma recovery coded in our genes. Second, it pointed to live exposure as the most potent therapeutic ingredient in behavioral treatment, thereby justifying the sharp focus of CFBT on anxiety cues and avoidance behaviors, excluding cognitive restructuring and other anxiety management strategies that characterize traditional cognitive-behavioral treatments. Furthermore, it made us realize that CFBT simply provides a motivational impetus for a naturally existing tendency in people to use self-exposure as a means of overcoming trauma-induced helplessness. In a sense the intervention merely imitated a key natural recovery process in humans. With such insight, we set out to search for other evidence pointing to exposure as an evolutionarily determined process in recovery from trauma. Indeed, such evidence eventually helped us conceive a self-help model of mental healthcare for survivors. This model incorporates several variants of CFBT, which were developed and routinely used with good results in more than 6000 earthquake survivors. Based on this experience we also developed tools designed to facilitate cost-effective dissemination of treatment knowledge to care providers as well as to survivors themselves.

This book brings together the knowledge and experience gained through two decades of work with torture, war, and earthquake survivors. Despite its broader scope, it could be regarded as a sequel to the 1992 book on torture (Başoğlu, 1992) in the sense that the hypotheses generated by a learning theory formulation of torture in the latter guided the entire research presented in this book. Although the book may appear to concern different trauma events, its focus is on mechanisms of traumatic stress and recovery common to all forms of trauma, whether of human design or due to natural causes. As such, it is designed to facilitate understanding of traumas of an apparently different nature around a unifying theory and how they may respond to brief behavioral interventions that closely match their underlying mechanisms of traumatic stress. As research guided by learning theory focuses on universals in animal and human behavior under duress, its findings cut across not only species but also cultures. This is an important point to bear in mind in evaluating the cross-cultural applicability of the findings reviewed in this book.

In view of the fact that CFBT is an exposure-based treatment, evidence of its efficacy reviewed in this book needs to be considered in the broader context of the robust evidence base for other exposure-based treatments (reviewed in American Psychiatric Association, 2004; National Institute of Clinical Excellence, 2005). We were initially reluctant to give it a different name to avoid cluttering the literature with yet another label for exposure-based treatments. However, considering the rather radical departure from habituation paradigm to anxiety tolerance and control and various procedural differences that distinguish it from traditional exposure treatment, Control-Focused Behavioral Treatment appeared to be an appropriate name for this intervention. We do not contend that it is an entirely novel intervention and it might well be regarded as a streamlined, simplified, and enhanced version of traditional behavioral treatment.

Evidence base

In this book we review findings from more than 20 studies that contributed to the development of CFBT and a mental healthcare model based on this intervention. As we refer to these studies throughout the book, their methodology is briefly summarized in Table 1, Table 2, and Table 3 to facilitate evaluation of their findings. These tables also provide some idea about the evidence base for CFBT. As part of the work covered in the book has already been published, some findings may be familiar to the reader. Nevertheless, as this is the first time we present our work in its entirety together with a detailed account of its theoretical

Table 1 Studies of survivors of torture, war, and earthquake with similar methodology

	Study	Trauma	Sample type	Sample size	Sampling method	Time since trauma (months)	Measures Assessor-rated	Measures Self-rated
1	Başoğlu, 2009; Başoğlu et al., 1997; Başoğlu et al., 1994c	Torture	Mixed group of political activists and non-activists	202	Consecutive referrals from human rights organizations and cases accessed using snowballing method in Istanbul, Turkey	44	SIST SCID CAPS	BDI
2	Başoğlu et al., 2007a	Torture	Veterans and civilian survivors of war	230[1]	Target sampling from two associations for war veterans and prisoners of war in Belgrade (Serbia), collective camps in Rijeka (Croatia), and community in Banja Luka (Republic of Srpska) and Sarajevo (Bosnia–Herzegovina)	95	SIST SCID CAPS RTSQ	SITSOW BDI DRS EBAW
3	Başoğlu et al., 2005a	War	Veterans, refugees, and internally displaced civilian survivors of war	1079	Cross-sectional survey through target sampling in Belgrade (Serbia), Rijeka (Croatia), Sarajevo (Bosnia-Herzegovina), and Banja Luka (Republic of Srpska)	77	SISOW SCID CAPS	SITSOW BDI DRS
4	Şalcıoğlu, 2004	Earthquake	Survivors in the community	387	Target sampling in the community (n =188) and among self-referrals for treatment (n = 199)	22	SISE SCID CAPS RTSQ	SITSES BDI FAQ EBAT

BDI = Beck Depression Inventory, DRS = Depression Rating Scale, CAPS = Clinician's Administered PTSD Scale, EBAT = Emotion and Beliefs after Trauma, EBAW = Emotions and Beliefs after War, FAQ = Fear and Avoidance Questionnaire, RTSQ = Redress for Trauma Survivors Questionnaire, SCID = Structured Clinical Interview for DSM-III-R/DSM-IV Disorders, SISE = Structured Interview for Survivors of Earthquake, SISOW = Structured Interview for Survivors of War, SIST = Structured Interview for Survivors of Torture, SITSES = Screening Instrument for Traumatic Stress in Earthquake Survivors, SITSOW = Screening Instrument for Traumatic Stress in War Survivors.
[1] In the original study the sample size was reported as 279, including 49 survivors whose psychological assessment was conducted in relation to a war stressor other than torture. The latter cases are excluded in the analyses reported in this book.

Table 2 Field surveys with earthquake survivors (N = 4332)

Study	n	Sampling method	Time since earthquake (months)	Measures
Başoğlu et al., 2002	1000	Consecutive screening in 5 survivor camps	10	SITSES
Başoğlu et al., 2004b	950	Random community sampling	14	SITSES, FAQ
Şalcıoğlu et al., 2003	586	Consecutive screening in 3 survivor camps	20	SITSES, FAQ
Şalcıoğlu et al., 2007	769	Consecutive screening among resettled homeless survivors	40	SITSES, FAQ
Livanou et al., 2002	1027	Consecutive self-referrals for treatment	14	SITSES

SITSES = Screening Instrument for Traumatic Stress in Earthquake Survivors, FAQ = Fear and Avoidance Questionnaire.

Table 3 Treatment studies

	Trauma	n	Treatment
Randomized controlled trials			
Başoğlu et al., 2005b	Earthquake	59	Single session CFBT
Başoğlu et al., 2007b	Earthquake	31	Earthquake Simulation Treatment + Single-session CFBT
Open trials			
Başoğlu et al., 2003b	Earthquake	231	Full-course CFBT
Başoğlu et al., 2003a	Earthquake	10	Earthquake Simulation Treatment
Şalcıoğlu & Başoğlu, 2008	Earthquake	23	Full-course CFBT with children
Şalcıoğlu & Başoğlu, 2008	Earthquake	8	Earthquake Simulation Treatment with children
Başoğlu & Şalcıoğlu, this volume	Earthquake	84	Self-help manual
Case studies			
Başoğlu & Aker, 1996	Torture	1	Exposure Treatment
Başoğlu et al., 2004a	Torture	1	Exposure Treatment
Başoğlu et al., 2009	Earthquake	8	Self-help manual
Başoğlu & Şalcıoğlu, this volume	War and torture	2	Full-course CFBT
Başoğlu & Şalcıoğlu, this volume	Earthquake	2	Full-course CFBT of prolonged grief

CFBT = Control-Focused Behavioral Treatment.

framework, the book might provide an opportunity to re-evaluate previously published findings around a unifying theory. We also present some previously unpublished findings based on pooled samples from previous studies. Table 1 shows the studies that examined mechanisms of traumatic stress in torture, war, and earthquake survivors using similar methodology.

The first study is a series of three consecutive studies designed to examine mechanisms of traumatic stress in torture survivors. A substantial part of the empirical evidence relating to mechanisms of traumatic stress in earthquake survivors originated from a study by Şalcıoğlu (2004). Table 2 shows the field surveys that examined PTSD prevalence and symptom profile and the risk factors for traumatic stress in earthquake survivors. Table 3 lists the treatment studies with torture and earthquake survivors. Other studies that examined psychometric properties of various questionnaires for assessment of earthquake, war, and torture trauma are reviewed in Chapter 3 and Chapter 5.

Preview of contents

Part 1 – theory

Chapter 1 presents a learning theory model of traumatic stress and some evidence in support of the model. It reviews the role of unpredictable and uncontrollable stressors in earthquake-related traumatic stress, cognitive and behavioral responses to earthquakes, natural recovery processes in earthquake survivors, and possible evolutionary processes that determine psychological responses to earthquake trauma. In addition, some research data are presented in support of the helplessness and hopelessness effects of earthquakes.

Chapter 2 is an updated version of a previous chapter (Başoğlu & Mineka, 1992) on the role of uncontrollable and unpredictable stressors in torture-induced traumatic stress, which appeared in our 1992 book on torture (Başoğlu, 1992). It presents a learning theory account of captivity, interrogation, and torture experiences and provides empirical evidence in support of this formulation. Also reviewed are various cognitive and behavioral coping responses during and after torture, the role of resilience and context of captivity in torture-induced distress, natural recovery processes in the post-captivity phase, and the role of cognitive factors in war and torture trauma.

Part 2 – assessment and treatment

Chapter 3 provides an assessment strategy for screening of mass trauma survivors and evaluation of intervention outcomes. The assessment instruments developed for this purpose are provided in Appendix A. We have also provided guidelines in determining treatment needs of survivors and priorities in treatment planning on the basis of data obtained using these instruments.

Chapter 4 includes a detailed description of CFBT as it would be delivered to war, torture, or earthquake survivors in a clinical or fieldwork setting. The treatment is described in a step by step how-to-do-it fashion with some case vignettes to facilitate understanding of various issues in behavioral assessment and treatment. The chapter includes a description of various

applications of CFBT in earthquake survivors, such as treatment of children, delivery of single-session CFBT individually and in groups, and using an earthquake simulator.

Chapter 5 details behavioral assessment of grief using two questionnaires developed for this purpose and describes application of CFBT in cases with prolonged grief problems. Case vignettes are provided, along with a discussion of various issues in treatment. Also presented are some evidence of treatment effectiveness from our studies and a comparison of CFBT with other treatments of prolonged grief.

Chapter 6 reviews the evidence from treatment studies that tested CFBT. This chapter is informative in demonstrating the developmental stages for CFBT and the various theoretical and practical considerations that went into development of its various applications, such as single-session CFBT, Earthquake Simulation Treatment, and self-administered CFBT. It also includes a discussion of mechanisms of improvement in CFBT (e.g. habituation versus increased sense of control) and available evidence pointing to the role of sense of control in recovery from traumatic stress. Also reviewed are various theoretical and procedural features of CFBT that distinguish it from other exposure treatments.

Part 3 – implications for care of mass trauma survivors

Chapter 7 reviews the implications of our work for a cost-effective mental healthcare model for earthquake survivors. The chapter is organized into three sections. The first section details a three-stage outreach treatment delivery program designed to deliver care to as many survivors as possible with minimal therapist involvement by utilizing single-session applications of CFBT and self-help tools. The second section reviews prospects for alternative methods of treatment dissemination through lay therapists, a self-help manual, and mass media. The third section outlines a mental healthcare model for earthquake survivors that incorporates all possible treatment dissemination methods and reviews procedures that need to be undertaken in pre- and post-disaster phases for large-scale implementation of the model in earthquake-prone countries.

Chapter 8 reviews the implications of our work for various issues concerning care of mass trauma survivors, including generally accepted guidelines regarding aims, levels, focus, and timing of interventions and the role of antidepressants in treatment of trauma survivors. This chapter casts a critical look at the current status of knowledge in trauma treatment, mental healthcare policies for mass trauma survivors, and the controversy that surrounds the concept of PTSD in the light of evidence from our work.

Chapter 9 reviews various controversial issues in rehabilitation of war and torture survivors, including the effectiveness of and justification for current lengthy and costly torture rehabilitation programs. As it is widely believed that torture is more severe than natural disaster trauma and therefore more difficult to treat, some comparative data from our studies testing this hypothesis are presented. Also included are two recent case studies of CFBT, which point to prospects for brief treatment of tortured asylum-seekers and refugees. Finally, the possible reasons for lack of progress in the field of torture rehabilitation are reviewed with some recommendations for effective rehabilitation of war and torture survivors.

Appendices: assessment instruments and treatment manuals

Appendix A provides various assessment instruments that might be of use to care providers in screening survivors for treatment needs and evaluation of intervention outcomes. These include the adult and child versions of the *Screening Instrument for Traumatic Stress in Earthquake Survivors, Fear and Avoidance Questionnaire, Depression Rating Scale, Screening Instrument for Traumatic Stress in War Survivors, Grief Assessment Scale, Behavior Checklist for Grief, Work and Adjustment Scale, Global Improvement Scale*, and *Sense of Control Scale*. Available psychometric data on as yet unpublished instruments are provided in Chapter 3 and Chapter 5. These instruments can be freely translated and used in their present form without permission from the publishers or the authors and with due reference to the authors in any publications based on them.

Appendix B includes a CFBT Delivery Manual (*Helping People Recover from Earthquake Trauma*), which is designed to assist health professionals (mental healthcare providers, general practitioners, nurses, social workers, etc.), as well as lay people with an adequate educational background in delivering CFBT to survivors. It is highly structured to provide step by step guidance in assessment and treatment. It also includes sections on treatment of children, delivery of treatment in a single session, and assessment and treatment of prolonged grief.

Appendix C includes a self-help manual (*Recovering from Earthquake Trauma*) designed to help earthquake survivors in administering CFBT by themselves. It is also highly structured to guide users at every stage of assessment and treatment. It includes sections on assessment, explanation of treatment and its rationale, overcoming earthquake-related fear and distress, evaluation of treatment progress, treating prolonged grief, and dealing with problems in treatment. This manual can be used after an initial assessment by a therapist or as a stand-alone tool with minimal or no therapist contact.

These manuals are prepared in the understanding that post-disaster circumstances, particularly in developing country settings, require psychological care dissemination to survivors in every way possible. It is worth noting here that while we piloted the self-help manual and used it in routine treatment delivery we did not yet have a chance to test the usefulness of the CFBT Delivery Manual in guiding lay therapists in delivery of the intervention. This is because we prepared this manual towards the end of the project in Turkey after we accumulated sufficient experience and observations (reviewed in Chapter 7) that made us think that such a manual may be a useful tool in treatment dissemination. Nevertheless, we decided to make the manual available so that it can be tested and used by others. At the very least it may be useful in disseminating treatment knowledge to mental health professionals involved in care of earthquake survivors. Considering the highly structured nature of the manual, it might perhaps be helpful in delivering the intervention without extensive prior training in CFBT, though this remains to be tested.

References

American Psychiatric Association (2004). *Practice Guideline for the Treatment of Patients with Acute Stress Disorder and Posttraumatic Stress Disorder*, Arlington, VA: American Psychiatric Association Practice Guidelines.

Amnesty International (2009). *Amnesty International Report 2009: The State of the World's Human Rights*. Accessed on May 10, 2010 at http://thereport.amnesty.org/.

Armenian, H. K., Morikawa, M., Melkonian, A. K., Hovanesian, A. P., Haroutunian, N., Saigh, P. A., Akiskal, K. and Akiskal, H. S. (2000). Loss as a determinant of PTSD in a cohort of adult survivors of the 1988 earthquake in Armenia: Implications for policy. *Acta Psychiatrica Scandinavica*, **102**, 58–64.

Barlow, D. H. (2002). *Anxiety and its Disorders: The Nature and Treatment of Anxiety and Panic*. New York: Guilford Press.

Başoğlu, M. (1992). *Torture and its Consequences: Current Treatment Approaches*. Cambridge: Cambridge University Press.

Başoğlu, M. (2009). A multivariate contextual analysis of torture and cruel, inhuman, and degrading treatments: Implications for an evidence-based definition of torture. *American Journal of Orthopsychiatry*, **79**, 135–145.

Başoğlu, M. and Aker, T. (1996). Cognitive-behavioural treatment of torture survivors: A case study. *Torture*, **6**, 61–65.

Başoğlu, M., Ekblad, S., Bäärnhielm, S. and Livanou, M. (2004a). Cognitive-behavioral treatment of tortured asylum seekers: A case study. *Journal of Anxiety Disorders*, **18**, 357–369.

Başoğlu, M., Jaranson, J. M., Mollica, R. F. and Kastrup, M. (2001). Torture and mental health: a research overview. In *The Mental Health Consequences of Torture*, ed. E. Gerrity, T. M. Keane and F. Tuma. Kluwer Academic / Plenum Publishers, 35–62.

Başoğlu, M., Kılıç, C., Şalcıoğlu, E. and Livanou, M. (2004b). Prevalence of posttraumatic stress disorder and comorbid depression in earthquake survivors in Turkey: An epidemiological study. *Journal of Traumatic Stress*, **17**, 133–141.

Başoğlu, M., Livanou, M. and Crnobarić, C. (2007a). Torture vs other cruel, inhuman, and degrading treatment: Is the distinction real or apparent? *Archives of General Psychiatry*, **64**, 277–285.

Başoğlu, M., Livanou, M., Crnobarić, C., Frančišković, T., Suljić, E., Đurić, D. and Vranešić, M. (2005a). Psychiatric and cognitive effects of war in former Yugoslavia: Association of lack of redress for trauma and posttraumatic stress reactions. *Journal of the American Medical Association*, **294**, 580–590.

Başoğlu, M., Livanou, M. and Şalcıoğlu, E. (2003a). A single session with an earthquake simulator for traumatic stress in earthquake survivors. *American Journal of Psychiatry*, **160**, 788–790.

Başoğlu, M., Livanou, M., Şalcıoğlu, E. and Kalender, D. (2003b). A brief behavioural treatment of chronic post-traumatic stress disorder in earthquake survivors: Results from an open clinical trial. *Psychological Medicine*, **33**, 647–654.

Başoğlu, M., Marks, I. M., Kılıç, C., Brewin, C. R. and Swinson, R. P. (1994a). Alprazolam and exposure for panic disorder with agoraphobia: Attribution of

improvement to medication predicts subsequent relapse. *British Journal of Psychiatry*, **164**, 652–659.

Başoğlu, M., Marks, I. M., Kılıç, C., Swinson, R. P., Noshirvani, H., Kuch, K. and O'Sullivan, G. (1994b). Relationship of panic, anticipatory anxiety, agoraphobia and global improvement in panic disorder with agoraphobia treated with alprazolam and exposure. *British Journal of Psychiatry*, **164**, 647–652.

Başoğlu, M. and Mineka, S. (1992). The role of uncontrollable and unpredictable stress in post-traumatic stress responses in torture survivors. In *Torture and its Consequences: Current Treatment Approaches*, ed. M. Başoğlu. Cambridge: Cambridge University Press, 182–225.

Başoğlu, M., Mineka, S., Paker, M., Aker, T., Livanou, M. and Gök, S. (1997). Psychological preparedness for trauma as a protective factor in survivors of torture. *Psychological Medicine*, **27**, 1421–1433.

Başoğlu, M., Paker, M., Paker, O., Özmen, E., Marks, I., İncesu, C., Şahin, D. and Sarımurat, N. (1994c). Psychological effects of torture: A comparison of tortured with nontortured political activists in Turkey. *American Journal of Psychiatry*, **151**, 76–81.

Başoğlu, M., Şalcıoğlu, E. and Livanou, M. (2002). Traumatic stress responses in earthquake survivors in Turkey. *Journal of Traumatic Stress*, **15**, 269–276.

Başoğlu, M., Şalcıoğlu, E. and Livanou, M. (2007b). A randomized controlled study of single-session behavioural treatment of earthquake-related post-traumatic stress disorder using an earthquake simulator. *Psychological Medicine*, **37**, 203–213.

Başoğlu, M., Şalcıoğlu, E. and Livanou, M. (2009). Single-case experimental studies of a self-help manual for traumatic stress in earthquake survivors. *Journal of Behavior Therapy and Experimental Psychiatry*, **40**, 50–58.

Başoğlu, M., Şalcıoğlu, E., Livanou, M., Kalender, D. and Acar, G. (2005b). Single-session behavioral treatment of earthquake-related posttraumatic stress disorder: A randomized waiting list controlled trial. *Journal of Traumatic Stress*, **18**, 1–11.

Campbell, T. A. (2007). Psychological assessment, diagnosis, and treatment of torture survivors: A review. *Clinical Psychology Review*, **27**, 628–641.

Craske, M. and Mystkowski, J. L. (2006). Exposure therapy and extinction: Clinical studies. In *Fear and Learning: From Basic Principles to Clinical Implications*, ed. M. G. Craske, D. Hermans and D. Vansteenwegen. Washington, DC: American Psychological Association, 217–233.

Craske, M. G., Kircanski, K., Zelikowsky, M., Mystkowski, J., Chowdhury, N. and Baker, A. (2008). Optimizing inhibitory learning during exposure therapy. *Behaviour Research and Therapy*, **46**, 5–27.

Durkin, M. E. (1993). Major depression and post-traumatic stress disorder following the Coalinga and Chile earthquakes: A cross-cultural comparison. *Journal of Social Behavior and Personality*, **8**, 405–420.

Guha-Sapir, D., Hargitt, D. and Hoyois, P. (2004). *Thirty years of natural disasters 1974–2003: the numbers.* Centre for Research on the Epidemiology of Disasters, UCL Presses, Universitaires de Louvain.

Johnson, H. and Thompson, A. (2008). The development and maintenance of post-traumatic stress disorder (PTSD) in civilian adult survivors of war trauma and torture: A review. *Clinical Psychology Review*, **28**, 36–47.

Lai, T.-J., Chang, C.-M., Connor, K. M., Lee, L.-C. and Davidson, J. R. T. (2004). Full and partial PTSD among earthquake survivors in rural Taiwan. *Journal of Psychiatric Research*, **38**, 313–322.

Livanou, M., Başoğlu, M., Şalcıoğlu, E. and Kalender, D. (2002). Traumatic stress responses in treatment-seeking earthquake survivors in Turkey. *Journal of Nervous and Mental Disease*, **190**, 816–823.

Marks, I. M., Lelliott, P., Başoğlu, M., Noshirvani, H., Monteiro, W., Cohen, D. and Kasvikis, Y. (1988). Clomipramine, self-exposure and therapist-aided exposure for obsessive-compulsive rituals. *British Journal of Psychiatry*, **152**, 522–534.

Marks, I. M., Swinson, R. P., Başoğlu, M., Kuch, K., Noshirvani, H., O'Sullivan, G., Lelliott, P. T., Kirby, M., McNamee, G. and Şengün, S. (1993). Alprazolam and exposure alone and combined in panic disorder with agoraphobia: A controlled study in London and Toronto. *British Journal of Psychiatry*, **162**, 776–787.

National Institute of Clinical Excellence (NICE) (2005). *Posttraumatic Stress Disorder (PTSD): The Management of PTSD in Adults and Children in Primary and Secondary Care.* London: Gaskel and the British Psychological Society.

Önder, E., Tural, Ü., Aker, T., Kılıç, C. and Erdoğan, S. (2006). Prevalence of psychiatric disorders three years after the 1999 earthquake in Turkey: Marmara Earthquake Survey (MES). *Social Psychiatry and Psychiatric Epidemiology*, **41**, 868–874.

Şalcıoğlu, E. (2004). *The effect of beliefs, attribution of responsibility, redress and compensation on posttraumatic stress disorder in earthquake survivors in Turkey.* PhD Dissertation. Institute of Psychiatry, King's College London, London.

Şalcıoğlu, E. and Başoğlu, M. (2008). Psychological effects of earthquakes in children: Prospects for brief behavioral treatment. *World Journal of Pediatrics*, **4**, 165–172.

Şalcıoğlu, E., Başoğlu, M. and Livanou, M. (2003). Long-term psychological outcome for non-treatment-seeking earthquake survivors in Turkey. *Journal of Nervous and Mental Disease*, **191**, 154–160.

Şalcıoğlu, E., Başoğlu, M. and Livanou, M. (2007). Post-traumatic stress disorder and comorbid depression among survivors of the 1999 earthquake in Turkey. *Disasters*, **31**, 115–129.

Steel, Z., Chey, T., Silove, D., Marnane, C., Bryant, R. A. and Van Ommeren, M. (2009). Association of torture and other potentially traumatic events with mental health outcomes among populations exposed to mass conflict and displacement: A systematic review and meta-analysis. *Journal of the American Medical Association*, **302**, 537–549.

United Nations High Commissioner for Refugees (UNHCR) (2009) 2008 Global Trends: Refugees, Asylum Seekers, Returnees, Internally Displaced and Stateless Persons.

Van Ommeren, M., Saxena, S. and Saraceno, B. (2005). Aid after disasters. *British Medical Journal*, **330**, 1160–1161.

Wang, X., Gao, L., Shinfuku, N., Zhang, H., Zhao, C. and Shen, Y. (2000). Longitudinal study of earthquake-related PTSD in a randomly selected community sample in North China. *American Journal of Psychiatry*, **157**, 1260–1266.

A learning theory formulation of earthquake trauma

Since the 1960s substantial experimental work with animals suggested that unpredictable and uncontrollable stressors play an important role in the development of anxiety and fear. Exposure to unpredictable and uncontrollable stressors is associated with certain associative, motivational, and emotional deficits in animals that closely resemble the effects of traumatic stress in humans (Mineka and Zinbarg, 2006). These deficits include learned helplessness, a phenomenon characterized by failure of animals initially exposed to uncontrollable shocks to later learn to escape or avoid shocks that were potentially controllable in a different situation (Overmier and Seligman, 1967; Seligman and Maier, 1967), and opiate-mediated analgesia (Maier et al., 1982; Maier et al., 1983). As detailed reviews of findings from experimental animal studies and their relevance to anxiety disorders are available elsewhere (Başoğlu and Mineka, 1992; Foa et al., 1992; Mineka and Zinbarg, 2006), such a review will not be attempted here. While much of the evidence concerning the role of unpredictable and uncontrollable stressors in anxiety is based on animals, evidence that emerged in the last two decades points to close parallels between animal and human responses to such stressors. In this chapter we present a learning theory model of traumatic stress and review the role of unpredictability and uncontrollability of stressors in the development of traumatic stress responses in people exposed to earthquakes. We also discuss various cognitive and behavioral responses to such stressors, which provide remarkable examples of how humans cope with unpredictable and uncontrollable stressors and recover from their effects. Finally, we present some data from our studies of earthquake survivors in support of the model.

A learning theory model of traumatic stress

Figure 1.1 illustrates how various factors or processes before, during, and after trauma lead to various post-trauma health outcomes. The model essentially reflects what we know about evolutionarily determined responses to life-threatening events in animals and humans. Animals have innate species-specific defense reactions against threatening events, such as fight, flight, or freezing (Bolles, 1970). Accordingly, during trauma exposure the model entails two types of stressor response sequences (or pathways) that broadly reflect fight and flight responses. Fight responses in humans involve various proactive cognitive, behavioral, and emotional responses aimed at removing the threat, minimizing its adverse effects, or reducing the distress associated with it. Flight responses (e.g. escape from the dangerous situation), on the other hand, are essentially avoidance processes aimed at self-protection (Bolles, 1970).

Appraisal of controllability of a threatening event determines whether a person engages in fight or flight responses. If the individual has not had previous learning of control over negative outcomes of stressor events, the event is perceived as uncontrollable, leading to flight responses. Loss of cognitive, behavioral, or emotional control over the event (e.g. inability to escape from the situation, avoid the occurrence of the event, or reduce its impact) is associated with distress, fear, or panic. Such loss of control confirms the uncontrollability of the stressor event and leads to a state of helplessness or anxiety with respect to possible future occurrences of the event. According to Alloy and colleagues (1990), individuals who are uncertain about their ability to control outcomes of future stressor events

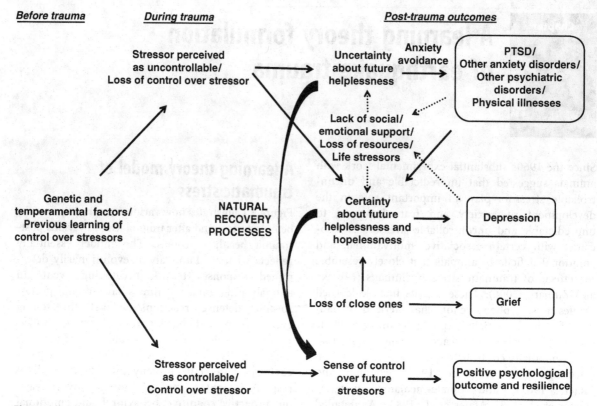

Figure 1.1 A learning theory model of traumatic stress.

are more likely to experience anxiety, whereas those who are more certain about their helplessness but still uncertain about whether a negative outcome will actually occur are likely to develop a mixed anxiety-depressive state. On the other hand, those who are certain of both their helplessness and the occurrence of negative outcomes are likely to develop hopelessness depression. In situations that involve multiple stressor events (e.g. recurring earthquakes, war violence, combat, political persecution, torture, etc.), future occurrences of the traumatic stressors may reinforce the learned helplessness effects of the initial event and may lead to more certain helplessness and even hopelessness. Several other factors may contribute to depression by increasing certainty about helplessness and hopelessness. These include uncontrollable stressor effects of various PTSD symptoms, such as intrusive thoughts, flashbacks, nightmares, etc. (Alloy et al., 1990), and additional uncontrollable life stressors caused by functional impairment secondary to PTSD symptoms (e.g. inability to find employment

due to severe behavioral avoidance, memory / concentration difficulties or serious family discord due to problems of irritability / anger outbursts, etc.) or other psychiatric / medical problems. In situations that involve a single traumatic event, certainty about helplessness and hopelessness may be enhanced by failed attempts at achieving control over re-experiencing symptoms of PTSD and / or overestimated probability of the same event occurring in the future. Learned helplessness might be facilitated by a pessimistic attributional style characterized by attributions of negative outcomes to internal, stable, and global causes (Abramson et al., 1978). Thus, the extent of certainty about the occurrence of future negative outcomes and helplessness are the two critical factors in anxiety and depression. While uncertainty about helplessness with respect to future threats is associated with anxiety, loss events are more likely to lead to hopelessness and depression (see Mineka et al., 1998 for a more detailed discussion of helplessness / hopelessness perspective in anxiety / depression).

Turning to the second pathway in Figure 1.1, if the individual has had previous learning of control over stressor events or the important aspects of their environment, they can utilize effective control strategies to secure safety (e.g. by removing or warding off threat), reduce the impact of the event if it cannot be avoided, and gain control over fear evoked by the stressor. Effective control might be achieved on cognitive, behavioral, or emotional levels. Such control often reduces anxiety or fear during exposure to the stressor event, facilitates recovery from the acute impact of trauma, and reinforces expectancies of control over future stressor events. Achieving effective control over stressor events also has protective or immunizing effects against future uncontrollable stressors (Hannum et al., 1976; Seligman and Maier, 1967; Williams and Maier, 1977).

The third pathway in Figure 1.1 represents *natural recovery processes* in trauma survivors. These processes involve various cognitive and behavioral control strategies that are utilized to reduce helplessness anxiety and hopelessness depression during both the trauma phase involving exposures to multiple ongoing stressor events and post-trauma phase. Recovery is likely to the extent that these strategies are effective in reducing helplessness and hopelessness. The model thus proposes an explanation as to why some people show 'spontaneous recovery' from traumatic stress, while others develop chronic traumatic stress. This issue will be clearer as we detail the various cognitive and behavioral control strategies most commonly employed by survivors and how they relate to natural recovery later in this chapter.

Mental and physical health outcomes of trauma exposure

Figure 1.1 shows an association between helplessness anxiety and various health outcomes of trauma exposure. These may include various psychiatric conditions (e.g. PTSD, other anxiety disorders, depression and suicide, substance abuse, psychotic illnesses, etc.) and physical health problems (e.g. cardiovascular disorders, psychosomatic illnesses, immune system disorders, etc.). In surveys that employed structured clinical interview forms for assessment of psychiatric disorders, PTSD and depression were the most common psychiatric outcomes of exposure to mass trauma events, including wars (Başoğlu et al., 2005; de Jong et al., 2003; Laban et al., 2004; Priebe et al., 2010; Steel

et al., 2002), torture (Başoğlu et al., 1994b; Van Ommeren et al., 2001), and natural disasters (Chou et al., 2005; Lai et al., 2004; McMillen et al., 2000; McMillen et al., 2002; Önder et al., 2006). In a study (Şalcıoğlu, 2004, see Table 1 in Introduction for methodological details) of 387 earthquake survivors that used structured interviews to assess all psychiatric disorders, while PTSD was the most common outcome (present in 41% of the cases), anxiety disorders other than PTSD were also quite common, at least one anxiety disorder occurring in 47% of treatment seekers and in 24% of non-treatment seekers. The rates of all other diagnoses (mood disorders other than depression, somatoform disorders, substance abuse / dependence disorders, adjustment disorder, and eating disorders) were 25% (less than 6% for each condition) among treatment seekers and 17% (less than 4% for each condition) among non-treatment-seekers.

The model could explain increased rates of suicidal ideas or acts among trauma survivors as a helplessness and hopelessness response to unpredictable and uncontrollable stressors. Indeed, studies (Chou et al., 2003; Yang et al., 2005) show an association between greater exposure to earthquake stressors and PTSD, depression, and increased suicide risk. In addition, analyses of pooled samples from our five surveys altogether (Başoğlu et al., 2002; Başoğlu et al., 2004; Livanou et al., 2002; Şalcıoğlu et al., 2003; Şalcıoğlu et al., 2007) involving 4299 earthquake survivors revealed a strong association between PTSD and suicidal ideas, the latter reported by 20.4% of survivors with PTSD, as opposed to 2.7% of the survivors without PTSD (p < 0.001). Survivors with depression had also higher rates of suicidal ideas than those without depression (27% versus 2.8%, respectively, p < 0.001). These findings lend support to an association between suicidal ideas and helplessness anxiety and hopelessness depression.

The effects of stress on physical health are well known. There are reports of an association between traumatic stress after earthquakes and increased blood pressure (Kario et al., 1997; Kario et al., 2001; Minami et al., 1997; Saito et al., 1997), myocardial infarction (Leor and Kloner, 1996; Suzuki et al., 1997; Tsai et al., 2004), deaths due to coronary heart disease (Kloner et al., 1997; Leor et al., 1996; Ogawa et al., 2000; Trichopoulos et al., 1983), increase in blood glucose levels in diabetic people (Inui et al., 1998), cerebrovascular stroke (Sokejima et al., 2004), increased incidence of gastric ulcer and bleeding ulcer (Aoyama et al., 1998;

Matsushima et al., 1999), and immune system dysregulation (Inoue-Sakurai et al., 2000; Segerstrom et al., 1998; Solomon et al., 1997). Furthermore, experimental studies show that perceived controllability of stressors is critical in modulating immune functioning in animals (Fleshner et al., 1998; Laudenslager et al., 1983) and in humans (Peters et al., 1999; Sieber et al., 1992).

Other factors contributing to traumatic stress reactions

The model includes lack of social / emotional support, loss of resources, and trauma-related or unrelated life stressors as mediating factors for all post-trauma health outcomes. Because of insufficient evidence regarding the role of these factors in particular post-trauma outcomes, these variables are included in the model only tentatively (hence the dotted arrows). Whether these mediating factors relate to all post-trauma outcomes or differentially to individual outcomes is not clear. Of particular interest is how these factors relate PTSD and depression as the two most common outcomes of trauma exposure. It is worth briefly reviewing the available evidence in this regard.

The association between stressful life events and depression is well documented in the life events literature (Tennant, 2002). This association may be mediated by the impact of additional stressor events on hopelessness. Impaired functioning resulting from debilitating traumatic stress may severely limit one's capacity to cope with stressful life events, which in turn may further undermine expectations of effective control over such events in general and contribute to hopelessness depression.

Loss of resources refer to loss of material possessions, employment, social status, employment / business / educational opportunities, ability to make future plans, access to health services, and lowered standard of life. Methodological issues in studies of the role of resource loss in post-trauma outcome preclude definitive conclusions. Such studies are generally characterized by an overly broad measurement of resource loss. In some studies (e.g. Freedy et al., 1994; Sattler et al., 2006) this construct included personal characteristics (e.g. sense of control, self-efficacy, optimism), external resources (e.g. material possessions, social support networks), and energy resources (e.g. money, time, skills). Findings of an association between this construct and psychological distress (Freedy et al., 1994) and PTSD (Asarnow et al., 1999) in earthquake

survivors are difficult to interpret because it is not clear which aspect of resource loss accounted for this association. Nevertheless, the critical mediating factor might be loss of control over traumatic stressors, as suggested by two other studies (Sattler et al., 2006), which found that loss of personal characteristic resources (largely characterized by sense of control over life) was the strongest predictor of Acute Stress Disorder and depression. In addition, such studies are not informative with regard to possible differential associations between resource loss and PTSD and depression, because of their failure to control for the effects of severity of trauma exposure in examining the impact of resource loss on post-trauma mental health status. In earthquake survivors, for example, resource loss may also mean greater exposure to trauma (e.g. collapse of house, being trapped under rubble, etc.). It is thus difficult to interpret the findings of some studies (Armenian et al., 2000) that reported an association between financial loss and PTSD and depression. Our studies (Başoğlu et al., 2002; Başoğlu et al., 2004; Şalcıoğlu et al., 2003; Şalcıoğlu et al., 2007) show no association between material loss and PTSD, when trauma severity is statistically controlled for.

Although social support is said to be a protective factor against traumatic stress (Hobfoll et al., 2007; Norris et al., 2002; Van Ommeren et al., 2005), studies have yielded conflicting findings in this regard. Furthermore, social support is a complex process and the mechanisms by which it might affect post-trauma outcome have not been extensively investigated in an empirical fashion. In addition, at least three major methodological problems preclude definitive conclusions on this issue. First, most studies have not made a distinction between *social* and *emotional* support, which may be different constructs with differential effects on helplessness and hopelessness responses. Second, in examining the effects of social support on traumatic stress reactions, most studies did not use multiple regression analysis to control for confounding variables. Findings based on bivariate analyses may be grossly misleading. Third, most studies did not examine how social support relates to PTSD and depression separately, and, when they did, they did not use uncorrelated measures of PTSD and depression. The latter issue is important, given the high rates of comorbidity between PTSD and depression.

It is important to note that the model in Figure 1.1 makes a distinction between *social* and *emotional* support. Social support includes, among others, emergency relief efforts in the immediate post-trauma phase, material aid, compensation for material loss, assistance in legal matters, and provision of various other forms of redress (e.g. restoration of justice). Emotional support, on the other hand, involves help and guidance in overcoming the disabling effects of fear and related traumatic stress symptoms, help with daily problems, and encouragement for problem-solving behaviors, and instilling courage and hope. In our studies we found no association between lack of social support and PTSD in survivors of earthquakes (Şalcıoğlu, 2004), war (Başoğlu et al., 2005), and torture (Başoğlu et al., 1994a), consistent with other studies (Bodvarsdottir and Elklit, 2004; Carr et al., 1995; Carr et al., 1997; Lai et al., 2004; Sattler et al., 2006) that used multiple regression analysis in examining risk factors for PTSD. Although a prospective study (Seplaki et al., 2006) of 1160 survivors of Chi Chi earthquake provided some support for an association between lack of social support and depression, this association was rather weak. These findings are consistent with a meta-analytic study (Ozer et al., 2003) of predictors of PTSD, which found that most studies reporting strong predictions with support variables emphasized emotional rather than other forms of support. Emotional support might perhaps reduce PTSD and depression through enhancing sense of control over traumatic stressors and / or anxiety and distress associated with them. Such support might play a role in natural recovery processes discussed later in this chapter and also has parallels with certain aspects of CFBT described in Chapter 4. It might be said that any form of support might mitigate the effects of traumatic stress to the extent that it directly or indirectly provides opportunities for learning of effective control in relation to stressor events, disabling effects of traumatic stress, and life in general.

The model also hypothesizes that functional impairment caused by health effects of trauma contributes to resource loss (e.g. loss of employment, social status, or employment / business / educational opportunities) and leads to additional life stressors. Similarly, traumatic stress reactions may lead to reduced social / emotional support, either by blocking the person's ability to process and utilize available support or by leading to an actual reduction in support through their alienating effects on people in a person's close social environment. Thus, there may be a two-way interaction between post-trauma stressors and health outcomes. As this issue needs to be confirmed

by further research, the contributions of PTSD and depression to loss of resources and social / emotional support, and stressful life events are represented by dotted arrows in Figure 1.1.

To summarize so far, available literature evidence does not allow reliable conclusions regarding the role of resource loss and lack of social / emotional support in traumatic stress reactions. Nevertheless, these variables are tentatively included in the model, because they may conceivably affect post-trauma health outcomes through their effects on sense of control over stressor events and / or life in general. Clearly, further research is needed to investigate this issue by more carefully defining and operationalizing these constructs. Such research also needs to examine how these factors relate to individual post-trauma outcomes, such as PTSD and depression. This issue is important, considering that differential stress-response associations have implications for treatment. For example, if social support relates to depression and not to PTSD, as one of our studies (Şalcıoğlu, 2004) suggests, this would imply that social support might be helpful in preventing or treating depression but it would not reduce PTSD, which would require interventions specifically targeting this problem.

Loss of close ones may lead to two distinct outcomes: grief and depression. Grief is a natural and time-limited reaction that is phenomenologically distinct from depression and PTSD (Bonanno et al., 2007). Whether loss of close ones relate to PTSD, depression, or both is not yet clear, as few studies examined these associations using uncorrelated measures of these conditions. Furthermore, most studies did not control for the effects of trauma severity in examining the effects of loss of close ones on post-trauma health outcomes. In mass trauma survivors loss of close ones is often associated with exposure to many other traumatic events. In the Şalcıoğlu (2004) study, for example, 52% of survivors who lost a family member were also trapped under rubble and 16% of them witnessed the death of family members trapped with them. In studies (Kılıç et al., 2006; Livanou et al., 2002; Şalcıoğlu et al., 2003; Şalcıoğlu et al., 2007) that circumvented these two methodological limitations, loss of a first-degree relative related to depression but not to PTSD. Loss of close ones might aggravate depression by increasing certainty about future helplessness and hopelessness. The latter effect might be mediated by loss of a significant source of emotional support.

Role of beliefs about safety, justice, and trust

Many psychological theories of trauma maintain that emotional responses to trauma are mediated by a change in beliefs about safety, justice, and trust (Ehlers and Clark, 2000; Foa et al., 1999; Horowitz, 1986; Janoff-Bulman, 1992). The few studies that examined this issue in trauma survivors failed to support the role of beliefs about justice and trust in traumatic stress. Although some studies (Başoğlu et al., 2005; Foa et al., 1999; Şalcıoğlu, 2004) found more negative beliefs about self and others and the world in trauma-exposed people, there is little evidence to suggest that such trauma effects on beliefs are associated with PTSD. In another study (Bodvarsdottir and Elklit, 2004) no difference was found between earthquake survivors and controls in their appraisal of the benevolence and meaningfulness of the world and self-worth. Furthermore, beliefs about these issues did not relate to PTSD. Similarly, in the Şalcıoğlu (2004) study loss of faith in people, beliefs about the benevolence of the world, just-world thinking, beliefs about justice, self-blame, fatalistic thinking, and attributions of responsibility for trauma, and emotional responses to perceived impunity for people held responsible for trauma showed no association with PTSD. PTSD and depression were most strongly associated with loss of control over fear of ongoing threat to safety. Findings from a study (Başoğlu et al., 2005) of war and torture survivors using similar measures of beliefs also suggested that fear-induced helplessness responses play a more important role in traumatic stress problems than do post-trauma beliefs about self and the world, though some trauma-altered beliefs may conceivably contribute to helplessness responses (see Chapter 2). In view of these findings the impact of trauma on beliefs is not included as a process variable in Figure 1.1.

Unpredictability and uncontrollability of earthquake stressors

Contrary to popular belief, earthquake trauma is not a single event but rather a prolonged trauma period of stressor events starting with the initial major shock and followed by hundreds of aftershocks that may last for months or even more than a year. The stressor events include (1) violent tremors during the initial major shock, (2) life-threatening events, such as collapse of buildings, being trapped under rubble, secondary fires, exposure to extreme weather conditions, etc., (3) exposure to grotesque scenes, such as people trapped under rubble, mutilated bodies, etc., (4) loss of close ones and resources, (5) stressful life events associated with the consequences of the disaster (e.g. relocation to shelters, hardships of post-disaster daily life, problems arising from loss of resources, etc.), and (6) ongoing aftershocks. The post-earthquake period characterized by these events lasted more than a year in Turkey. Hence, the DSM-IV definition of acute trauma phase as 1 month after the traumatic event does not apply to earthquake trauma. We use the term trauma phase to refer to the period of continued exposure to unpredictable and uncontrollable stressors and post-trauma phase to refer to the period after cessation of these stressor events. These considerations also apply to war and torture trauma, as these events occur over an extended period of time and pose a realistic threat to safety. Furthermore, the DSM-IV distinction between acute and chronic trauma phase does not make much sense from a learning theory perspective, as the mechanisms of traumatic stress are the same in both phases.

The initial major shock

Exposure to earthquakes is an intensely frightening experience, as anyone with such an experience would know. The intensity of fear experienced during an earthquake and associated physiological responses may indeed explain the increased rates of myocardial infarction, abortions, premature births, and normal deliveries after earthquakes (Noji, 1997). While a typical earthquake lasts about 30 seconds, durations up to 10 minutes have also been recorded. The first major shock is most often unexpected, catching people by surprise. Much of the devastation caused by earthquakes most commonly occurs during the initial major shock. The first shock is often followed by thousands of aftershocks, which may last for months. Unlike the first major shock, their occurrence is often expected but they occur in unpredictable time intervals.

The August 17, 1999 earthquake in Turkey occurred at 3 am, catching most people asleep in their homes. It lasted 45 seconds. Most people were unable to leave their homes and some did not even feel the tremors, because their house collapsed within the first few seconds of the earthquake. Turkey is an

Table 1.1 Endorsement rates of and intensity of distress associated with stressors during the initial major shock

	Endorsement	Mean[1]	SD
Walls moving	53%	3.2	1.1
The rumbling noise of the earthquake	61%	3.1	1.2
Sound of buildings collapsing and other noises	50%	3.1	1.2
Being thrown about during the earthquake	24%	3.0	1.3
Furniture moving	57%	2.7	1.3
Cracks on the walls	35%	2.7	1.3
Falling during the tremors	27%	2.6	1.5
Being left in darkness during the earthquake	81%	2.2	1.6

[1] 0 = no fear / distress, 1 = slight, 2 = marked, 3 = severe, 4 = very severe fear / distress.

earthquake-prone country and many people have a previous experience of earthquakes. Nevertheless, the tremors were so violent that some people at the epicenter, failing to recognize it as an earthquake, thought that it was judgment day.

What is it about earthquakes that make them so frightening? It is worth examining some of the stressors during an earthquake that might explain the frightening nature of earthquake tremors. These stressors fall mainly into three groups: visual and auditory stimuli and loss of postural control. Table 1.1 shows the intensity of distress associated with these stressor events rated on a 0–4 scale. These data are based on an *Exposure to Earthquake Stressors Scale* (EESS; Şalcıoğlu, 2004) that we used to obtain information about the relative stressfulness of 44 events during the earthquake and its early aftermath.

What are the reasons that might account for the intensely distressing nature of these stressors? Perceptually, a moving physical environment is quite an extraordinary phenomenon, well out of the range of ordinary human experience. This is perhaps because spatial or proprioceptive orientation in humans (and possibly in other sub-human living organisms) is defined in reference to a stable physical environment. The extremely alien nature of this perceptual experience might indeed explain why earthquake survivors have a very high rate of re-experiencing

symptoms (74%) in the early aftermath of the disaster (Başoğlu et al., 2001), many of which (e.g. nightmares, flashbacks, intrusive thoughts) involve such visual images. The distressing nature of this experience might be further enhanced by equally alien auditory stimuli, such as the rumbling noise that comes from under the ground and the noise made by moving structures and objects in the environment. A shaking physical environment is also a physiologically aversive experience, which perhaps might be due in part to a transient disturbance in the vestibular system. While there are no systematic studies of physiological responses during an earthquake, survivor reports (consistent with the first author's own experience of the same earthquake) suggest that cardiovascular responses, such as tachycardia, are quite common. An increased heart rate may be accompanied by a subjective experience of fear in some people, whereas in others it may occur on its own. Such cardiovascular responses might indeed explain increased rates of death from cardiac events after an earthquake (Kloner et al., 1997; Leor et al., 1996; Ogawa et al., 2000; Trichopoulos et al., 1983). Given that vestibular dysfunction is associated with autonomic nervous system stimulation (Balaban, 1996; Yates, 1992; Yates, 1996), this might perhaps explain such cardiovascular responses in some people.

Lack of control over the events during the earthquake is an important mediator of distress, particularly when the tremors are sufficiently violent to render postural control impossible. Loss of postural control is a particularly distressing situation, as it makes any self-protective action very difficult. Indeed, survivor accounts of an experience of a 7.4-magnitude earthquake indicate that it is quite difficult to stand up, walk, and engage in any meaningful self-protective action during the tremors. Findings from the Şalcıoğlu (2004) study regarding coping responses during the earthquake are meaningful in this regard. The responses reported by the 280 survivors from the epicenter region were attempts to reach close ones in the house (39%), attempts to leave the building (38%), freezing or panic (38%), passive waiting for the tremors to end (21%), seeking a safe place in the house (16%), praying (15%), crying for help (8%), and jumping off the balcony (3%). Given that the recommended action during an earthquake in Turkey is to seek 'life saving spaces' in the house (e.g. next to solid metal objects, such as refrigerators, washing machines, metal cupboards, etc.) that are said to afford some protection in a collapsing building, most survivors could not engage in any rational self-protective behaviors. While this might be due in part to lack of training in earthquake-preparedness, it also reflects fear-induced disorganized behavior. Indeed, 76% of the survivors described severe / very severe fear and 40% reported marked to total loss of control during the earthquake (based on 0–4 ratings of fear and loss of control during the earthquake). A significant correlation between these measures ($r = 0.27$, $p < 0.001$) supports the point that fear is closely associated with the uncontrollability of earthquake stressors.

The aftermath

Post-earthquake stressors are best examined under two headings: stressor events caused by devastation and aftershocks. The devastating impact of the earthquake is most intensely experienced in the early aftermath of the disaster, lasting a few days or perhaps a week or two. This period is characterized by rescue and relief efforts and involves intense exposure to a wide range of stressors, including frequent aftershocks.

Stressors caused by devastation

Table 1.2 shows the EESS data (Şalcıoğlu, 2004) on the most common stressors in the early aftermath of an earthquake and their relative psychological impact. Note that the events with highest distress ratings are those that would evoke feelings of helplessness in most people. Indeed, most survivors, being unable to save their close ones from rubble, found themselves in a state of total helplessness. Many people made frantic but often futile efforts to save their close ones, digging through rubble with primitive tools or even bare hands. Perceptions of delayed or inadequate rescue efforts aggravated feelings of helplessness. These findings provide further evidence showing that the intensity of distress during a traumatic event is closely associated with the uncontrollability of stressors. It is worth noting that witnessing grotesque scenes such as sights of people trapped under rubble dead or alive, mutilated bodies, or smell of rotting bodies was also among the most distressing experiences.

Aftershocks

As noted earlier, major earthquakes are often followed by numerous aftershocks that usually last several months or sometimes much longer. Following the August 17 earthquake in Turkey, 2000 aftershocks were registered until October 2, their magnitude ranging from 2 to 5.8 on the Richter scale (Ito et al., 2002). There are striking similarities between exposure to aftershocks and inescapable shock experiments in animals; both situations involve repetitive stressors that are unpredictable and uncontrollable and they lead to similar psychological responses, i.e. anxiety, fear, and helplessness. Several factors contribute to appraisal of risk of threat and consequent anticipatory fear in earthquake survivors. The initial shock demonstrates the nature and extent of devastation that can be caused by major earthquakes. This is particularly true for developing countries, where earthquakes cause extensive devastation because of poor quality of constructions and lack of preparedness for earthquakes. People whose houses collapse during the earthquake are directly exposed to the devastating impact of the earthquake, while others are indirectly affected by witnessing its destructive effects on other people. Everyone knows the same events could happen again. Second, the aftershocks, although usually less strong than the initial shock, demonstrate that further devastation is possible, however limited it might be. Third, as the second (November 12) earthquake in Turkey demonstrated, there is always a risk of further major earthquakes in a seismically active region and not necessarily in the too distant future. Finally, as noted earlier, aftershocks occur at variable intervals in an unpredictable fashion. They can catch people while they are asleep, in the bathroom, having sexual intercourse, or in an enclosed space from which escape is difficult. Thus, 'protection' from a possible earthquake requires high levels of constant vigilance.

Cognitive and behavioral responses to earthquakes

In this section we review some observations on individual and collective responses to earthquakes and various cognitive and behavioral strategies that people commonly utilize in coping with fear. These observations highlight the prevalent and pervasive nature of fear among earthquake survivors and provide remarkable examples of how humans respond to unpredictable and uncontrollable stressors.

Quest for safety

As noted earlier, the August 17 earthquake occurred at 3 am. Most people outside the epicenter region (e.g. in Istanbul) thought it was just one of the many

Table 1.2 Endorsement rates of and intensity of distress associated with common stressors in the early aftermath of the earthquake

	Percent endorsement	Mean[1]	SD
Waiting helplessly near rubble unable to save close ones	21	3.8	0.6
Waiting without knowing whether close ones trapped under rubble were alive	22	3.7	0.8
Close ones dying because of rescue teams arriving late	11	3.6	0.7
Close ones dying under rubble despite rescue efforts	14	3.6	0.8
Sights of rubble under which close ones were trapped	42	3.5	1.1
People dying because of rescue teams arriving late	21	3.5	0.8
Sights of close ones' dead bodies under rubble	15	3.5	1.1
Slow death of close ones under rubble (e.g. voices fading)	7	3.4	1.2
Rescue teams arriving late while close ones trapped under rubble	14	3.4	1.0
Rescue teams not making sufficient efforts to save close ones	9	3.4	1.0
Waiting helplessly near rubble unable to save people	38	3.3	1.0
Slow death of people under rubble (e.g. voices fading)	21	3.3	1.2
People's indifference to one's close ones being trapped under rubble	19	3.3	1.1
People dying under rubble despite rescue efforts	28	3.3	1.0
Close ones' dead bodies being taken out from rubble	22	3.2	1.2
Mutilated bodies	29	3.2	1.2
Rescue teams not making sufficient efforts to save people	13	3.2	0.9
Rescue teams not arriving while close ones trapped under rubble	11	3.2	1.2
Collapsed buildings	86	3.2	1.1
Smell of rotting bodies under rubble	68	3.1	1.1
Dead bodies being taken out from rubble	46	3.1	1.2
Sight of dead bodies under rubble	38	3.1	1.2
People's indifference to others being trapped under rubble	35	3.1	1.2
Voices coming from rubble	43	3.0	1.2
Close ones' voices coming from rubble	12	2.8	1.5
Witnessing rescue work for close ones	22	2.7	1.5
People screaming	79	2.7	1.3
Sight of fire in destroyed buildings	23	2.6	1.4
People in panic	73	2.5	1.3
Injured people	68	2.5	1.4
Sights of people trapped alive under rubble	31	2.3	1.6
Sights of close ones trapped alive under rubble	10	2.3	1.7
Witnessing rescue work	50	2.2	1.4
People being taken out of rubble alive	37	1.3	1.5
Close ones being taken out of rubble alive	12	1.3	1.7

[1] 0 = no fear / distress, 1 = slight, 2 = marked, 3 = severe, 4 = very severe fear / distress.

earthquakes that occur in the country. This response, however, began to change dramatically when the TV channels began to broadcast images of devastation in the disaster region at around noon the same day. The realization of the extent of devastation caused by the earthquake led to a noticeable increase in people's fear, consistent with the view that re-appraisal of an already experienced traumatic event as dangerous enhances its traumatic impact (Foa et al., 1989). In the days and weeks that followed, public fear was aggravated by the appearance of seismology experts on TV screens, predicting yet another major earthquake (with a likely magnitude of 7.0+) in the region, this time much closer to Istanbul. Although these seismologists emphasized that this earthquake could occur anytime in the next 30 years, many people perceived these predictions as a warning of an impending earthquake. This is consistent with what we already know about cognitive effects of trauma; people exposed to a traumatic event tend to overestimate the probability of a similar event and other aversive events occurring in the near future (Foa et al., 1989; Smith and Bryant, 2000; Warda and Bryant, 1998).

The aftershocks were quite frequent in the early weeks and months of the disaster, occurring at variable intervals and variable times of the day. Many people used various coping strategies to reduce their fear. A typical behavioral pattern involved a search for any information that would help them assess the extent of danger they were facing. Millions of people were glued to their TV sets, watching earthquake-related programs and listening to seismologists, trying to understand where the active fault lines are located and the risks they posed for various locations in the region. Some people were relatively relieved to find out that they were not living in the first-degree threat zones. Many people living in such zones moved to relatively safer locations. Consequently, property prices plummeted in first-degree earthquake zones and rose sharply in others said to be safer.

Some people rushed to get an expert assessment of their house and felt relatively relieved if the experts concluded that the building was safe. If they felt that the assessment was not conducted reliably, they sought private firms to do the assessment. Others engaged in an eager search to find out whether their house was originally built according to building regulations. If the house was built before the early 1990s when the current building regulations came to force, they tried to find out whether the building regulations of the

time conformed to the current ones. Those people who could not afford to have an expert damage assessment tried to make the assessment themselves as best as they could. They felt more secure if they heard from their neighbors, for example, that their house was sitting on a solid rocky terrain, rather than on soft ground. Some people traced the building contractor who had built their house and sought reassurance from them about the quality of the construction. People who knew or discovered that the contractor who built their house was living in the same building felt safer, as they reckoned that the contractor would not have lived there if the building were not safe. At the bottom of this pyramid were people who faced no uncertainty about the state of their house, as experts had already confirmed serious structural damage (e.g. cracks in supporting columns or walls). Some of those who could not afford to have the building repaired or to move to a new place simply had the walls plastered to hide away the cracks (visual fear cues for many survivors) and went on with their lives.

Some people who could not find comforting information about their safety simply created them. For example, some tried to estimate how their house would collapse during an earthquake and, if they decided, for example, it was likely to go to the left, then they would sleep in a room that was on the right side of the building. Some people who lived in the upper floors of a building tended to believe that they were safer because they had easy access to the roof where they felt they would stand a better chance of surviving in case the building collapsed. Others who lived in the lower floors were comforted by the thought that they had a better chance of getting out of the building during an earthquake. Such estimations were in stark contrast to the fact that the overwhelming majority of the people could not get out of their home in 45 seconds during the August 17 earthquake (including the first author who was fully awake and dressed on the second floor of a building when the earthquake started). Some people conducted drills to find out how many seconds it took them to get out of their house; the shorter the time, the safer they felt.

Reliance on safety signals

Many people developed safety signals that seemed to reduce their fear. Safety signals are cues, objects, or situations that reduce anxiety by virtue of their safety value (Rachman, 1984a; Rachman, 1984b). Use of safety signals to ward off danger is a characteristic behavior of people with anxiety disorders. For example, agoraphobics carry anxiolytic tablets in case they find themselves in a feared situation. Particular behaviors of animals (e.g. birds making a noise or dogs barking), a particular color of the sea, clear visibility of the stars at night, or an unusually hot and windless day were perceived as signaling danger and their absence signaling safety. Some people sought the company of their close ones or friends during times of heightened fears, feeling safer with them. People visited relatives and friends more often and spent more time with them, particularly when rumors about an impending earthquake were going around. Such behavior was not necessarily motivated by a belief that the presence of others during an earthquake might facilitate survival. Rather, other people's presence appeared to have a safety signal value. For example, a woman felt less anxious staying at home with her 1-year-old child. Many people stayed with their next-door neighbors in the same building on the day of an expected earthquake, simply because the company of others made them feel safer.

Many people displayed a remarkable tendency to believe in frequently emerging rumors of a major earthquake that was going to occur on a particular date. Endless public reassurances by seismologists who repeatedly emphasized the fact that there was no way of predicting the timing of earthquakes did not prevent such rumors from spreading widely throughout the country. Both the media and the public were particularly interested in the opinion of a seismologist, who had become a household name due to his frequent TV appearances. This seismologist, the then head of a university institute of seismology, became a well-known public figure after the earthquake. A few days after the earthquake, he reported unusual seismic activity in the region, which he thought might be signaling an impending major aftershock. He therefore advised the people to stay outdoors for the next 24 hours and millions of Istanbul residents spent the (uneventful) night on the streets. After this event the public closely watched his statements for any clues or predictions about future aftershocks. When rumors about an impending earthquake broke out, reporters closely watched his actions to find out whether he was staying in his house on the day of the expected earthquake. His actions were perceived as signaling danger or safety and people wanted to know if he was staying outdoors that day so that they could do the same. At

times he came under so much public pressure that he had to make public announcements on TV channels, reassuring the public about his intention to stay in his house on that day.

These rumors appeared to serve an important psychological function by making unpredictable shocks predictable and thereby controllable. The 'certainty' about the timing of the next earthquake seemed to reduce people's fear because it also signaled safety until that day. When the expected date came, many people simply avoided the danger by spending the day outside. Interestingly, when the rumors were eventually disconfirmed by an eventless day, this did not appear to reduce people's tendency to believe in future rumors. Soon enough, another rumor appeared, which in effect postponed the expected disaster to a later date. This process continued for some years, albeit with reduced frequency.

These observations are consistent with findings from experimental work with animals. When given a choice, animals generally show a strong preference for predictable or signaled aversive events in comparison to unpredictable or unsignaled aversive events (Badia et al., 1979). According to Seligman's safety signal theory (Seligman, 1968; Seligman and Binik, 1977), preference for predictability derives from the fact that having a signal when the event is going to happen also means functionally that when the signal is not on, the organism can relax and feel safe. In other words, when the organism has a reliable signal for when bad things are going to happen, the absence of the signal can be used as a safety signal. For organisms experiencing unsignaled or unpredictable aversive events, the absence of a reliable signal also means the absence of a reliable safety signal. If the organism is in a context where aversive events are occurring unpredictably, this means that they may be in a state of chronic fear (Seligman, 1968; Seligman and Binik, 1977). Another theory accounting for the preference for predictability is that it reduces uncertainty (Imada and Nageishi, 1982), which may in and of itself be rewarding. Evidence in support of the safety signal theory in humans has largely been drawn from clinical cases with anxiety disorders. As noted earlier, characteristic examples of reliance on safety signals have been observed in agoraphobic patients. What is interesting with our observations is the fact that the safety signal theory appears to be able to account for a social phenomenon or the collective behavior of large masses of people.

Fatalistic thinking and Tawakkul

Another commonly observed attempt to reduce fear was to resort to philosophical, religious, or fatalistic beliefs. Thinking in the form of "*There is no running away from earthquakes*" or "*If death is fated to happen, it will happen*" became increasingly more common among people. A taxi driver told the first author that his intense fear of earthquakes disappeared when his father, a religious man, told him "*Son, there is no escape from earthquakes; you have to accept it.*" Total acceptance of helplessness in uncontrollable situations reflects a particular state of mind described and reinforced by Islamic philosophy, namely 'tevekkül' in Turkish or 'Tawakkul' in Arabic. Although this concept does not have an exact equivalent in English, it can be loosely translated as 'to resign oneself unto God.' Essentially, it denotes passive acceptance of fate by 'putting one's trust in God.' The case of the taxi driver described above is an illustrative example of this phenomenon. Some bereaved survivors also resorted to this form of thinking to cope with the grief and pain associated with their loss (e.g. "*It was God's will*").

A tendency in people to resort to religious thinking or an increase in religious faith after traumatic events has been reported by other studies (Carmil and Breznitz, 1991; Falsetti et al., 2003; Valentine and Feinauer, 1993). Nevertheless, whether this form of thinking has a direct fear-reducing effect remains unclear. In our studies fatalistic thinking related to either greater trauma exposure (Şalcıoğlu, 2004) or more severe PTSD (Başoğlu et al., 2005). It might thus well be a cognitive coping process secondary to severe traumatic stress. Such coping is unlikely to have much effect on conditioned fears, considering their irrational nature that makes them resistant to cognitive processes (Öhman and Mineka, 2001). On the other hand, fatalistic thinking might perhaps have an indirect effect on traumatic stress by prescribing total acceptance of an anticipated threat event. Such acceptance implies more risk-taking behaviors, less behavioral avoidance, and therefore greater opportunities for learning of control over fear cues. In the case of the taxi driver, for example, the father's words might have encouraged him not to avoid earthquakes and his fear might have reduced *after* having done so. Fatalistic thinking might also make it easier to accept the consequences of disasters (e.g. loss of close ones, loss of resources, personal injury, disability, etc.) *after* they have occurred. Nevertheless, available evidence does not allow definitive conclusions on the causal relationship between fatalistic thinking and traumatic stress. Prospective controlled studies would be needed to examine whether it has a direct effect on fear and other psychological responses to trauma. It would also be interesting to examine in future research whether fatalistic thinking reduces avoidance and facilitates exposure to feared situations.

Avoidance

Avoidance of various earthquake-related situations was one of the most common psychological responses among survivors. In five field surveys (Başoğlu et al., 2002; Başoğlu et al., 2004; Livanou et al., 2002; Şalcıoğlu et al., 2003; Şalcıoğlu et al., 2007) conducted at different stages after the earthquake (range mean 8 to 40 months), the rates of cognitive and behavioral avoidance ranged from 41% to 70%. In these studies the survivors avoided a mean of 7 to 11 different trauma-related situations or activities (measured by a 35-item *Fear and Avoidance Questionnaire*, see Appendix A). Avoidance behaviors related to two types of situations: (a) those that signaled danger in case of a future earthquake and (b) those that acted as distressing reminders of the past earthquake. The most common example of the first type of avoidance related to concrete buildings. Many people avoided entering buildings, even when they knew that a particular building was safe. This reflected realistic fears to a certain extent, because information on the safety of the surviving buildings was not available in the early months of the disaster. These fears were also reinforced by certain slogans repeatedly broadcast by seismologists on TV screens (presumably to alleviate public fear of earthquakes!), such as "*Earthquakes don't kill. Buildings do.*" As expert assessment of the buildings became increasingly available in time, many people still continued to avoid their houses, even when the experts reported them as safe. This reflected in part their mistrust of expert assessments, which were sometimes conducted in a rather cursory fashion. The extent of avoidance among earthquake survivors is best demonstrated by the fact that 58% of the 15 000 people who were living in shelters 6 months after the earthquake had a safe and inhabitable house (Committee for Tent Cities in Kocaeli, 2000). Similarly, behavioral avoidance due to fear was the strongest predictor of relocation to shelters in our three field surveys conducted a mean of 1.3

years after the earthquake (Şalcıoğlu et al., 2008). Many survivors preferred to live under difficult conditions in camps rather than moving back to their homes or alternative accommodation.

Other common examples of the first type of avoided situations included staying alone at home, staying in the dark, taking a shower, getting undressed before going to bed, sleeping with lights off, sleeping with the bedroom door closed, or sleeping before 3 am (the time of the night when the earthquake happened), having sexual intercourse, or being in places from which escape during an earthquake would be difficult. Some people could not go near the sea, because parts of the land near the sea had sunk during the earthquake, causing many people to drown. Many people devised a rota at home to have a family member stay awake and keep vigil during the night, while the others slept. This type of avoidance clearly reflected a state of constant vigilance caused by the unpredictable nature of aftershocks. Indeed, one needs to be vigilant all the time if the exact timing of a threatening event cannot be predicted. Such avoidance often caused significant social and occupational disability, because it interfered with normal daily functioning.

The second type of avoidance reflected conditioned fears or distress with respect to a wide range of trauma reminders. For example, some people stopped sleeping in the room where they had experienced the earthquake and slept in another room. Others avoided sights of rubble or destroyed buildings, which were distressing reminders of the earthquake. Some survivors could not go to work, because that meant having to go through the devastated neighborhoods. Others stopped reading newspapers or watching TV news to avoid being reminded of the earthquake. Conditioned fears often generalized to a wide range of situations. For example, some people avoided wearing the same clothes they had on during the earthquake. A woman who was brushing her teeth during the earthquake had to change the toothbrush and the brand of the toothpaste she was using, because they evoked fear. She complained to her therapist that she was also distressed by the presence of her husband (whom she had married recently and who was with her during the earthquake), because he served as a reminder of the earthquake. Many people avoided places where they experienced shaking sensations, such as hung floors in shops that shook when people walked over them or other locations where the ground vibrations created by passing trucks could be felt.

Fear of earthquakes: an evolutionary perspective

Evidence reviewed so far suggests that exposure to earthquakes leads to high rates of fear and avoidance responses that are quite resistant to extinction in the long term. This might perhaps reflect an evolutionarily determined response geared towards self-preservation. It is long known that defensive responses such as heightened vigilance, flight or fight, and avoidance of threat have played a fundamental role in the survival of the species for millions of years (Marks, 1987). Several lines of evidence suggest that earthquakes have an evolutionary significance for living organisms. For example, there are close parallels between human and animal responses to earthquakes. Snarr (2005) has noted that animal responses to earthquakes have been observed as far back as 3000 years ago, including responses before, during, and after the earthquake. Among the documented responses of non-human primates to earthquakes are increased restlessness and changes in space utilization in chimpanzees (Shaw, 1977), freezing responses in langur monkeys (*Presbytis entellus*; Krusko et al., 1986), and stress, nervousness, and fear in orangutans (Antilla, 2001). In a study Snarr (2005) documented the response of a group of wild mantled howlers (*Alouatta palliata*) on the north coast of Honduras to an earthquake that occurred 341 kilometers away in El Salvador. The response of the howlers to the coseismic activity was very similar to a ground threat, such as the appearance of a dog or an unknown human. Following the seismic event and at the approximate time when the body waves arrived at the study site, the howlers rapidly moved from mid-canopy to the higher inner canopy and showed signs of restlessness and alertness.

Another line of evidence concerns anecdotal and retrospective reports of seismic-escape behavior in some animals living in seismically active regions (see Tributsch, 1982 for a review). As an explanation for such behavior, Kirschvink (2000) suggested that evolutionary processes might have led to tilt, hygroreception (humidity), electric, and magnetic sensory systems in animals that enable them to detect certain earthquake precursors, such as P waves. Tectonic plate activities have existed for at least the past two billion years on Earth, giving rise to sufficiently frequent earthquakes to allow living organisms to develop a capacity for self-preservation. In this connection, Kirschvink (2000) noted that

... we now realize that great earthquakes occur with average repeat intervals of 100 years or so ... Although moderate earthquakes of M ~ 6 + affect smaller geographic areas, they are more numerous and may dominate the local seismic hazards for an area. Furthermore, zones of high seismic activity have existed on Earth for at least the past two billion years or more, as they are a by product of plate tectonic processes. A small selection pressure acting over a vast interval of geological time can be just as effective at gene fixation as is stronger selection acting over a shorter time interval. Second, evasive action can, in many instances, reduce mortality during an earthquake. Earthquakes can kill animals or reduce their fitness in a variety of ways, from direct physical shaking (e.g. causing burrows to collapse, shaking eggs out of nests, breaking honeycomb, etc.) to indirect action of mudslides and tsunamis. Fitness can also be reduced in the interval after an earthquake as a result of the disruption of normal behavior from aftershocks. For many organisms, behavioral action taken prior to an earthquake could reduce mortality: fish and cetaceans leaving coastal zones, rodents exiting from collapsible burrows or dwellings, bees swarming, parents delaying egg-laying, etc.

(pp. 313)

Preparedness theory in fear acquisition

Further evidence on the evolutionary significance of fear comes from experimental work with animals. It has been suggested that primates may have a preparedness to acquire fear of certain kinds of objects or situations that have evolutionary significance (Öhman and Mineka, 2001; Seligman, 1971). Mineka and Zinbarg (2006) noted that

... people are much more likely to have phobias of snakes, water, heights, and enclosed spaces than of bicycles, guns, or cars, even though the latter objects (not present in our early evolutionary history) may be as likely to be associated with trauma ... this is because there may have been a selective advantage in the course of evolution for primates who rapidly acquired fear of certain objects or situations that posed threats to humans' early ancestors ... Thus, prepared fears are not seen as inborn or innate but rather as very easily acquired and / or especially resistant to extinction.

(pp. 4)

In a series of experiments using mild shock as the unconditioned stimulus (US), Öhman and his

colleagues found superior conditioning effects with fear-relevant conditioned stimuli (CS) such as snakes and spiders than with fear-irrelevant CSs, such as slides of flowers, mushrooms, or electric outlets (see a review by Öhman and Mineka, 2001). In addition, using videotaped model monkeys, Cook and Mineka (1989; 1990) showed that naïve monkeys can easily learn to fear fear-relevant stimuli (e.g. a toy snake or a toy crocodile) but not fear-irrelevant stimuli, such as flowers or a toy rabbit. In their review of the evidence in support of this issue, Mineka and Zinbarg (2006) concluded that

In both monkeys and humans, therefore, evolutionary fear-relevant stimuli more readily enter into selective associations with aversive events, and these same stimuli seem more likely than others to become the objects of human phobias. Moreover, the special characteristics of fear learning seen with fear-relevant (but not fear-irrelevant) stimuli (e.g. its automaticity and its resistance to higher cognitive control) suggest that the acquisition of phobias involves a primitive basic emotional level of learning that humans share with many other mammalian species (Öhman and Mineka, 2001).

(pp. 5)

The preparedness theory might thus explain why people respond to earthquakes with such intense fear, rapidly acquire conditioned fears and avoidance in relation to a wide range of situations or activities, and why such fear is resistant to extinction in the long term. This theory would predict a higher rate of fear and avoidance responses associated with earthquakes than with other life-threatening events without an evolutionary significance (e.g. road traffic accidents). This hypothesis seems to be well worth testing in future research.

Observational learning of fear

While the prevalent nature of conditioned fears and avoidance among earthquake-exposed people is consistent with evidence of an association between inescapable shocks and conditioned fears (Desiderato and Newman, 1971; Mineka et al., 1984; Warren et al., 1989), another contributing factor might be acquisition of fear through observational learning. Experiments with animal and human subjects showed that observing others experiencing a traumatic event or acting fearfully could lead to the development of phobias (Mineka and Öhman, 2002; Mineka and Zinbarg, 2006; Öhman and Mineka, 2001). Mineka and Zinbarg (2006) also noted that humans are susceptible to acquiring fear vicariously through watching movies and TV. Our observations provide some indirect support for the role of observational learning in fear and avoidance. Devastating earthquakes affecting millions of people indeed provide ample opportunities for observational learning of fear. In the early aftermath of the disaster survivors often witnessed people suffering, horrified, panicking, screaming, etc. Those who participated in rescue efforts in the early days of the disaster had even more intense exposure to such scenes. In addition, throughout the period of aftershocks, people observed others acting fearfully in anticipation of future earthquakes, panicking during aftershocks, and avoiding a wide range of situations in daily life. Various examples of pervasive fear that gripped the public were provided earlier.

The possible role of the media in promoting observational learning also deserves attention. Following the disaster more than 20 national TV channels endlessly (and rather irresponsibly) broadcast graphic images of severely injured, distressed or bereaved survivors, people trapped alive under rubble (some of them for days), and rescue teams recovering survivors from rubble. Evidence from the Şalcıoğlu (2004) study suggests that such exposure did have an impact on public fear of earthquakes. This issue was examined in 273 survivors who did not have a personal experience with the kind of events displayed on TV screens (e.g. collapse of house, being trapped under rubble, etc.). In response to a question about whether watching TV in the early days of the disaster led to an increase in their anticipatory fear of earthquakes, 51% of the survivors reported marked to very much increase, with a further 17% reporting only slight increase. This study also showed that women and those who experienced greater fear and loss of control during the earthquake were more vulnerable to the impact of such TV broadcasts. The effect of TV on fear is further supported by another analysis showing an association between self-reported increase in fears and more severe and extensive avoidance behaviors (as measured by the *Fear and Avoidance Questionnaire*) at the time of assessment. While such increase in fear might have been due in part to a re-appraisal of the danger posed by the earthquake (e.g. *it could have happened to me / my close ones* or *it may happen to me / my close ones next time*), consistent with an

unconditioned stimulus re-evaluation process (Davey, 2006), it might also reflect the direct observational learning effects of watching people's expressions of distress or fear in response to their traumatic experiences. These findings are consistent with reports (Blanchard et al., 2004; Schlenger et al., 2002) of an association between exposure to TV images of 9/11 events and subsequent PTSD.

Natural recovery processes and associated factors

In a review of the evidence on the role of evolutionarily determined defensive responses in PTSD, Cantor (2005) noted that vigilant avoidance was the most commonly used strategy early in our evolutionary history, because of reptilian energy limitations. The use of this strategy, however, is said to be dependent on an appraisal of the relative costs and benefits of avoidance behavior or the 'cost-benefit ratio' (Kavaliers and Choleris, 2001). In other words, avoidance has a survival value in animals as long as it does not interfere with feeding and mating opportunities. There is indeed evidence (Lima, 1998) to suggest that animals are prepared to take greater risks with predators when they are hungry. It has also been suggested that hunger might cause a transient decrease in post-traumatic stress (Cantor, 2005).

This theory would predict that the development or persistence of avoidance of concrete buildings (the primary cause of death during earthquakes) following an earthquake would be dependent on an appraisal of the relative costs and benefits of living out of buildings (e.g. in tents or other shelters). The study by Şalcıoğlu (2004) provided an opportunity to examine this issue. Some survivors had left their home immediately after the earthquake but then had gone back to live in the same place, either within the same day or soon after the earthquake. Others were relocated to a shelter (camps, tents, makeshift barracks, etc.), either because they had lost their house or were too afraid to go back home. These survivors had moved out of the shelters at some stage to go back to their home or other alternative accommodation. Home or alternative accommodation meant concrete buildings in all cases. We examined the reasons why these survivors (n = 156) did not avoid concrete buildings from the outset or stopped avoiding them in the longer term. The mean time it took them to move back home or to an alternative accommodation (i.e. resettlement) was 126 days

(SD = 162, range 1–905). The most commonly stated reason for resettlement was the inconvenience or hardships of living in shelters (67%). Other reasons that reflected a voluntary decision for resettlement included the belief that their house was safe enough (8%), having built or found a safe house to live in (6%), to overcome fear of earthquakes (4%), and feeling no longer frightened (4%). Only 8% of the survivors resettled involuntarily for reasons outside their control (e.g. pressure from the family, closure of camps). It is of interest to note that resettlement took place about 4 months after the August 17 earthquake, when the particularly harsh winter of 1999 began to set in. These findings are indeed consistent with the cost-benefit theory of avoidance. What is not clear from these findings, however, is whether the survivors experienced a reduction in their fear and related stress problems for some reason *before* resettlement. The fact that only 4% of the survivors reported a reduction in their fear before resettlement suggests that this is unlikely. This is also supported by a field survey (Şalcıoğlu et al., 2007) that found high levels of fear and avoidance in survivors shortly after resettlement, reducing in time with increased opportunities for exposure to fear cues.

The foregoing account of possible evolutionary factors in fear and avoidance suggests an important role for risk-taking behaviors in natural recovery processes.[1] Evidence indeed supports this point. Several factors counteract avoidance by reinforcing motivation to confront fear. An important factor is the inconvenience of living in the shelters, as noted above. We observed that many survivors whose houses survived the earthquake needed to enter their house at some stage to fetch various items, such as clothes, blankets, electric heaters, etc., even though that meant taking a risk of being caught up in the building during an aftershock. In the Şalcıoğlu (2004) study, among 80 survivors who avoided going back to their house for at least one day after the earthquake, 94% entered their house for the first time within the first month,

thus displaying risk-taking behavior at a time when the aftershocks were most frequent. The reasons for doing so were mainly to fetch various essential items, to go to the bathroom, to take a shower, etc. This is yet another finding that supports the cost-benefit theory of avoidance (Kavaliers and Choleris, 2001). The time taken to enter the house for the first time was not associated with the intensity of fear experienced during the initial major shock (the strongest predictor of PTSD), suggesting that the survivors took risks regardless of the severity of their fear and related traumatic stress reactions.

We also observed that some survivors, also motivated by the inconvenience of living away from their homes, made attempts to overcome their fear of earthquakes by entering their homes in a graduated fashion. A common feature of these survivors was a realization of the fact that letting fear take control of their lives and, consequently, having to live in a state of total helplessness and under difficult conditions away from home was too high a price to pay for the relative safety of shelters. Thus, many eventually came to the conclusion "*I cannot continue to live like this. I've got to do something to overcome my fear. I will go back home and take the risk. If it is fated to happen, it will happen anyway.*" Such cognitive change did not necessarily reduce fear initially. Faced with intense fear at the first attempt, many could not do this at once and thus employed a graduated approach in moving back to their house, in pretty much the same way it would be prescribed by a therapist delivering CFBT (see Chapter 4). For example, they first spent a couple of hours in their home, cleaning the debris and tidying up things. Feeling more confident, they spent more time in the house next time, drinking tea or coffee, for example. Then they started spending the whole day in the house, going back to the camp for the night. At the next step they started spending one night a week in the house and so on. This continued until they felt comfortable with the idea of staying in the house. The following case vignette illustrates this process.

---

[1] It is also worth noting in this connection that certain forms of risk-taking behaviors in some trauma survivors with PTSD, such as reckless driving or getting themselves into other dangerous situations (often labelled as 'trauma addiction') might simply be a manifestation of evolutionary processes designed to overcome fear by challenging it. The fact that such behavior is regarded as maladaptive in our modern world does not necessarily rule out this possibility, as in ancient times it might have been adaptive. It would be interesting to examine the impact of such behaviors on PTSD symptoms.

Case vignette

We met Semra in a café in the epicenter region about 1 month after the earthquake. She and her family had experienced the earthquake in her lower ground flat in a six-story building, which had survived the earthquake with minimal damage. The family had been living in a tent city that had been set up locally for survivors. After a month of living under difficult circumstances in the camp and facing serious limitations in her daily functioning because of pervasive fear and extensive avoidance of a variety of situations, she had finally decided to do something about this problem. When we met her in the café, she was about to go back to her home for the first time after the earthquake and try to overcome her fear by entering her flat. She did not care about the possibility of an aftershock happening while she was in the building and thought it was about time she started taking risks. We asked whether we could accompany her to videotape this process and she agreed. To avoid 'contaminating' the natural self-help process, we refrained from encouraging her or answering any questions that would imply approval of what she was about to do. When we arrived at her place, we waited outside the building, while she made her first attempt to enter the building. Initially, she displayed signs of intense anxiety but then summoned up sufficient courage to go into the building. Half an hour later, she signaled to us from the balcony asking us to come in. When we went in, she was in a state of joy for having accomplished the dreaded task and wanted to share it with us. She repeatedly said "I've done it! I have beaten my fear!" She went around the flat focusing her attention on the plaster cracks on the wall and pieces of broken objects and glass strewn across the floor (fear-evoking cues for many earthquake survivors) in an effort to challenge fear, in exactly the same way that would be prescribed during a therapist-aided exposure session. She said she would come back again and stay longer in her flat and clean up the place. She also said she would invite us for coffee when she was permanently resettled. When we visited her a month later, she was indeed living in her flat with her family, almost completely free of fear and other traumatic stress problems.

Our observations suggest that such risk-taking behavior is the most important factor that reverses the traumatization process and protects against the traumatic effects of earthquakes. In fact, it is such observations that led us to focus on a largely self-help approach in care of disaster survivors (detailed in Chapter 7) that essentially capitalizes on people's naturally existing potential for risk-taking behaviors. Risk-taking behaviors might also be initiated by certain life changes. For example, resettlement in concrete buildings often becomes unavoidable when survivor camps are eventually closed down. Evidence from our studies (Şalcıoğlu et al., 2007; Şalcıoğlu et al., 2008)

shows that resettlement is associated with some improvement in traumatic stress symptoms, possibly due to the beneficial effects of exposure to fear cues.

We have also seen survivors who discovered the beneficial effects of exposure after an unintended or unavoidable exposure to a particular feared situation and then went on to use this strategy intentionally to overcome their fear of other situations. Indeed, total avoidance of all earthquake-related cues is practically impossible, because of the pervasive nature of earthquake-related fears that permeate almost every aspect of life. Avoidance of sexual intercourse for fear of being caught unprepared (e.g. naked) in an earthquake, a common problem in earthquake survivors, is a case in point. Social and occupational obligations that necessitate certain activities (e.g. travelling, visiting friends or relatives in their homes, etc.) also render total avoidance difficult. Such occasions provide opportunities for testing risk-taking behaviors, which may then lead to the discovery of exposure as an effective method of overcoming fear. In some cases this strategy, once discovered, might even be used to overcome earthquake-unrelated fears. For example, we have seen a woman who told us that, after having successfully utilized exposure to overcome her fear of earthquakes, she went on to treat her snake phobia by searching for snakes in the region. She eventually found some and came back home free of her phobia.

Another factor in natural recovery from fear that deserves attention is possible immunization against traumatic stress through repeated exposures to earthquakes. In the Şalcıoğlu (2004) study, when the participants were asked (mean 21 months after the earthquake) if they experienced any change in their fear of earthquakes, 60% reported some decrease (slight to very much), 25% no change, and 15% slight to very much increase. This suggests that fear reduction is possible despite continuing earthquakes. Although the mechanisms of such change are not entirely clear, some evidence (reviewed later in this chapter) from our studies suggest that such fear reduction occurs with learning of coping with earthquake tremors and increased sense of control over fear. A regression analysis showed that increased sense of control over aftershocks and fear reduction were associated with prior experiences with earthquake-like shaking sensations (e.g. as in sailors or people living near a busy road used by heavy trucks or a railway bridge). The latter finding is consistent with findings from stress immunization experiments, which showed that animals (dogs or rats) that were first exposed to a short series of escapable (controllable) shocks prior to receiving a long series of inescapable shocks did not show the learned helplessness deficits (Seligman and Maier, 1967; Williams and Maier, 1977). Interestingly, in the Williams and Maier experiment (1977) these immunization effects occurred even when different kinds of aversive stimuli were used in the immunization and helplessness induction phases (e.g. experience of escaping from cold water immunized rats against the effects of exposure to uncontrollable foot shocks). This might explain why repeated exposures to earthquake-like shaking, which bears only some resemblance to real earthquake tremors, was sufficient in producing a protective effect against fear of real earthquakes. This is indeed one of the findings from our studies that inspired the idea of using an earthquake simulator in enhancing survivors' resilience against the traumatic effects of earthquake tremors (see Chapter 4). Consistent with previous evidence (Başoğlu et al., 1997) pointing to the protective role of psychological preparedness for trauma in torture survivors, this finding also suggests that immunization against traumatic stress is possible in humans through repeated exposures to a traumatic stressor, provided that such experience allows learning of control over the stressor event.

Mechanisms of traumatic stress in earthquake trauma

Earlier in this chapter we described the unpredictable and uncontrollable nature of various earthquake-related stressors and how such stressors lead to various cognitive and behavioral coping responses in survivors. These stressors include the initial major shock, stressor events in the early aftermath of an earthquake, and aftershocks. In this section we review further evidence regarding the role of these stressors in helplessness and hopelessness responses and how these responses relate to traumatic stress reactions, such as PTSD and depression.

In our field surveys (Başoğlu et al., 2002; Başoğlu et al., 2004; Livanou et al., 2002; Şalcıoğlu et al., 2003; Şalcıoğlu et al., 2007) we investigated the role of fear experienced during the initial major shock in the development of traumatic stress reactions, using a 0–4 rating of fear intensity. This measure was validated in our previous studies (Başoğlu et al., 2002; Livanou

et al., 2002; Şalcıoğlu et al., 2003) and demonstrated to reflect actual fear during the earthquake, independent of PTSD-related recall bias in retrospective assessment. In all studies this measure was the strongest predictor of PTSD and comorbid depression, explaining more variance in symptoms than all other trauma exposure variables combined, including collapse of house, being trapped under rubble, loss of close ones, and participation in rescue work. Similar findings were reported by other studies in Turkey (Kılıç et al., 2006; Kılıç and Ulusoy, 2003), Greece (Bergiannaki et al., 2003; Livanou et al., 2005), and the United States (Asarnow et al., 1999). These findings support our earlier discussion regarding the intensely frightening nature of earthquakes and their helplessness effects.

Helplessness and hopelessness effects of earthquakes

Şalcıoğlu (2004) examined the cumulative helplessness effects of the initial major earthquake and subsequent aftershocks at mean 21 months post-disaster (range 13–32 months) using an 11-item *Fear and Loss of Control Scale*. Table 1.3 shows the item endorsement rates (i.e. items rated as markedly to very true) in two groups of survivors. The group with 'low' earthquake exposure includes survivors who experienced the earthquakes with no damage to their house, whereas the group with 'high' earthquake exposure includes survivors with additional trauma experiences, such as the collapse of their house or being trapped under rubble.

Both groups had fairly high rates of anticipatory fear and feelings of helplessness that persisted well beyond the cessation of the aftershocks. The groups did not significantly differ in their mean total scale scores, suggesting that additional trauma events did not contribute to fear and helplessness responses in the long term. The fear and loss of control items were strongly intercorrelated, suggesting that anticipatory fear of earthquakes was the primary factor in generalized feelings of helplessness.

The hopelessness effects of earthquakes are evidenced by the fact that 69% of the survivors reported hopelessness (as assessed by the *Traumatic Stress Symptom Checklist*; Başoğlu et al., 2001). Furthermore, the presence of hopelessness was associated with 10-fold increase in risk of major depression (95% CI = 4.8–21.7, p < 0.001). These findings were

Table 1.3 Comparison of fear and helplessness responses in survivors with high versus low earthquake exposure (Fear and Loss of Control Scale[1])

	High EE (n = 169) %	Low EE (n = 210) %[2]
Fear responses		
I fear for my life.	37	37
I feel I am in danger.	31	39
I feel my loved ones are in danger.	53	56
I have developed fears that I did not have before.	52	41
I cannot lead my normal life for fear of earthquakes.	46	31**
Helplessness responses		
I feel helpless about future earthquakes.	78	70
I think I cannot change anything in my life.	42	42
I feel I have no control over my life.	45	40
I learned how to cope with aftershocks.	49	57
I can control my fear during the aftershocks.	53	60
I got used to the aftershocks.	62	66

High EE = High earthquake exposure (severe structural damage to home, partial or total collapse, having been trapped under rubble); Low EE = Low earthquake exposure (no severe damage to home).
[1] Item scale: 0 = not at all true, 2 = slightly, 4 = moderately, 6 = markedly, 8 = very true.
[2] Chi-square comparison of endorsement rates (moderately to very true); Bonferroni adjusted p value = 0.005
** p = 0.003.

corroborated in a much larger sample of survivors. In a pooled sample of 4332 survivors from five field surveys, hopelessness was present in 63% of the cases and associated with a 22-fold increase in comorbid depression (95% CI = 16.7–28.4, p < 0.001). These findings point to a strong association between hopelessness and depression.

Evidence from experimental work with animals shows that exposure to uncontrollable electric shocks is associated with various associative, motivational, and emotional deficits (Overmier and Seligman, 1967; Seligman and Maier, 1967). Associative deficit involves an impaired ability to detect response-outcome contingencies in future situations where responses do exert control over outcomes (Seligman et al., 1971). Animals initially exposed to uncontrollable shocks later fail to learn to escape or avoid shocks that are potentially controllable in a different situation, because they learn to expect that they have no control over outcomes. The items *I feel I have no control over my life* and *I think I cannot change anything in my life* may reflect such an associative deficit. A motivational deficit involves a reduced incentive to attempt to gain control in future situations resulting from a belief that responses would be ineffective in producing relief. Emotional deficits, on the other hand, include decreased aggressiveness and decreased competitiveness (Rapaport and Maier, 1978; Williams, 1982), loss of appetite and / or weight (Desan et al., 1988; Weiss, 1968), anhedonia (Bowers et al., 1987), and stress induced ulceration (Weiss, 1971a; Weiss, 1971b; Weiss, 1971c; Weiss, 1977). Although the *Fear and Loss of Control Scale* did not specifically tap motivational and emotional deficits, the fact that it correlated highly with *Beck Depression Inventory* (Beck et al., 1979)(r = 0.62) and symptoms of depressed mood, loss of interest, loss of pleasure, hopelessness, loss of appetite, fatigue, and loss of libido (Pearson correlation coefficients ranging from 0.26 to 0.52, all p's < 0.001) was suggestive of such deficits among the survivors.

Consistent with the integrated helplessness / hopelessness model of anxiety and depression (Alloy et al., 1990; Mineka et al., 1998), PTSD and depression were closely associated in all our studies. In the pooled sample of 4332 survivors from five field surveys, 72% of the survivors who had PTSD also had depression. Among the survivors with PTSD in the Şalcıoğlu (2004) study, 53% also had current depression, whereas among those without PTSD, only 15% had depression (odds ratio = 6.4, 95% CI = 4.0–10.4, p < 0.001). Thus, the presence of PTSD was associated with more than a 6-fold increase in the risk of depression. In addition, among the survivors with depression, only 14% had 'pure' depression without any comorbid anxiety disorder (including PTSD), whereas among the cases with at least one anxiety disorder 53% had 'pure' anxiety without depression. This finding accords with Alloy and colleagues' (1990) review of the evidence showing that cases of pure depression without concomitant anxiety are rarer than cases of pure anxiety without concomitant depression. This might be explained by the fact that people who are hopeless also perceive that they are helpless but the reverse is not necessarily true (Alloy et al., 1990; Mineka et al., 1998). It is worth noting that

Table 1.4 Correlations among measures of helplessness, avoidance, PTSD, and depression

		1	2	3	4
1	Loss of control during initial shock	–			
2	Anticipatory fear and helplessness	0.25	–		
3	Avoidance behaviors	0.29	0.70	–	
4	PTSD symptoms	0.31	0.64	0.73	–
5	Depression symptoms	0.26	0.62	0.65	0.69

All p's < 0.001.

depression in the Şalcıoğlu (2004) study did not overlap with grief reactions due to bereavement, as the diagnosis of depression ruled out bereavement in the last 2 months as a possible cause.

Associations among helplessness, avoidance, and traumatic stress reactions

The model in Figure 1.1 hypothesizes that helplessness and avoidance are the underlying causal processes in PTSD. Testing of this hypothesis requires prospective studies examining the temporal sequence of these processes. Although correlations based on cross-sectional data do not allow inferences regarding causality, they nevertheless provide some idea about the associations among the variables. Table 1.4 shows the correlations among the measures of helplessness, avoidance, PTSD, and depression in the Şalcıoğlu (2004) study. Helplessness during the initial major shock was measured by a 0–4 assessor-rated scale (0 = completely in control, 4 = total loss of control / completely helpless). Avoidance behaviors were assessed by the *Fear and Avoidance Questionnaire*. This scale measures only avoidance behaviors and not fear, whereas the *Fear and Loss of Control Scale* measures only fear and helplessness but not avoidance behaviors. As such, the two scales do not tap the same constructs. PTSD was assessed using the *Clinician-Administered PTSD Scale* (CAPS; Blake et al., 1990). The items relating to cognitive and behavioral avoidance were omitted in calculation of total CAPS scores to avoid overlapping between the CAPS and the *Fear and Avoidance Questionnaire* in their measurement of avoidance.

The correlation between these scales thus reflects the association between avoidance and all other PTSD symptoms. The correlations in Table 1.4 point to strong associations among helplessness, avoidance, PTSD, and depression.

A multiple regression analysis (Table 1.5) was conducted to examine the relative contributions of helplessness and avoidance to PTSD and depression. Background variables were entered at step 1, followed by loss of control during the earthquake at step 2, other trauma exposure variables at step 3, and helplessness and avoidance measures at step 4.

Controlling for all other variables, helplessness and avoidance explained 31% and 27% of the total variance in PTSD and depression symptoms, respectively. Trauma exposure variables accounted for a much smaller portion of the variance in PTSD and depression. In the full regression model avoidance was the strongest predictor of both PTSD and depression, followed by helplessness. Helplessness measured in the long term was a stronger predictor of PTSD than loss of control during the earthquake, possibly reflecting the cumulative impact of exposures to aftershocks during the first year of the disaster. The impact of stressors in the early aftermath of the earthquake (EESS distress score) was a relatively weak predictor of PTSD and did not relate to depression.

To examine the relative contributions of helplessness and avoidance to PTSD, the analysis was repeated twice, first entering helplessness variable at step 3 and the avoidance variable at step 4 and then entering them in reverse order. When the helplessness variable was entered first, it explained 21% of the variance in PTSD scores, while avoidance explained a further 10%. When the avoidance variable was entered first, it explained 28% of the variance, whereas the helplessness variable explained a further 3%. The same analyses using depression score as the dependent variable revealed similar findings. These findings point to the important role of avoidance in earthquake-related PTSD and depression, consistent with findings from other studies (Başoğlu et al., 2001; Pynoos et al., 1993).

The direction of causality between helplessness and avoidance is difficult to ascertain. While avoidance might be regarded as a coping response to helplessness anxiety, this does not explain why blocking avoidance responses to feared situations (e.g. as in exposure treatment) reduce helplessness (see Chapter 6 for discussion of mechanisms of change during treatment). Perhaps there is a two-way interaction between the

Table 1.5 Multiple regression analysis of factors associated with PTSD and depression in earthquake survivors

	PTSD[a]		Depression[b]	
	R^2	Change statistics	R^2	Change statistics
Step 1[c]	0.14	$F_{6,334} = 9.4^{***}$	0.16	$F_{6,334} = 10.2^{***}$
Step 2[d]	0.06	$F_{1,333} = 23.6^{***}$	0.04	$F_{1,333} = 16.0^{***}$
Step 3[e]	0.09	$F_{5,328} = 7.8^{***}$	0.05	$F_{5,328} = 4.1^{***}$
Step 4[f]	0.31	$F_{2,326} = 125.2^{***}$	0.27	$F_{2,326} = 90.5^{***}$
Overall model	0.60	$F_{14,326} = 34.4^{***}$	0.51	$F_{14,326} = 24.4^{***}$
		β		β
Age		0.05		0.07
Male gender		0.01		0.03
Single marital status		0.00		0.07
Lower education		0.01		0.03
History of past psychiatric illness		−0.01		0.09*
Family history of psychiatric illness		−0.01		0.02
Control during earthquake (0–4)[g]		0.11**		0.07
Damage to home (0–4)[h]		−0.04		0.00
Trapped under rubble		0.08		−0.04
Lost family members		0.05		0.08
Participated in rescue work		0.02		0.01
EESS total distress scores		0.10*		0.04
Fear and Loss of Control Scale score		0.27***		0.28***
Fear and Avoidance Questionnaire score		0.49***		0.44***

[a] Clinician-Administered PTSD Scale total score.
[b] Beck Depression Inventory total score.
[c] Age, gender, education, marital status, personal and family history of psychiatric illness.
[d] Degree of control during the initial major shock.
[e] Extent of damage to home, trapped under rubble, lost family members, participated in rescue work, Exposure to Earthquake Stressors Scale total distress scores.
[f] Fear and Loss of Control Scale and Fear and Avoidance Questionnaire total scores.
[g] 0 = completely in control, 1 = slight loss of control, 2 = marked loss of control, 3 = severe loss of control, 4 = total loss of control / helplessness.
[h] 0 = no damage, 1 = minimal, 2 = moderate (uninhabitable until structural repair), 3 = severe (serious structural damage beyond repair), 4 = total collapse.
* $p < 0.05$, ** $p < 0.01$, *** $p < 0.001$.

two phenomena, each having reinforcing effects on the other.

Role of catastrophic cognitions in traumatic stress

Cognitive theory of trauma (Ehlers and Clark, 2000) views PTSD as resulting from appraisal of trauma and / or its consequences in a way that produces a sense of serious current threat. In other anxiety disorders catastrophic cognitions are viewed as mediators of fear responses. For example, agoraphobic patients avoid crowded places often for fear of fainting, losing control, or embarrassment. In people with panic disorder various bodily sensations, such as dizziness, chest pain, or shortness of breath, might evoke panic because they are interpreted as signaling an impending heart attack. Thus, when applied to earthquake trauma, cognitive theory would predict a close association between perceived threat to safety arising from anticipated catastrophic consequences of future earthquakes and PTSD. As this hypothesis has treatment implications, it was tested in the Şalcıoğlu (2004) study by using an *Anticipatory Fears Scale* to obtain anticipatory fear ratings (0 = no fear, 4 = very severe fear) in relation to 14 stressor events during an earthquake. These included (1) exposure to earthquake sensations (e.g. tremors, walls and furniture moving, the rumbling noise from the ground), (2) the devastating impact of earthquake on buildings (e.g. dying under collapsing house, dying and leaving close ones behind, suffering while trapped under rubble, close ones suffering or dying under rubble, being left physically disabled), and (3) catastrophic events, such as being engulfed by the sea, disappearing in large cracks appearing in the ground, or the arrival of judgment day. More than 50% of the survivors had marked to severe fear of catastrophic events and exposure to earthquake sensations, while more than 70% had fear of harm to self and close ones. Fear of catastrophic events reflected in part memory of certain geological events in the region, such as the sinking of part of the coastline into the sea, taking away half of the central town park and some buildings on the coast, and fault line cracks in the land.

A principal components analysis of the scale items yielded three components (66% of the total variance), which represented *fear of earthquake sensations*, *fear of harm to self and close ones*, and *fear of catastrophic events*. These components closely paralleled the item groupings indicated above. To examine the relative contributions of these fears to PTSD symptoms (total CAPS score), a multiple regression analysis was conducted, entering the background variables at step 1, loss of control during the earthquake at step 2, trauma exposure variables at step 3, and the *Anticipatory Fears Scale* component scores at step 4. The variance explained in PTSD symptoms at each step (15%, 6%, 7%, and 8%, respectively) was significant. In the full regression model, significant predictors were fear of earthquake sensations ($\beta = 0.30$, p < 0.001), greater distress associated with stressors in the early aftermath of the earthquake (EESS score, $\beta = 0.20$, p < 0.001), loss of control during the earthquake ($\beta = 0.19$, p < 0.001), and fear of catastrophic events ($\beta = 0.10$, p < 0.05). Thus, controlling for other trauma exposure variables, loss of control during the earthquake, and fear of earthquake sensations were more closely associated with traumatic stress than fear of devastating consequences of earthquakes.

Why were fears of possible disastrous consequences of earthquakes not so strongly associated with traumatic stress, given the extent of devastation caused by the earthquake? A possible explanation is that the likely outcomes of an earthquake were not perceived as entirely unpredictable and uncontrollable. As described earlier, people use various cognitive and behavioral strategies to avoid the devastating consequences of earthquakes or reduce anticipatory fear associated with catastrophic thoughts (e.g. by avoiding buildings, strengthening their homes, keeping survival kits at home, moving to a safer location, reliance on safety signals, unrealistic beliefs in safety, etc.). Earthquake tremors, on the other hand, are totally unpredictable and uncontrollable, hence with intensely distressing effects. Furthermore, earthquake tremors have strong fear conditioning effects, which are quite resistant to cognitive control. Indeed, we have seen many examples of irrational fear that cannot be explained by appraisal of threat to safety alone. In survivor camps we frequently observed people displaying intense fear during aftershocks, rushing out of their tents in panic or running around in the field aimlessly. When asked about why they were frightened later, they were often unable to state a plausible reason for their fear and acknowledged the irrational nature of their behavior (e.g. '*I know it is silly but I couldn't help it*'). The irrational nature of fears can also be observed in some people who jump out of windows in panic during even mild aftershocks, breaking limbs or seriously endangering themselves. Another demonstrative example is the fear that survivors experience in an earthquake simulator (see Chapter 4), even when they know that the tremors are not real and that there is no real danger involved.

There is similar evidence from other studies to suggest that earthquakes cause considerable fear and helplessness, even when they do not lead to devastation and casualties. Indeed, the 2000 Hella earthquakes in Iceland – the first major earthquakes occurring in the last 88 years of the country – provided almost experimental evidence in this regard. These two 6.6-magnitude earthquakes occurring 4 days apart caused no structural damage or casualties. Yet, in a study (Bodvarsdottir and Elklit, 2004), 60% of the participants reported fear and helplessness during the tremors and 24% developed PTSD. Fifty-four percent of the participants experienced fear during aftershocks and 44% had anticipatory fear of another large earthquake. Such anticipatory fear was the strongest predictor of PTSD, whereas fear of dying during the earthquake did not relate to PTSD. Interestingly, none of the control group subjects who did not experience the earthquakes developed PTSD.

Concluding remarks

Perhaps the most striking and informative aspect of our experience with earthquake survivors was observations of collective responses to unpredictable and uncontrollable earthquake stressors. These observations, together with other evidence reviewed in this chapter, lend support to the role of unpredictability and uncontrollability of stressors in the development of fear, helplessness, avoidance, and traumatic stress responses, such as PTSD and depression. Our observations also provide valuable insights into some natural recovery processes in trauma survivors. While fear and avoidance of life-threatening events may have their origins in the evolution of living organisms, evolutionary processes also appear to have gifted us with a capacity for risk-taking behaviors to ensure that our survival is not threatened by such avoidance itself. Repeated exposures to earthquake tremors appear to play a more important role in traumatic stress than direct exposure to the devastating impact of an earthquake. Consistent with preparedness theory (Öhman and Mineka, 2001), fear conditioning effects of earthquakes might reflect a preparedness to acquire fears of situations that have evolutionary significance. These findings have important public health implications in the aftermath of major earthquakes (reviewed in Chapter 7). They also shed light on aspects of earthquake trauma that need focus in treatment and interventions likely to be effective in reducing fear and helplessness.

References

Abramson, L. Y., Seligman, M. E. and Teasdale, J. D. (1978). Learned helplessness in humans: Critique and reformulation. *Journal of Abnormal Psychology*, **87**, 49–74.

Alloy, L., Kelly, K., Mineka, S. and Clements, C. (1990). Comorbidity in anxiety and depressive disorders: A helplessness / hopelessness perspective. In *Comorbidity of Mood and Anxiety Disorders*, ed. J. D. Maser and C. R. Cloninger. Washington: American Psychiatric Press, 499–543.

Antilla, A. (2001). Orangutans react to earthquake in Seattle. *Long Call*, **6**, 4.

Aoyama, N., Kinoshita, Y., Fujimoto, S., Himeno, S., Todo, A., Kasuga, M. and Chiba, T. (1998). Peptic ulcers after the Hanshin-Awaji earthquake: Increased incidence of bleeding gastric ulcers. *The American Journal of Gastroenterology*, **93**, 311–316.

Armenian, H. K., Morikawa, M., Melkonian, A. K., Hovanesian, A. P., Haroutunian, N., Saigh, P. A., Akiskal, K. and Akiskal, H. S. (2000). Loss as a determinant of PTSD in a cohort of adult survivors of the 1988 earthquake in Armenia: Implications for policy. *Acta Psychiatrica Scandinavica*, **102**, 58–64.

Asarnow, J. R., Glynn, S., Pynoos, R. S., Nahum, J., Guthrie, D., Cantwell, D. P. and Franklin, B. (1999). When the earth stops shaking: Earthquake sequelae among children diagnosed for pre-earthquake psychopathology. *Journal of the American Academy of Child and Adolescent Psychiatry*, **38**, 1016–1023.

Badia, P., Harsh, J. and Abbott, B. (1979). Choosing between predictable and unpredictable shock conditions: Data and theory. *Psychological Bulletin*, **86**, 1107–1131.

Balaban, C. D. (1996). Vestibular nucleus projections to the parabrachial nucleus in rabbits: Implications for vestibular influences on the autonomic nervous system. *Experimental Brain Research*, **108**, 367–381.

Başoğlu, M., Kılıç, C., Şalcıoğlu, E. and Livanou, M. (2004). Prevalence of posttraumatic stress disorder and comorbid depression in earthquake survivors in Turkey: An epidemiological study. *Journal of Traumatic Stress*, **17**, 133–141.

Başoğlu, M., Livanou, M., Crnobarić, C., Frančišković, T., Suljić, E., Đurić, D. and Vranešić, M. (2005). Psychiatric and cognitive effects of war in former Yugoslavia – Association of lack of redress for trauma and posttraumatic stress reactions. *Journal of the American Medical Association*, **294**, 580–590.

Başoğlu, M. and Mineka, S. (1992). The role of uncontrollable and unpredictable stress in post-traumatic stress responses in torture survivors. In *Torture and its Consequences: Current Treatment Approaches*, ed. M. Başoğlu. Cambridge: Cambridge University Press, 182–225.

Başoğlu, M., Mineka, S., Paker, M., Aker, T., Livanou, M. and Gök, S. (1997). Psychological preparedness for trauma as a protective factor in survivors of torture. *Psychological Medicine*, **27**, 1421–1433.

Başoğlu, M., Paker, M., Özmen, E., Taşdemir, O. and Şahin, D. (1994a). Factors related to long-term traumatic stress responses in survivors of torture in Turkey. *Journal of the American Medical Association*, **272**, 357–363.

Başoğlu, M., Paker, M., Paker, O., Özmen, E., Marks, I., İncesu, C., Şahin, D. and Sarımurat, N. (1994b). Psychological effects of torture: A comparison of tortured with nontortured political activists in Turkey. *American Journal of Psychiatry*, **151**, 76–81.

Başoğlu, M., Şalcıoğlu, E. and Livanou, M. (2002). Traumatic stress responses in earthquake survivors in Turkey. *Journal of Traumatic Stress*, **15**, 269–276.

Başoğlu, M., Şalcıoğlu, E., Livanou, M., Özeren, M., Aker, T., Kılıç, C. and Mestçioğlu, Ö. (2001). A study of the validity of a Screening Instrument for Traumatic Stress in Earthquake Survivors in Turkey. *Journal of Traumatic Stress*, **14**, 491–509.

Beck, A. T., Rush, A. J., Shaw, B. F. and Emery, G. (1979). *Cognitive Therapy of Depression*. New York: Guilford Press.

Bergiannaki, J. D., Psarros, C., Varsou, E., Paparrigopoulos, T. and Soldatos, C. R. (2003). Protracted acute stress reaction following an earthquake. *Acta Psychiatrica Scandinavica*, **107**, 18–24.

Blake, D. D., Weathers, F. W., Nagy, L. M., Kaloupek, D. G., Charney, D. S. and Keane, T. M. (1990). *Clinician-Administered PTSD Scale (CAPS) – Current and Lifetime Diagnostic Version*. Boston: National Center for Posttraumatic Stress Disorder, Behavioral Science Division.

Blanchard, E. B., Kuhn, E., Rowell, D. L., Hickling, E. J., Wittrock, D., Rogers, R. L., Johnson, M. R. and Steckler, D. C. (2004). Studies of the vicarious traumatization of college students by the September 11th attacks: Effects of proximity, exposure and connectedness. *Behaviour Research and Therapy*, **42**, 191–205.

Bodvarsdottir, I. and Elklit, A. (2004). Psychological reactions in Icelandic earthquake survivors. *Scandinavian Journal of Psychology*, **45**, 3–13.

Bolles, R. C. (1970). Species-specific defense reactions and avoidance learning. *Psychological Review*, **77**, 32–48.

Bonanno, G. A., Neria, Y., Mancini, A., Coifman, K. G., Litz, B. and Insel, B. (2007). Is there more to complicated grief than depression and posttraumatic stress disorder? A test of incremental validity. *Journal of Abnormal Psychology*, **116**, 342–351.

Bowers, W., Zacharko, R. and Anisman, H. (1987). Evaluation of stressor effects on intracranial self stimulation from the nucleus accumbens and the substantia nigra in a current intensity paradigm. *Behavioral Brain Research*, **23**, 85–93.

Cantor, C. (2005). *Evolution and Posttraumatic Stress: Disorders of Vigilance and Defence*. New York: Routledge.

Carmil, D. and Breznitz, S. (1991). Personal trauma and world view: Are extremely stressful experiences related to political attitudes, religious beliefs, and future orientation? *Journal of Traumatic Stress*, **4**, 393–405.

Carr, V. J., Lewin, T. J., Webster, R. A., Hazell, P. L., Kenardy, J. A. and Carter, G. L. (1995). Psychological sequelae of the 1989 Newcastle earthquake: I. Community disaster experiences and psychological morbidity 6 months post-disaster. *Psychological Medicine*, **25**, 539–555.

Carr, V. J., Lewin, T. J., Webster, R. A., Kenardy, J. A., Hazell, P. L. and Carter, G. L. (1997). Psychological sequelae of the 1989 Newcastle earthquake: II. Exposure and morbidity profiles during the first 2 years post-disaster. *Psychological Medicine*, **27**, 167–178.

Chou, F. H.-C., Su, T. T.-P., Chou, P., Ou-Yang, W.-C., Lu, M.-K. and Chien, I.-C. (2005). Survey of psychiatric disorders in a Taiwanese village population six months after a major earthquake. *Journal of the Formosan Medical Association*, **104**, 308–317.

Chou, Y.-J., Huang, N., Lee, C.-H., Tsai, S.-L., Tsay, J.-H., Chen, L.-S. and Chou, P. (2003). Suicides after the 1999 Taiwan earthquake. *International Journal of Epidemiology*, **32**, 1007–1014.

Committee for Tent Cities in Kocaeli: Report on the status of tent cities in Kocaeli, March 8, 2000.

Cook, M. and Mineka, S. (1989). Observational conditioning of fear to fear-relevant versus fear-irrelevant stimuli in rhesus-monkeys. *Journal of Abnormal Psychology*, **98**, 448–459.

Cook, M. and Mineka, S. (1990). Selective associations in the observational conditioning of fear in rhesus-monkeys. *Journal of Experimental Psychology: Animal Behavior Processes*, **16**, 372–389.

Davey, G. C. L. (2006). Cognitive mechanisms in fear acquisition and maintenance. In *Fear and Learning: From Basic Processes to Clinical Implications*, ed. M. G. Craske, D. Hermans and D. Vansteenwegen. Washington, DC: American Psychological Association.

de Jong, J. T. V. M., Komproe, I. H. and Van Ommeren, M. (2003). Common mental disorders in postconflict settings. *The Lancet*, **361**, 2128–2130.

Desan, P., Silbert, L. and Maier, S. (1988). Long term effects of inescapable stress on daily running activity and antagonism by desipramine. *Pharmacology, Biochemistry, and Behaviour*, **30**, 21–29.

Desiderato, O. and Newman, A. (1971). Conditioned suppression produced in rats by tones paired with escapable or inescapable shock. *Journal of Comparative and Physiological Psychology*, **96**, 427–431.

Ehlers, A. and Clark, D. M. (2000). A cognitive model of posttraumatic stress disorder. *Behaviour Research and Therapy*, **38**, 319–345.

Falsetti, S. A., Resick, P. A. and Davis, J. L. (2003). Changes in religious beliefs following trauma. *Journal of Traumatic Stress*, **16**, 391–398.

Fleshner, M., Nguyen, K. T., Cotter, C. S., Watkins, L. R. and Maier, S. F. (1998). Acute stressor exposure both suppresses acquired immunity and potentiates innate immunity. *American Journal of Physiology – Regulatory, Integrative and Comparative Physiology*, **275**, R870–878.

Foa, E. B., Ehlers, A., Clark, D. M., Tolin, D. F. and Orsillo, S. M. (1999). The Posttraumatic Cognitions Inventory (PTCI): Development and validation. *Psychological Assessment*, **11**, 303–314.

Foa, E. B., Steketee, G. and Rothbaum, B. O. (1989). Behavioral and cognitive conceptualizations of post-traumatic stress disorder. *Behavior Therapy*, **20**, 155–176.

Foa, E. B., Zinbarg, R. and Rothbaum, B. O. (1992). Uncontrollability and unpredictability in posttraumatic stress disorder: An animal-model. *Psychological Bulletin*, **112**, 218–238.

Freedy, J. R., Saladin, M. E., Kilpatrick, D. G., Resnick, H. S. and Saunders, B. E. (1994). Understanding acute psychological distress following natural disaster. *Journal of Traumatic Stress*, **7**, 257–273.

Hannum, R., Rosellini, R. and Seligman, M. (1976). Retention of learned helplessness and immunization in the rat from weaning to adulthood. *Developmental Psychology*, **12**, 449–454.

Hobfoll, S. E., Watson, P., Bell, C. C., Bryant, R. A., Brymer, M. J., Friedman, M. J., Friedman, M., Gersons, B. P. R., de Jong, J. T. V. M., Layne, C. M., Maguen, S., Neria, Y., Norwood, A. E., Pynoos, R. S., Reissman, D., Ruzek, J. I., Shalev, A. Y., Solomon, Z., Steinberg, A. M. and Ursano, R. J. (2007). Five essential elements of immediate and mid-term mass trauma intervention: Empirical evidence. *Psychiatry*, **70**, 283–315.

Horowitz, M. J. (1986). *Stress Response Syndromes*. New Jersey: Jason Aronson.

Imada, H. and Nageishi, Y. (1982). The concept of uncertainty in animal experiments using aversive stimulation. *Psychological Bulletin*, **91**, 573–588.

Inoue-Sakurai, C., Maruyama, S. and Morimoto, K. (2000). Posttraumatic stress and lifestyles are associated with natural killer cell activity in victims of the Hanshin-Awaji earthquake in Japan. *Preventive Medicine*, **31**, 467–473.

Inui, A., Kitaoka, H., Majima, M., Takamiya, S., Uemoto, M., Yonenaga, C., Honda, M., Shirakawa, K., Ueno, N., Amano, K., Morita, S., Kawara, A., Yokono, K., Kasuga, M. and Taniguchi, H. (1998). Effect of the Kobe earthquake on stress and glycemic control in patients with diabetes mellitus. *Archives of Internal Medicine*, **158**, 274–278.

Ito, A., Ucer, B., Baris, S., Nakamura, A., Honkura, Y., Kono, T., Hori, S., Hasegawa, A., Pektas, R. and Isikara, A. M. (2002). Aftershock activity of the 1999 Izmit, Turkey, Earthquake revealed from microearthquake observations. *Bulletin of the Seismological Society of America*, **92**, 418–427.

Janoff-Bulman, R. (1992). *Shattered Assumptions: Towards a New Psychology of Trauma*. New York: Free Press.

Kario, K., Matsuo, T., Kobayashi, H., Yamamoto, K. and Shimada, K. (1997). Earthquake-induced potentiation of acute risk factors in hypertensive elderly patients: Possible triggering of cardiovascular events after a major earthquake. *Journal of the American College of Cardiology*, **29**, 926–933.

Kario, K., Matsuo, T., Shimada, K. and Pickering, T. G. (2001). Factors associated with the occurrence and magnitude of earthquake-induced increases in blood pressure. *The American Journal of Medicine*, **111**, 379–384.

Kavaliers, M. and Choleris, E. (2001). Antipredator responses and defensive behavior: Ecological and ethological approaches for the neurosciences. *Neuroscience and Biobehavioral Reviews*, **25**, 577–586.

Kılıç, C., Aydın, I., Taşkıntuna, N., Özçürümez, G., Kurt, G., Eren, E., Lale, T., Özel, S. and Zileli, L. (2006). Predictors of psychological distress in survivors of the 1999 earthquakes in Turkey: Effects of relocation after the disaster. *Acta Psychiatrica Scandinavica*, **114**, 194–202.

Kılıç, C. and Ulusoy, M. (2003). Psychological effects of the November 1999 earthquake in Turkey: An epidemiological study. *Acta Psychiatrica Scandinavica*, **108**, 232–238.

Kirschvink, J. L. (2000). Earthquake prediction by animals: Evolution and sensory perception. *Bulletin of the Seismological Society of America*, **90**, 312–323.

Kloner, R. A., Leor, J., Poole, W. K. and Perritt, R. (1997). Population-based analysis of the effect of the Northridge earthquake on cardiac death in Los Angeles County, California. *Journal of the American College of Cardiology*, **30**, 1174–1180.

Krusko, N., Dolhinov, P., Anderson, C., Bortz, W., Kastlen, J., Flesher, K., Flood, M., Howe, R., Kelly, A., Favour, N. E., Leydorf, C., Limbach, C. and Read, E.

(1986). Earthquake: Langur monkey's response. *Laboratory Primate Newsletter*, **25**, 6–7.

Laban, C. J., Gernaat, H. B. P. E., Komproe, I. H., Schreuders, B. A. and de Jong, J. T. V. M. (2004). Impact of a long asylum procedure on the prevalence of psychiatric disorders in Iraqi asylum seekers in the Netherlands. *Journal of Nervous and Mental Disease*, **192**, 843–851.

Lai, T.-J., Chang, C.-M., Connor, K. M., Lee, L.-C. and Davidson, J. R. T. (2004). Full and partial PTSD among earthquake survivors in rural Taiwan. *Journal of Psychiatric Research*, **38**, 313–322.

Laudenslager, M. L., Ryan, S. M., Drugan, R. C., Hyson, R. L. and Maier, S. F. (1983). Coping and immunosuppression: Inescapable but not escapable shock: Stability under varying conditions. *Science*, **221**, 568–570.

Leor, J. and Kloner, R. A. (1996). The Northridge earthquake as a trigger for acute myocardial infarction. *The American Journal of Cardiology*, **77**, 1230–1232.

Leor, J., Poole, W. K. and Kloner, R. A. (1996). Sudden cardiac death triggered by an earthquake. *New England Journal of Medicine*, **334**, 413–419.

Lima, S. L. (1998). Stress and decision-making under the risk of predation: Recent developments from behavioral, reproductive and ecological perspectives. *Advances in the Study of Behavior*, **27**, 215–290.

Livanou, M., Başoğlu, M., Şalcıoğlu, E. and Kalender, D. (2002). Traumatic stress responses in treatment-seeking earthquake survivors in Turkey. *Journal of Nervous and Mental Disease*, **190**, 816–823.

Livanou, M., Kasvikis, Y., Başoğlu, M., Mytskidou, P., Sotiropoulou, V., Spanea, E., Mitsopoulou, T. and Voutsa, N. (2005). Earthquake-related psychological distress and associated factors 4 years after the Parnitha earthquake in Greece. *European Psychiatry*, **20**, 137–144.

Maier, S., Drugan, R. and Grau, J. (1982). Controllability, coping behavior, and stress induced analgesia in the rat. *Pain*, **12**, 47–56.

Maier, S., Sherman, J. J., Lewis, J., Terman, G. and Liebeskind, J. (1983). The opioid / nonopioid nature of stress induced analgesia and learned helplessness. *Journal of Experimental Psychology: Animal Behavior Processes*, **9**, 80–90.

Marks, I. M. (1987). *Fears, Phobias, and Rituals*. Oxford: Oxford University Press.

Matsushima, Y., Aoyama, N., Fukuda, H., Kinoshita, Y., Todo, A., Himeno, S., Fujimoto, S., Kasuga, M., Nakase, H. and Chiba, T. (1999). Gastric ulcer formation after the Hanshin-Awaji earthquake: A case study of helicobacter pylori infection and stress-induced gastric ulcers. *Helicobacter*, **4**, 94–99.

McMillen, C., North, C., Mosley, M. and Smith, E. (2002). Untangling the psychiatric comorbidity of posttraumatic stress disorder in a sample of flood survivors. *Comprehensive Psychiatry*, **43**, 478–485.

McMillen, C. J., North, C. S. and Smith, E. M. (2000). What parts of PTSD are normal: Intrusion, avoidance, or arousal? Data from the Northridge, California, earthquake. *Journal of Traumatic Stress*, **13**, 57–75.

Minami, J., Kawano, Y., Ishimitsu, T., Yoshimi, H. and Takishita, S. (1997). Effect of the Hanhin-Awaji earthquake on home blood pressure in patients with essential hypertension. *American Journal of Hypertension*, **10**, 222–225.

Mineka, S., Cook, M. and Miller, S. (1984). Fear conditioned with escapable and inescapable shock: Effects of a feedback stimulus. *Journal of Experimental Psychology: Animal Behavior Processes*, **10**, 307–323.

Mineka, S. and Öhman, A. (2002). Phobias and preparedness: The selective, automatic, and encapsulated nature of fear. *Biological Psychiatry*, **52**, 927–937.

Mineka, S., Watson, D. and Clark, L. A. (1998). Comorbidity of anxiety and unipolar mood disorders. *Annual Review of Psychology*, **49**, 377–412.

Mineka, S. and Zinbarg, R. (2006). A contemporary learning theory perspective on the etiology of anxiety disorders – It's not what you thought it was. *American Psychologist*, **61**, 10–26.

Noji, E. K. (1997). Earthquakes. In *The Public Health Consequences of Disasters*, ed. E. K. Noji. New York: Oxford University Press, 135–178.

Norris, F. H., Friedman, M. J. and Watson, P. J. (2002). 60,000 disaster victims speak. Part II: Summary and implications of the disaster mental health research. *Psychiatry*, **65**, 240–260.

Ogawa, K., Tsuji, I., Shiono, K. and Hisamichi, S. (2000). Increased acute myocardial infarction mortality following the 1995 Great Hanshin-Awaji earthquake in Japan. *International Journal of Epidemiology*, **29**, 449–455.

Öhman, A. and Mineka, S. (2001). Fears, phobias, and preparedness: Toward an evolved module of fear and fear learning. *Psychological Review*, **108**, 483–522.

Önder, E., Tural, Ü., Aker, T., Kılıç, C. and Erdoğan, S. (2006). Prevalence of psychiatric disorders three years after the 1999 earthquake in Turkey: Marmara Earthquake Survey (MES). *Social Psychiatry and Psychiatric Epidemiology*, **41**, 868–874.

Overmier, J. B. and Seligman, M. E. P. (1967). Effects of inescapable shock upon subsequent escape and avoidance responding. *Journal of Comparative and Physiological Psychology*, **63**, 28–33.

Ozer, E. J., Best, S. R., Lipsey, T. L. and Weiss, D. S. (2003). Predictors of posttraumatic stress disorder and symptoms in adults: A meta-analysis. *Psychological Bulletin*, **129**, 52–73.

Peters, M. L., Godaert, G. L. R., Ballieux, R. E., Brosschot, J. F., Sweep, F. C. G. J., Swinkels, L. M. J. W., Van Vliet, M. and Heijnen, C. J. (1999). Immune responses to experimental stress: Effects of mental effort and uncontrollability. *Psychosomatic Medicine*, **61**, 513–524.

Priebe, S., Bogic, M., Ajdukovic, D., Franciskovic, T., Galeazzi, G. M., Kucukalic, A., Lecic-Tosevski, D., Morina, N., Popovski, M., Wang, D. and Schutzwohl, M. (2010). Mental disorders following war in the Balkans: A study in 5 countries. *Archives of General Psychiatry*, **67**, 518–528.

Pynoos, R. S., Goenjian, A. K., Tashjian, M., Karakashian, M., Manjikian, R., Manoukian, G., Steinberg, A. M. and Fairbanks, L. A. (1993). Post-traumatic stress reactions in children after the 1988 Armenian earthquake. *British Journal of Psychiatry*, **163**, 239–247.

Rachman, S. (1984a). Agoraphobia – A safety-signal perspective. *Behaviour Research and Therapy*, **22**, 59–70.

Rachman, S. (1984b). The experimental analysis of agoraphobia. *Behaviour Research and Therapy*, **22**, 631–640.

Rapaport, P. and Maier, S. (1978). Inescapable shock and food competition dominance in rats. *Animal Learning and Behavior*, **6**, 160–165.

Saito, K., Kim, J. I., Maekawa, K., Ikeda, Y. and Yokoyama, M. (1997). The great Hanshin-Awaji earthquake aggravates blood pressure control in treated hypertensive patients. *American Journal of Hypertension*, **10**, 217–221.

Şalcıoğlu, E. (2004). *The effect of beliefs, attribution of responsibility, redress and compensation on posttraumatic stress disorder in earthquake survivors in Turkey*. PhD Dissertation. Institute of Psychiatry, King's College London, London.

Şalcıoğlu, E., Başoğlu, M. and Livanou, M. (2003). Long-term psychological outcome for non-treatment-seeking earthquake survivors in Turkey. *Journal of Nervous and Mental Disease*, **191**, 154–160.

Şalcıoğlu, E., Başoğlu, M. and Livanou, M. (2007). Post-traumatic stress disorder and comorbid depression among survivors of the 1999 earthquake in Turkey. *Disasters*, **31**, 115–129.

Şalcıoğlu, E., Başoğlu, M. and Livanou, M. (2008). Psychosocial determinants of relocation in survivors of the 1999 earthquake in Turkey. *Journal of Nervous and Mental Disease*, **196**, 55–61.

Sattler, D. N., De Alvarado, A. M. G., De Castro, N. B., Van Male, R., Zetino, A. M. and Vega, R. (2006). El Salvador earthquakes: Relationships among acute stress disorder symptoms, depression, traumatic event exposure, and resource loss. *Journal of Traumatic Stress*, **19**, 879–893.

Schlenger, W. E., Caddell, J. M., Ebert, L., Jordan, B. K., Rourke, K. M., Wilson, D., Thalji, L., Dennis, J. M., Fairbank, J. A. and Kulka, R. A. (2002). Psychological reactions to terrorist attacks: Findings from the national study of Americans' reactions to September 11. *Journal of the American Medical Association*, **288**, 581–588.

Segerstrom, S. C., Solomon, G. F., Kemeny, M. E. and Fahey, J. L. (1998). Relationship of worry to immune sequelae of the Northridge earthquake. *Journal of Behavioral Medicine*, **21**, 433–450.

Seligman, M. (1971). Phobias and preparedness. *Behavior Therapy*, **2**, 307–320.

Seligman, M. E. P. (1968). Chronic fear produced by unpredictable shock. *Journal of Comparative and Physiological Psychology*, **66**, 402–411.

Seligman, M. E. P. and Binik, Y. (1977). The safety-signal hypothesis. In *Operant-Pavlonian Interactions*, ed. H. Davis and H. Hurwitz. Hillsdale, NJ: Erlbaum, 165–187.

Seligman, M. E. P., Maier, S. and Solomon, R. (1971). Consequences of unpredictable and uncontrollable trauma. In *Aversive Conditioning and Learning*, ed. F. R. Brush. New York: Academic Press.

Seligman, M. E. P. and Maier, S. F. (1967). Failure to escape traumatic shock. *Journal of Experimental Psychology: Animal Behavior Processes*, **74**, 1–9.

Seplaki, C. L., Goldman, N., Weinstein, M. and Lin, Y.-H. (2006). Before and after the 1999 Chi-Chi earthquake: Traumatic events and depressive symptoms in an older population. *Social Science and Medicine*, **62**, 3121–3132.

Shaw, E. (1977). Can animals anticipate earthquakes? *Natural History*, **86**, 14–20.

Sieber, W. J., Rodin, J., Larson, L., Ortega, S., Cummings, N., Levy, S., Whiteside, T. and Herberman, R. (1992). Modulation of human natural killer cell activity by exposure to uncontrollable stress. *Brain, Behavior, and Immunity*, **6**, 141–156.

Smith, K. and Bryant, R. A. (2000). The generality of cognitive bias in acute stress disorder. *Behaviour Research and Therapy*, **38**, 709–715.

Snarr, K. A. (2005). Seismic activity response as observed in mantled howlers (Alouatta palliate), Cuero y Salado Wildlife Refuge, Honduras. *Primates*, **46**.

Sokejima, S., Nakatani, Y., Kario, K., Kayaba, K., Minowa, M. and Kagamimori, S. (2004). Seismic intensity and risk of cerebrovascular stroke: 1995 Hanshin-Awaji earthquake. *Prehospital and Disaster Medicine*, **19**, 297–306.

Solomon, G. F., Segerstrom, S. C., Grohr, P., Kemeny, M. and Fahey, J. (1997). Shaking up immunity: Psychological and immunologic changes after a natural disaster. *Psychosomatic Medicine*, **59**, 114–127.

Steel, Z., Silove, D., Phan, T. and Bauman, A. (2002). Long-term effect of psychological trauma on the mental health of Vietnamese refugees resettled in Australia: A population-based study. *The Lancet*, **360**, 1056–1062.

Suzuki, S., Sakamoto, S., Koide, M., Fujita, H., Sakuramoto, H., Kuroda, T., Kintaka, T. and Matsuo, T. (1997). Hanshin-Awaji earthquake as a trigger for acute myocardial infarction. *American Heart Journal*, **134**, 974–977.

Tennant, C. (2002). Life events, stress and depression: A review of recent findings. *Australian and New Zealand Journal of Psychiatry*, **36**, 173–182.

Tributsch, H. (1982). *When the Snakes Awake: Animals and Earthquake Prediction*. London: The MIT Press.

Trichopoulos, D., Zavitsanos, X., Katsouyanni, K., Tzonou, A. and Dalla-Vorgia, P. (1983). Psychological stress and fatal heart attack: The Athens (1981) earthquake natural experiment. *The Lancet*, **321**, 441–444.

Tsai, C.-H., Lung, F.-W. and Wang, S.-Y. (2004). The 1999 Ji-Ji (Taiwan) earthquake as a trigger for acute myocardial infarction. *Psychosomatics*, **45**, 477–482.

Valentine, L. and Feinauer, L. L. (1993). Resilience factors associated with female survivors of childhood sexual abuse. *The American Journal of Family Therapy*, **21**, 216–224.

Van Ommeren, M., de Jong, J. T. V. M., Sharma, B., Komproe, I., Thapa S. B. and Cardena, E. (2001). Psychiatric disorders among tortured Bhutanese refugees in Nepal. *Archives of General Psychiatry*, **58**, 475–482.

Van Ommeren, M., Saxena S. and Saraceno, B. (2005). Mental and social health during and after acute emergencies: Emerging consensus? *Bulletin of the World Health Organization*, **83**, 71–75.

Warda, G. and Bryant, R. A. (1998). Cognitive bias in acute stress disorder. *Behaviour Research and Therapy*, **36**, 1177–1183.

Warren, D., Rosellini, R. and Maier,S. (1989). Fear, stimulus feedback, and stressor controllability. In *Psychology of Learning and Motivation*, ed. G. Bower. New York: Academic Press, 167–205.

Weiss, J. (1968). Effects of coping response on stress. *Journal of Comparative and Physiological Psychology*, **65**, 251–260.

Weiss, J. (1971a). Effects of coping behavior in different warning signal conditions on stress pathology in rats. *Journal of Comparative and Physiological Psychology*, **77**, 1–13.

Weiss, J. (1971b). Effects of coping behavior with and without a feedback signal on stress pathology in rats. *Journal of Comparative and Physiological Psychology*, **77**, 22–30.

Weiss, J. (1971c). Effects of punishing the coping response (conflict) on stress pathology in rats. *Journal of Comparative and Physiological Psychology*, **77**, 14–21.

Weiss, J. (1977). Psychological and behavioral influences on gastrointestinal lesions in animal models. In *Psychopathology: Experimental Models*, ed. J. D. Maser and M. E. P. Seligman. San Francisco: Freeman, 232–269.

Williams, J. (1982). Influence of shock controllability by dominant rats on subsequent attack and defensive behaviors toward colony intruders. *Animal Learning and Behavior*, **10**, 240–252.

Williams, J. and Maier, S. (1977). Transsituational immunisation and therapy of learned helplessness in the rat. *Journal of Experimental Psychology: Animal Behavior Processes*, **3**, 240–252.

Yang, C. H., Xirasagar, S., Chung, H. C., Huang, Y. T. and Lin, H. C. (2005). Suicide trends following the Taiwan earthquake of 1999: Empirical evidence and policy implications. *Acta Psychiatrica Scandinavica*, **112**, 442–448.

Yates, B. J. (1992). Vestibular influence on the sympathetic nervous system. *Brain Research Reviews*, **17**, 51–59.

Yates, B. J. (1996). Vestibular influences on autonomic control. *Annals of the New York Academy of Science*, **781**, 458–473.

A learning theory formulation of torture and war trauma

Wars or armed conflicts involve a wide range of traumatic events, including exposure to various forms of war violence and life-threatening events, witnessing atrocities, massacres, or grotesque scenes, combat, captivity, rape, torture, displacement, and refugee experience. A learning theory formulation of war trauma postulates that these events exert their traumatic impact on people through their helplessness effects. In this chapter we review some observational and research evidence in support of this theoretical formulation. As torture provides the most striking examples of the parallels between animal and human responses to extreme stressors, we first focus on torture trauma and review features of unpredictability and uncontrollability in captivity and torture events and various cognitive and behavioral strategies employed in coping with such experiences. We then present some evidence from our studies of war and torture survivors that lend support to the learning theory of traumatic stress.

The observational evidence reviewed in this chapter was largely gleaned from in-depth interviews with left-wing political activists who were detained, imprisoned, and tortured during the years that followed the military coup in Turkey in 1980. Political activists provide more demonstrative examples of successful coping with torture, because they are generally more psychologically prepared for such an event. They are often part of a political group or organization that resembles military structures in providing ideological and military training as well as a shared value system, goals, and life style for their members. Some political groups also train their members in coping with captivity and related events. These groups often prescribe total commitment to their goals to the point of self-sacrifice and regard captivity, torture, or even death as merely a price to pay for higher ideals. In such an environmental context captivity or torture is not unexpected and, when it occurs for the first time, it does not have a strong element of unpredictability.

Captivity, interrogation, and torture

Several stressor categories associated with captivity experience can be identified: (1) falling captive to an enemy, (2) interrogation and manipulations designed to induce distress, fear, and helplessness, (3) acts designed to inflict physical discomfort or pain, and (4) deprivation of basic needs. While these stressor events overlap considerably in terms of their occurrence and psychological effects, we will examine them separately for the purposes of our review.

Falling captive to an enemy: contextual factors

Captivity by definition involves substantial loss of control over one's life. A sudden shift from normal life routines to a captivity situation which allows little personal autonomy or control over various aspects of life is possibly one of the most distressing aspects of captivity. This is supported by evidence showing that 20% of the suspects detained for ordinary police interrogation experience abnormally high levels of anxiety because of uncertainty and lack of control over the environment (Gudjonsson, 2003) and that some people develop post-traumatic stress disorder after such an experience (Gudjonsson and MacKeith, 1982). Such intense anxiety is also known to lead to increased suggestibility in detainees (Gudjonsson, 1991; Gudjonsson and Clark, 1986) and might also explain suicides that occur during detention or imprisonment (Hayes and Rowan, 1988; Royal College of Psychiatrists, 2002; Stuart, 2003). This phenomenon might perhaps reflect an evolutionarily determined need of living organisms to exert control over a potentially threatening social and physical environment. Indeed, survival could not have been possible without sufficient control over a potentially dangerous environment.

In war or armed conflict settings where hostilities are relatively less restrained and many people get killed every day, falling captive to the enemy entails greater perceived threat to life. Such threat appraisal may be further augmented by various events in the early phases of capture, such as verbal insults, threats of death, beating, blindfolding, hooding, handcuffing, or rope bondage. This is the phase when people are likely to be most vulnerable to traumatic stress, because of strong elements of unpredictability and uncontrollability in such stressor events. Anticipatory fear may be particularly intense if the detainee is transferred to an interrogation center notorious for its treatment of detainees or an unknown and isolated location where no access to outside help is possible.

Availability of access to outside help (e.g. from family, friends, lawyers, etc.) is an important contextual factor that modulates the traumatic impact of captivity, as knowledge and confidence that help is available serve as safety signals to the detainee. That is, if the detainee feels confident that help is available, distress is attenuated relative to what is seen when the detainee believes their disappearance has not been noticed or attended to. Isolation from the outside world and lack of access to lawyers and due process of law deprive the detainee of such safety signals and maximize fear and helplessness. Detention incommunicado also allows the captors total control over the situation without any pressure or interference from the outside world.

Interrogation and helplessness-inducing psychological manipulations

The helplessness-inducing effects of captivity are further augmented by interrogation procedures, particularly in settings where due process of law is not observed. Implicit in such situations is that relief from fear, helplessness, and further aversive events is contingent on cooperation with the interrogators. Failure to cooperate may imply indefinite captivity, ill-treatment, torture, or even death. Thus, such context is likely to involve substantial threat appraisal and anticipatory fear independently from the effects of interrogators' behaviors.

The interrogator–captive relationship is characterized by a struggle for control between the two sides. The captors employ various strategies to remove total control from the captive so that they can achieve their aims (e.g. extracting information or confession, punishment, etc.), while the captive struggles to maintain control to avoid total helplessness. The latter can be achieved by behaviors designed to ward off danger,

avoid aversive events, or reduce pain or distress associated with the event or by anxiety-reducing thoughts or beliefs. Emotional control, on the other hand, involves an ability to maintain organized and meaningful coping behaviors during an experience of intense distress or fear.

The effects of interrogation are compounded by verbal induction of helplessness and hopelessness. The interrogators often attempt to undermine any sense of hope or self-reassurance in the detainees by suggestions, threats, and bluffs during interrogation (e.g. they are completely alone; no one can come to their rescue; their captured associates have already talked; they shouldn't count on walking out of here alive because they will be tortured to death if necessary, and this will be made to look like a suicide, etc.). These threats usually have a significant impact in settings where many people are known to have died during captivity. Suicides during this period are not uncommon, which may not be too surprising given that hopelessness is a common precursor of suicide (Abramson et al., 1989; Beck et al., 1975).

A common technique used during interrogation is the 'good cop / bad cop' strategy. The 'good cop' behaviors serve to produce a transient sense of safety in the detainee, thereby maximizing the distressing impact of the 'bad cop' behaviors when they are introduced next time around. Variable use of these behaviors maximizes their unpredictability, while also preventing the detainee from developing psychological defenses against or habituation to aversive 'bad cop' behaviors. Indeed, animals are also known to show some attenuation in their physiological responses to uncontrollable shocks when the latter are presented in identical (15 daily) sessions (Weiss et al., 1976).

There are also other psychological manipulations that are used either by themselves or in combination with physical torture. For example, blindfolding or hooding is a common practice, which not only helps the interrogators remain unidentified, but also increases the impact of torture. Blindfolding is highly distressing even when not combined with other forms of torture. Loss of visual control over the environment intensifies feelings of helplessness and introduces a significant element of unpredictability regarding imminent aversive events. When blindfolding is combined with other forms of torture, it potentiates their effects. Certain combinations are reported to be particularly distressing. For instance, the interrogators sometimes form a ring around the blindfolded detainee, and randomly take turns serving blows to the detainee's face, often varying the intervals between blows. The detainee is thus unable to know when and from which direction the blows will come. There is some evidence in animals that unpredictability about where on the body an aversive stimulus is to be applied can be highly stressful (Mineka and Kihlstrom, 1978). Another combination involves making the blindfolded detainee walk and give them the false impression that they are about to hit their head against a hard object. They are repeatedly subjected to false alarms by shouting "mind your head," the effect of which is intensified by occasionally not warning the detainee when the feared collision is actually about to occur. Unpredictability and helplessness appear to be maximized by this procedure. Blindfolding is also used to intensify the terror induced by apparent threats to life. For example, the blindfolded detainee is first made to stand on a table and then given a push after being led to believe that they are dangerously close to an open window that is at considerable height from the ground; they are then given a push out of the window which is actually only a few feet from the ground. Thus, for the detainee the blindfolding magnifies a realistically minor threat into an apparently life endangering situation.

Stripping the detainee naked is another common practice during captivity. Nakedness seems to induce a sense of helplessness and danger in the face of imminent danger by depriving the detainee of the sense of protection and illusory security that clothing affords. Because of the sexual connotations of nakedness, stripping also raises a possible but uncertain threat of sexual assault. Nakedness also potentiates the effects of exposure to extreme temperatures or hot or cold showers.

Sham executions are also a widely practiced form of torture. Sometimes the detainee is subjected to a prolonged threat of execution. For instance, they are told that they are going to be shot the next morning. The next day they are taken from their cell, blindfolded and taken to another room where someone holds an unloaded gun at their head and pulls the trigger. The same procedure may be repeated for days or weeks on end. The fact that the threat has not been realized after several occasions provides no disconfirmation of the threat because the detainee is aware of the real possibility that execution may occur one day. Thus, the detainee is repeatedly subjected to an unreliable signal of the ultimate uncontrollable threat – their own death. This chronic high level of uncertainty over an

uncontrollable threat might be expected to result in greater distress and anxiety than would be seen in an uncontrollable but predictable situation, e.g. being certain of one's execution the next day. The latter might be expected to induce a sense of hopelessness and hence depression (Abramson et al., 1989; Alloy et al., 1990; Mineka et al., 1998).

Another common form of torture is confronting the detainee with an impossible choice. For example, the detainee is told that if they refuse to comply, close relatives will be arrested, raped, and tortured in front of them. If the detainee speaks, they will save themselves and loved ones but will have to reveal information about associates leading to their arrest, torture, or even death. In animals, it is known that inducing conflict of this sort (e.g. being punished with a mild shock for choosing to exert control and avoid a strong shock) is highly stressful (Weiss, 1971).

Survivors often report as one of the most distressing aspects of their past experience being forced to witness other people being tortured. Other people may include friends, close relatives, or even total strangers. A variation of this method is forced engagement of the captive in the torture of others. Some state such treatment is even more distressing than being tortured oneself. This vulnerability, obviously well-known to the torturers, is sometimes exploited by also having the detainees listen to audio- or videotape recordings of torture sessions of others. Survivors also report this as distressing as oneself being tortured. The distressing nature of this event is not surprising given that other non-human primates also react with high levels of distress when observing fear and distress in conspecifics (Mineka, 1987; Mineka and Öhman, 2002). This is perhaps because the conditioned release of endogenous opiates which may mediate habituation and the numbing experience during physical torture (see below) may not occur simply in response to the sight of torture in others. This may help to account for why witnessing torture may be more distressing than physical torture itself which causes release of these endogenous opiates.

Certain forms of torture seem to have a much greater impact than others in inducing loss of control and feelings of helplessness in the detainee. Those that involve a perceived risk of death during the process appear to be more traumatic than the ones that merely involve physical pain but no real threat to life. Submersion of the head under water until near asphyxiation and sham execution is an example of such methods. Indeed, unpublished data from a study (Başoğlu et al., 1994b) of tortured political activists showed that suffocation or asphyxiation was not only among the most distressing stressor events but also associated with chronic PTSD in the long term.

Another commonly reported method is humiliation of the detainee. Humiliation is usually achieved by attacking the individual's integrity and by violating taboos, political or religious beliefs or other values upheld by the detainee. In the case of a male detainee, inserting a baton into the anus, for instance, is not only extremely painful but also a powerful insult to his 'manhood.' Near drowning is not only exposure to an uncontrollable threat to life but also profoundly humiliating when it is carried out in a bucket full of vomit and feces, as is sometimes the case. Threats of rape or actual rape are not only a form of uncontrollable violence but also an attack on the individual's social standing, particularly in traditional societies. Torture of loved ones is not only an extremely distressing sight to witness but also a powerful assault on his/her sense of responsibility for others. Verbal abuse and insults often damage the individual's sense of identity and self-esteem. Numerous examples of such treatment can be given which all induce feelings of helplessness in the detainee through not being able to act on anger and hostility generated by such aversive treatment. There is a substantial body of evidence that animals and humans respond with anger, hostility, and aggression to threats to physical and psychological well-being (Averill, 1982; Baron, 1977).

Another particularly stressful experience is the anticipation of torture. This vulnerability is often exploited by the interrogators who make verbal threats of torture. Many survivors report that having to wait to be taken from their cell to the torture chamber can be even more distressing than torture itself. For example, one survivor stated that he almost felt relieved once electrical torture had started. He had learned to cope with it after several occasions and every time the session started, he realized it was not as bad as he feared it would be. The anticipatory distress seems to be greater if the intervals between sessions are variable and / or if there is an uncertainty about the nature of the next torture session; both of these factors obviously maximize unpredictability. Such observations are corroborated by research in animals showing that shocks delivered at variable intervals (as opposed to fixed intervals) produce greater heart rate elevations (Bersh et al., 1953) and more ulceration (Guile, 1987).

Physical torture

Among the physical forms of torture, brutal beatings are most common. Beating might be regarded as an ordinary event, as it occurs in many other settings. In a detention or captivity context, however, it often acquires a different meaning. As it is often the first torture event encountered after capture at a time when the person is least psychologically prepared for such an event, it has a strong element of unpredictability and uncontrollability. It also evokes considerable anticipatory fear, because it signals threat of further torture. In addition, survivors often describe it as a humiliating experience.

More refined torture methods include prolonged application of electricity to mouth, ears, nipples, and genitals. Experienced torturers often vary the intensity of the current. At other times they intermittently turn the shock off, pretending the session is over, but then start it up again with no warning. This can be seen to maximize the unpredictability of the already uncontrollable shock torture experience, and indeed survivors' testimonies confirm the added effect of this element. This is consistent with animal research reviewed earlier showing that unpredictability potentiates at least some of the deleterious consequences of uncontrollable shock (e.g. Overmier, 1985; Weiss, 1977).

Falaqa is another common form of physical torture which involves the beating of the soles of the feet with cables, iron rods, sticks or other instruments of wood or metal (Skylv, 1992). Conventionally, the detainee is laid on their back on the floor while the feet are lifted up and the exposed soles beaten up with a baton. The upper half of the body is left free to move. A variation of this method said to maximize the pain involves seating the detainee in the middle of a few automobile tires placed on top of each other such that they are completely immobilized while the beating takes place. Restraint in animals is thought to potentiate the effects of exposure to uncontrollable stressors (Mineka and Kihlstrom, 1978). Another version of the technique that is reported to increase the perceived pain is serving the blows at irregular intervals rather than in a rhythmic fashion. This can be seen as maximizing unpredictability of the uncontrollable stressor.

Forced stress positions, such as rope bondage, forced standing, restriction of movement (e.g. in a small cage) are essentially physical forms of torture, as they can create excruciating bodily pain after a while and may even lead to life-threatening complications. Such positions also serve to increase helplessness, particularly when combined with other forms of physical torture, such as beating or electrical torture. Palestinian hanging (hanging by the wrists with hands tied at the back) is one of the most extreme forms of stress positions, which causes excruciating pain at shoulder joints and becomes unbearable after 10–15 minutes. Survivors often describe this position as one of the most helplessness-inducing forms of torture, as there is not much that can be done to avoid or reduce the pain. Even the slightest movement increases the strain on shoulder joints and aggravates the pain.

The impact of torture in inducing a sense of helplessness is often compounded by suggestions that the effects of torture will be irreversible. Indeed, it seems that situations of extreme stress or pain may increase suggestibility. Evidence suggests that detainees can show increased suggestibility even during ordinary police interrogation without physical torture (Gudjonsson, 1991; Gudjonsson and Clark, 1986). One detainee, for example, was told during electrical torture that she would never be able to get pregnant again. Although she knew this did not make any sense, she was nevertheless horrified at the thought and had obsessive thoughts of this comment for 2 years after her release until she actually gave birth to a healthy baby. Similarly, a male detainee was told while a baton was being inserted into his anus that he had now lost his 'manhood' and that he would never be able to return to normal sexual functioning again. This again became a theme for recurrent nightmares later. Such threats of irreversible damage to sexual organs (or any other part of the body) are not always merely bluffs as serious damage is known to have been inflicted on sexual organs through mutilation, venereal disease, and forced abortions (Lunde and Ortmann, 1992).

Deprivation of basic needs

Sleep deprivation is often designed to maximize helplessness through its various effects, such as fatigue, cognitive disorientation, and concentration difficulty. These effects make clear thinking and meaningful self-protective action difficult in the face of threatening events. As such, they are anxiety-evoking in and of themselves. Because of reduced ability to maintain cognitive and behavioral control over threatening events, they also augment anxiety during interrogation and reduce the person's ability to withstand intense psychological pressure.

Solitary confinement is probably one of the few stressor situations that induce almost total helplessness. Combined with additional stressors of social isolation and reduced environmental stimulation, loss of control over almost all aspects of life is associated with a wide range of psychiatric consequences, including anxiety, panic, depression, outbursts of anger and violence, poor memory and concentration, cognitive disorientation, hallucinations, psychotic episodes, self-harm, and suicide (Shalev, 2008). While social isolation and reduced environmental stimulation may explain some of these phenomena, there is some evidence [McCleery, 1961 and Toch, 1992 cited in Shalev, 2008 pp. 21] to suggest that prior knowledge of duration of solitary confinement mitigates the effects of the latter. Thus, the element of uncertainty appears to augment the helplessness effects of uncontrollable stressors during solitary confinement. Indeed, the effects of control and prediction are known to be closely intertwined, both functionally and operationally (Mineka and Hendersen, 1985).

Deprivation of other basic needs, such as water, food, personal hygiene, or medical care, not only promotes helplessness but may also involve a threat to life. The consequences of prevention of urination or defecation may be intensely humiliating for the person. Similarly, female ex-detainees often report deprivation of personal hygiene during menstruation as being particularly distressing and humiliating. Adverse living conditions, such as overcrowding, lack of privacy, and infested surroundings constitute additional stressors that contribute to helplessness.

Psychological responses to torture

Psychological responses during captivity broadly fall into two groups: those occurring between episodes of torture and those in response to the infliction of physical pain during torture. Not surprisingly, anticipation of the next torture episode provokes intense fear and anxiety. Animal research leads one to predict that this anticipatory fear and anxiety may be particularly intense if the waiting occurs in a dangerous context relative to in a safe context (e.g. Overmier and Murison, 1989). Hyperarousal, hypervigilance, startle responses, restlessness, increased auditory acuity, and reduced sleep are characteristic of this phase. Many of these symptoms have also been observed in animals that have undergone prolonged exposure to uncontrollable and unpredictable aversive events (Mineka and Hendersen, 1985; Mineka and Kihlstrom, 1978). Intense terror and panic may lead to serious suicide attempts. Near catatonic reactions or milder forms of negativistic behavior may also occur. Acute cognitive impairment such as disorientation may also be observed, perhaps paralleling attentional and learning deficits seen in animals following exposure to unpredictable and uncontrollable aversive events (Jackson et al., 1980; Lee and Maier, 1988; Maier et al., 1987; Minor et al., 1984). Torture may also induce extremely submissive behavior or dependency on the torturers (Suedfeld, 1990). This may be functionally analogous to the defeatist postures adopted by formerly dominant mice that have been exposed to uncontrollable shock prior to being placed with an unfamiliar conspecific (e.g. Fleshner et al., 1989).

Coping with captivity and torture

The struggle for control to avoid threats to physical and psychological well-being starts during the very early stages of captivity. Attempts at re-establishing contact with the outside world are common, when such contact is perceived as reducing the likelihood of indefinite captivity, torture, or death. Such attempts have also been frequently observed in prisoners of war (Sherwood, 1986). Experienced political activists often use every possible means to contact other detained comrades (or those outside) to find out what exactly the captors want from them, who else has been arrested, who has said what during interrogation and so on. Special codes of communication may be developed and used to smuggle out messages via other inmates or bribed wardens, or through verbal or non-verbal communication with other inmates during brief outings to the lavatory. A realistic appraisal of the risk of torture reduces the unpredictability of the situation and consequent stress even when the perceived likelihood approaches certainty.

Responses to interrogation and torture show significant variation from one individual to another, depending on their level of psychological preparedness for such stressor events. Ordinary civilians with no prior experience with similar situations often find it very difficult to cope with interrogation. For example,

a young man who accidentally got into trouble with the police had so severe cognitive disorientation after his detention that he was not able to understand even simple questions about his name and identity. The interrogators, misinterpreting his lack of response as a sign of resistance, tortured him for several weeks just to get him to tell his name, which made his confusion only worse. When he finally understood what was expected of him, he readily cooperated with the interrogators, asking them why they did not say what they wanted from him before. The distress associated with interrogation and torture is so intense that ordinary people are most likely to avoid it by simply cooperating with the interrogators, even when this means providing information they do not have or confessing to an alleged crime they have not committed.

Experienced political activists, on the other hand, experience generally less loss of control and less distress in such situations (Başoğlu et al., 1997). As noted earlier, captivity and torture may not have a strong element of unpredictability for them. Furthermore, many regard such events as a natural consequence of their struggle for a better world. Their behavior during captivity and torture is largely governed by internalized peer group norms and values, which dictate resilience, resistance, and commitment to their political cause, and condemn submission to or cooperation with the captors as betrayal of cause. Such a value system helps many political activists tolerate extremely severe torture, physical or otherwise, without giving in to the interrogators. Nevertheless, they often use various strategies to avoid torture, whenever possible. For example, when asked for information about people involved in particular political activities or missions, they may successfully mislead the interrogators into thinking that they do not have information of any importance or they may simply provide false information. Or they may convincingly pretend to be cooperative by divulging information that they know is already known to the interrogators or by providing the names of those who would not be endangered by this information because they are in a safe location or they have already left the country and so on. When torture cannot be avoided they resort to other coping strategies, some of which are detailed below.

In situations where the captive is kept together with other inmates, coping may be relatively easier because of access to various forms of emotional and other support from others. Isolation is common practice in the early stages of captivity, however, mainly because it maximizes the impact of interrogation. Coping strategies during isolation may vary, depending on its duration and the extent of reduced environmental stimulation. It has also long been known that an effective way of coping with prolonged isolation is to follow a structured program of activities and engage in some mental or behavioral exercises that help retain control over some areas of life (Suedfeld, 1990). Various responses to prolonged isolation reported in the literature (reviewed by Shalev, 2008), such as talking to oneself and frequent daydreaming or fantasizing, appear to be attempts at maintaining control over reduced environmental stimulation. Perhaps even visual or auditory hallucinations that are reported to occur during prolonged isolation serve a similar purpose. An ex-detainee reported that knocking on the wall of the neighboring cell was helpful in reducing the effect of isolation, even when the only message he could convey by doing so was no more than *"I'm alive."*

Coping with physical torture takes place on three overlapping levels: psychophysiological, behavioral, and cognitive. Psychophysiological responses include depersonalization (*"this is not happening to me, this is not my body"*), derealization (*"this is not real"*), and analgesia (feeling numb all over). For example, one survivor said the difficult part of electrical torture was the beginning; after a while he felt numb all over his body and completely dissociated from the situation. It is quite possible that such numbness is mediated by conditioned release of endogenous opiates as seen in animals exposed to uncontrollable shock that later show opiate release following the first few shocks, which have become conditioned stimuli controlling the conditioned response of opiate release (Maier et al., 1982; Maier et al., 1983a; Maier et al., 1983b). Dissociative states have also been reported in other traumatic situations (Spiegel and Fink, 1979).

Behavioral and cognitive coping strategies seem to be geared towards maintaining a sense of perceived control. The availability of behavioral defenses against physical pain depends largely on the form of torture used. If pain is inflicted while parts of the body are left free to move, such as in beating while untied or in falaqa with the upper part of the body mobile, the self defensive body movements, however ineffective they might be, seem to be useful in reducing pain and preserving a sense of control. As noted earlier, no defensive bodily movement is possible during Palestinian hanging. Even then certain gestures can be

helpful in reducing the frustration caused by helplessness. For example, one female survivor urinated forcefully while hanging naked from the ceiling – an act which she perceived to spoil the interrogators' fun who were mocking and laughing at her.

Some survivors try to maintain control over the torture events by misleading the torturers to think that certain forms of torture are likely to be more painful or distressing than others. For example, a female detainee who was being beaten while also subjected to sexual advances (e.g. fondling of her breasts) at the same time was able to avoid the latter by displaying signs of distress during beating but not during sexual advances. Similarly, during beating a male detainee avoided blows to the most sensitive parts of his body by remaining silent during blows to those parts but displaying signs of pain during blows to less sensitive parts of his body.

Survivors often point to the importance of exerting some control over events even when this is most likely to incur further punishment. For instance, deliberate disobedience or refusal to display any sign of distress during torture is designed to frustrate the torturers. To do so may be a gratifying (or anger / frustration reducing) experience in the sense that one ceases to be a passive recipient of others' actions. For example, one survivor noted that, during torture when blindfolded, his senses were acutely tuned in to the torturer's responses for signs of frustration which he could 'turn on and off' at will.

Certain cognitive factors, such as an awareness of the broader political dynamics that lead to use of torture as an instrument of repression, seem to have a protective effect against the cognitive impact of torture (Başoğlu et al., 1996). Politically aware individuals tend to regard their torturers as merely instruments of a repressive political regime and attribute blame to the regime or 'the establishment' rather than to their torturers *per se*. They also often maintain a sense of moral superiority over their torturers, regarding them as uneducated and politically unaware individuals who are merely executing orders. These cognitions seem to have protective effects, particularly against humiliating treatment during torture. Such 'de-personalization' of torture experience may sometimes lead to seemingly bizarre interactions between the detainee and the torturers. For example, after the termination of a torture session, a female survivor embarked on a conversation with one of her torturers, who asked her for advice about his marital problems at home. Feeling sorry for him, she tried to help him as much as she could. Similar stories about chatting with the torturers over a cup of tea during a break in the torture session are also not uncommon.

Certain coping processes can be better understood within the context of the captor-captive relationship and of the group processes in which systematic torture takes place. The torturers are also often part of an ideological system, with shared values, goals, a common jargon, and a common enemy. They often perceive their captives as fanatic extremists or terrorists committed to destroying the captors' way of life, values, morality, and everything else they stand for. The captives therefore deserve the treatment they get. The torturers' duty is to obey orders and serve their country by annihilating the enemy. They get credit for executing their job successfully. In such a context successful coping with torture may assume a special meaning for a person, particularly when the detainees are kept in groups and when the power struggle generalizes to the larger group of captors and captives. The captives may come to view any hint of surrender on their part as the personal success of the captors. Thus, resisting torture may be an effective way of retaliation when the interrogators' failure to break the 'tough nut' is likely to cause embarrassment and loss of prestige among their colleagues. Such dynamics explain why some interrogators develop personal vendettas against certain detainees and also why some 'accidental' deaths occur during torture.

Life in captivity is often regulated by extremely oppressive measures. Indoctrination procedures, daily beatings, and other forms of punishment such as solitary confinement, banning visitors, and withholding mail are common. Such treatments, however, become a predictable feature of daily life in the longer term and the captives learn ways of coping with them. Coping becomes easier if the detainees with similar belief systems are kept in groups. Sharing torture experiences with each other and use of humor in doing so are common coping strategies that alleviate the impact of torture. A sense of solidarity in such groups helps their members maintain a sense of control over stressor events. Collective hunger strikes are a prime example of exercising control over the captors, when all other attempts fail. Such action often attracts national or international media attention, thereby putting intense pressure on the captors. Solidarity among the captives and collective resistance means loss of authority and control for the captors and this is indeed why prisoners are kept in isolated cells in some prisons.

Natural recovery from captivity and torture trauma

Release from captivity does not necessarily imply safety for many political activists, as they often face the possibility of further arrest and torture. Acceptance by comrades is critical during this phase for several reasons. Most importantly, it enables them to re-establish contact with their political group and return to political activity. Those who have passed the litmus test of torture and demonstrated strength, integrity, and commitment to the cause by not cooperating with the torturers often enjoy considerable prestige and credibility in later political life. Indeed, we have come across a survivor who was perceived as a hero by his comrades because he broke the group record by being able to tolerate Palestinian hanging for 17 minutes. Fear or submission, on the other hand, is regarded as a sign of cowardice or personality weakness. We have seen a survivor who felt guilty long after her release from detention, because she accepted a cup of tea from her torturers during a brief break in the torture session – an act that she regarded as defeat and submission. Such group culture facilitates recovery by its strong emphasis on resilience and discouragement of fear, avoidance, and helplessness responses. Furthermore, after release from captivity, tortured group members are expected to resume political activity, which provides ample opportunities for exposure to trauma cues or reminders (e.g. police or army officers) or other situations that pose a risk of further captivity and torture (e.g. political demonstrations, various political missions, etc.). Such repeated exposures to trauma cues and risk-taking behaviors appear to have resilience-building effects. Being part of a group also affords some protection from further threats of persecution and harassment, though this may not always prevent further occasions of capture and torture.

We have observed similar recovery processes in other survivors of torture who were not part of a political group. For example, a young journalist who developed PTSD after his torture experience had considerable difficulty in maintaining his job because of extensive fear and avoidance of situations where he thought he might come across police officers. At some point he decided that he had to overcome his fear and went into a police station with an excuse and chatted with the police officers until he no longer felt anxious in their presence. With continued exposure to similar fear-evoking situations, he completely recovered from PTSD. Another example concerns an ex-Guantanamo detainee, who returned to his country after his release from prison. He was intensely distressed whenever he heard English being spoken, as this acted as a trigger that brought back memories of his trauma. He decided that he had to overcome this problem and started taking English courses. These anecdotes are consistent with our observations of similar natural recovery processes in earthquake survivors.

The role of social or emotional support in recovery from PTSD is unclear. In our study (Başoğlu et al., 1994a) of political activists, perceived support from close ones did not relate to PTSD. Considering the conditioned nature of fears in tortured individuals (as in earthquake survivors), social support in relation to various trauma-related or unrelated life problems are not likely to have much impact on fear-related traumatic stress problems. This is illustrated by the fact that 18% of the tortured political activists had PTSD, despite strong support from their close ones and peers in their political group. Yet, with its emphasis on resilience, the social environment of political groups might be regarded as providing strong emotional support and encouragement for risk-taking behaviors that are conducive to recovery from trauma. Indeed, emotional support of this kind might have contributed to the relatively low rates of PTSD among the political activists in our study.

In summary, resilience factors such as immunization against traumatic stress appear to be the most important factor that determines successful coping with torture as well as recovery from its traumatic effects. Resilience in humans has an obvious analogue in animal experiments on immunization against learned helplessness where it has been shown that prior exposure to controllable or escapable aversive events may immunize the animals against the deleterious effects of subsequent exposure to uncontrollable aversive events (Seligman and Maier, 1967; Williams and Maier, 1977). It is worth noting that certain military training methods also involve procedures designed to enhance resilience. For example, the SERE (Survival, Evasion, Resistance, and Escape) program in the Unites States used in the training of some soldiers involves controlled exposure to torture-like procedures to increase resilience against brutal interrogation techniques or torture.

Evidence from studies of torture survivors

The foregoing account of torture trauma implies several important hypotheses regarding the development of traumatic stress in survivors: (1) anxiety, fear, or distress experienced during a stressor event is closely associated with its unpredictability and uncontrollability, (2) perceived uncontrollability of stressor events or loss of control during the event is associated with helplessness responses, (3) individuals who are more psychologically prepared for torture experience less loss of control and distress during torture and develop less traumatic stress reactions following the trauma events, and (4) contextual factors during captivity play an important role in the development of helplessness and other traumatic stress responses. The latter hypothesis implies that captivity and torture taking place in the context of a war or armed conflict where hostilities are relatively less restrained is likely to be associated with more severe traumatic stress responses than similar events occurring in a non-war setting. We tested these hypotheses using pooled data from our studies of 202 torture survivors in Turkey (Başoğlu, 2009; Başoğlu et al., 1997; Başoğlu et al., 1994b) and 230 tortured war survivors in former Yugoslavia (Başoğlu et al., 2005) (see Table 1 in Introduction for methodological details). Having conducted these studies in two different socio-political contexts using similar methodology, we were able to examine some of the contextual characteristics of the captivity setting and their effect on psychological outcomes in survivors. The survivors from former Yugoslavia countries had experienced torture in the context of war captivity, whereas the survivors in Turkey were tortured during detention or imprisonment by the authorities for political and other reasons in a non-war setting.

Psychological preparedness for trauma (hereafter resilience) in the study in Turkey was measured using a *Psychological Preparedness for Torture Scale* (0 = very well psychologically prepared, 4 = not at all psychologically prepared), which was based on an evaluation of the survivor's political activities, prior knowledge of torture events, threat of arrest / torture prior to detention, commitment to a political cause and group, and any training in physical and mental stoicism as part of the political group activity. The measure of resilience in the study in former Yugoslavia was based on an assessment of (a) the extent of prior training in endurance (e.g. military, paramilitary, commando, survival or other forms of training designed to enhance physical or mental stoicism), (b) coping (e.g. training in ways of coping with emergency situations, self-protection, etc. or previous experience with certain stressors such as witnessing people dying or dealing with mutilated or charred bodies as part of one's occupational training, as in the case of doctors, nurses, paramedics, ambulance drivers, or firemen), and (c) commitment to a war cause, which referred to goals such as a sovereign or independent state, a multi-ethnic and democratic society, preserving the country's unity, assertion of ethnic identity and values, reclaim of lost land, etc.

Data on captivity and torture experiences in both studies were gathered using an assessor-rated 46-item *Exposure to Torture Scale*. The scale items were rated for perceived distress (0 = not at all distressing, 4 = extremely distressing) and loss of control (0 = completely in control, 4 = not at all in control / entirely helpless). The latter ratings were based on a detailed assessment of various coping strategies employed during the stressor events. Evidence pertaining to the validity of these scales can be found in the main reports of these studies.

Sample characteristics

The mean age of the study participants in Turkey was 30 (SD = 8); 63% were male. Forty-three percent of the survivors were rated as fairly to very psychologically prepared for torture. The mean duration of detention was 35 (SD = 58) days. Fifty-nine percent had an experience of imprisonment; the mean duration of stay in prison was 35 (SD = 44) months. The participants reported a mean of 22 (SD = 8) torture events during captivity. Time since last torture was 44 (SD = 47) months. Fifty-three percent of the participants had a diagnosis of lifetime PTSD, while 37% had current PTSD and 13% had major depression.

It is worth highlighting further the remarkable severity of the torture experienced by some of the survivors in Turkey. In 21 survivors data were available on the number of times each stressor event was experienced on different occasions. These survivors endured on average 24 (SD = 6, range 16–35) different types of torture, with a mean total of 305 (SD = 169,

range 65–719) exposures to different stressor events (excluding beating and verbal abuse that were too many to count), during a mean of 85 (SD = 60) months of captivity. Eighty-six percent of these survivors endured electrical torture (mean = 14 times, SD = 13), 48% hanging by the hands (mean = 12 times, SD = 10), and 67% falaqa (mean = 15 times, SD = 12). Despite such severe torture, only two (10%) had moderately severe PTSD at the time of assessment.

The mean age of the study participants in former Yugoslavia was 45 (SD = 10); 85% were male. Fourteen percent of the survivors were rated as fairly to very psychologically prepared for torture. Seventy-one percent of the survivors were volunteer army conscripts or draftees, while 24% were civilian ex-detainees. Sixty-seven percent had active combat, 63% had prisoner-of-war, and 73% had detention camp experience. The participants reported a mean of 19 (SD = 7) torture events during captivity. Time since last torture was 95 (SD = 25) months. Seventy-seven percent of the participants had a diagnosis of lifetime PTSD, while 57% had current PTSD and 17% had major depression. Thus, relative to the study participants in Turkey, those in former Yugoslavia were older, more likely to be male, less likely to be psychologically prepared for torture, had experienced fewer number of torture events, had longer time since last torture, and had more lifetime and current PTSD (all p's < 0.001).

Role of resilience and context of captivity in torture-induced distress

Table 2.1 compares three groups of survivors from Turkey and former Yugoslavia in terms of their perceived distress ratings with respect to various captivity stressors. Group 1 includes 86 political activists with high levels of resilience, whereas Group 2 and Group 3 include survivors with relatively low resilience. Group 2 included ordinary civilians who were tortured for non-political reasons in Turkey. These two groups were similar in age, gender, and duration of detention but Group 1 survivors had higher education, less imprisonment experience but longer stay in prison, more severe torture, and longer time since last torture than did Group 2 survivors. The 32 survivors with high resilience from former Yugoslavia were not included in the comparison, because of too few cases reporting various stressor events. Post hoc comparisons between Group 1 versus Group 2 represent

Table 2.1 Comparison of study samples in distress associated with torture stressors[1]

| | Turkey | | | | Former Yugoslavia | | |
| | Group 1 High resilience (N = 86) | | Group 2 Low resilience (N = 116) | | Group 3 Low resilience (N = 198) | | Multiple comparisons |
Stressor categories and events	n	Mean (SD)	n	Mean (SD)	n	Mean (SD)	
Physical pain / discomfort							
Palestinian hanging	28	3.5 (0.6)	29	3.7 (0.5)	3	3.7 (0.6)	NA
Hanging by the hands	45	3.3 (0.7)	45	3.5 (0.7)	14	3.6 (0.5)	–
Stretching of extremities	13	3.2 (0.7)	19	3.3 (0.9)	17	3.4 (1.1)	–
Electrical torture	65	3.3 (0.9)	57	3.5 (0.8)	17	3.7 (0.6)	–
Burning parts of body	16	2.3 (1.0)	13	2.6 (1.1)	15	3.6 (0.6)***	1 and 2 < 3
Needles under toenails or fingernails	6	3.2 (0.8)	6	2.8 (1.0)	4	3.8 (0.5)	NA
Forced extraction of teeth	0	–	2	3.0 (1.4)	7	3.6 (0.8)	NA
Beating	86	2.4 (1.0)	109	2.9 (0.9)	177	3.5 (0.7)***	1 < 2 < 3
Falaqa (beating of the soles of the feet)	53	2.9 (0.9)	53	2.9 (0.9)	36	3.6 (0.6)***	1 and 2 < 3
Beating over the ears with cupped hands	35	2.3 (1.0)	44	2.9 (0.8)	79	3.5 (0.7)***	1 < 2 < 3
Pulling / dragging by hair	77	2.0 (1.0)	84	2.6 (0.8)	118	3.2 (0.8)***	1 < 2 < 3
Rope bondage	13	2.5 (1.1)	18	3.0 (1.0)	96	3.3 (0.7)**	1 < 3
Forced standing with weight on	25	2.8 (1.0)	22	2.7 (1.1)	22	3.1 (0.9)	–
Forced standing	80	2.2 (1.1)	74	2.4 (1.1)	149	3.0 (0.9)***	1 and 2 < 3
Restriction of movement	48	2.4 (1.1)	29	2.5 (1.1)	182	2.9 (1.0)**	1 < 3
Exposure to extreme hot / cold	52	2.0 (1.1)	64	2.5 (0.9)	80	3.0 (0.9)***	1 < 2 < 3
Cold showers	51	2.5 (1.0)	54	2.7 (1.1)	64	2.8 (1.1)	–
Exposure to bright light	29	1.7 (1.0)	24	2.1 (1.0)	45	2.9 (0.9)***	1 and 2 < 3
Exposure to loud music	55	2.2 (1.2)	58	2.4 (1.0)	67	2.6 (0.9)	–
Asphyxiation / suffocation	24	2.6 (1.2)	32	3.2 (0.9)	38	3.7 (0.6)***	1 < 2 < 3
Fear-inducing manipulations							
Sham executions	35	2.3 (1.4)	27	2.3 (1.4)	67	3.7 (0.7)***	1 and 2 < 3
Threats of rape	54	2.7 (1.1)	61	3.1 (1.0)	38	3.6 (0.6)***	1 < 2 < 3
Threats against family	60	2.6 (1.2)	70	2.8 (1.1)	106	3.4 (0.9)***	1 and 2 < 3
Witnessing torture	66	3.2 (0.8)	80	3.5 (0.6)	149	3.5 (0.6)*	1 < 2 and 3
Threats of death	78	1.7 (1.1)	87	2.3 (1.1)	179	3.4 (0.8)***	1 < 2 < 3
Threats of torture	77	1.9 (1.0)	92	2.5 (1.0)	150	3.3 (0.8)***	1 < 2 < 3
Fluctuating interrogator attitude	77	1.2 (1.1)	81	1.9 (1.2)	127	3.0 (1.0)***	1 < 2 < 3
Blindfolding	83	2.3 (1.1)	97	2.7 (1.0)	50	3.3 (0.8)***	1 < 2 < 3

Table 2.1 (cont)

| Stressor categories and events | Turkey | | | | Former Yugoslavia | | Multiple comparisons |
| | Group 1 High resilience (N = 86) | | Group 2 Low resilience (N = 116) | | Group 3 Low resilience (N = 198) | | |
	n	Mean (SD)	n	Mean (SD)	n	Mean (SD)	
Sexual torture							
Rape	10	3.0 (1.3)	8	3.9 (0.4)	15	3.9 (0.5)*	1 < 2 and 3
Fondling of genitals	31	2.9 (1.2)	37	3.6 (0.6)	27	3.7 (0.5)***	1 < 2 and 3
Sexual advances	29	3.1 (1.0)	31	3.4 (0.8)	36	3.5 (0.8)	—
Humiliating treatment							
Throwing feces / urine at detainee	8	1.5 (1.6)	4	3.3 (1.5)	30	3.5 (0.7)	NA
Excrement in food	8	1.9 (1.6)	30	2.4 (1.2)	10	3.1 (0.9)	–
Stripping naked	65	2.1 (1.1)	59	2.7 (1.1)	73	3.2 (0.9)***	1 < 2 < 3
Verbal abuse	86	1.7 (1.2)	113	2.2 (1.2)	190	3.1 (0.9)***	1 < 2 < 3
Humiliating treatment	50	1.7 (1.1)	62	2.1 (1.1)	184	3.1 (0.9)***	1 < 2 < 3
Deprivation of basic needs							
Isolation / solitary confinement	61	2.3 (1.1)	54	2.4 (1.1)	60	3.6 (0.8)***	1 and 2 < 3
Sleep deprivation	68	2.0 (1.0)	73	2.5 (0.9)	139	3.2 (0.7)***	1 < 2 < 3
Water deprivation	53	2.1 (1.2)	57	2.3 (1.0)	124	3.0 (0.9)***	1 and 2 < 3
Food deprivation	56	1.5 (1.0)	58	1.9 (1.1)	154	2.7 (0.8)***	1 < 2 < 3
Deprivation of medical care	63	1.6 (0.9)	71	2.1 (1.0)	102	2.9 (1.0)***	1 < 2 < 3
Prevention of urination / defecation	61	1.7 (1.0)	63	1.9 (1.1)	87	3.4 (0.7)***	1 and 2 < 3
Prevention of hygiene	68	1.6 (0.9)	76	2.1 (1.1)	159	2.8 (0.9)***	1 < 2 < 3
Denial of privacy	60	1.9 (1.2)	52	2.5 (1.2)	161	2.7 (1.0)***	1 < 2 and 3
Exposure to infested surroundings	33	1.4 (1.1)	31	2.1 (1.0)	141	2.7 (1.0)***	1 < 2 < 3

Note: statistical testing not conducted for comparisons involving cell sizes less than 5.
* p < 0.05, ** p < 0.01, *** p < 0.001.
[1] Distress scale: 0 = not at all distressing, 1 = slightly distressing, 2 = moderately distressing, 3 = fairly distressing, 4 = extremely distressing.

resilience effects, whereas Group 2 versus Group 3 comparisons reflect captivity context effects.

Several findings are worth noting. The three groups significantly differed in their Mean Distress Scores (i.e. distress ratings averaged across all stressor events reported; mean = 2.2, SD = 0.6 vs. mean = 2.6, SD = 0.7 vs. mean = 3.1, SD = 0.6, respectively, p < 0.001). Thus, despite having experienced more severe torture, more resilient survivors in Turkey had significantly lower Mean Distress Scores than did less resilient survivors. They perceived less distress in relation to various forms of beating (except falaqa), asphyxiation / suffocation, fear-inducing manipulations (except sham executions and threats against family), humiliating treatments, sexual torture, and deprivation of basic needs (except solitary confinement, water deprivation, and prevention of urination / defecation). The fact that their mean distress rating in relation to asphyxiation / suffocation was 2.6 (moderately to fairly distressing) is most remarkable, considering that this is one of the most traumatic torture events for an ordinary person. Equally remarkable is the finding of significant resilience effects in relation to sexual torture, including rape, despite the negative cultural connotations of these events. Overall, these findings reflect the effects of various behavioral and cognitive control strategies reviewed earlier. On the other hand, no resilience effects were noted in relation to most events that involve extreme physical pain or discomfort, possibly reflecting the fact that these forms of torture are conducted in ways that make them more uncontrollable.[1]

Group 2 versus Group 3 comparisons revealed captivity context effects in relation to 27 of the 41 torture events on which between-group comparisons were conducted. As noted above, the survivors from former Yugoslavia countries had significantly higher Mean Distress Scores than did the two Turkish survivor groups. On the other hand, consistent with similar findings pertaining to resilience effects, perceived

distress associated with events involving extreme physical pain or discomfort was independent of the captivity context. Sexual torture events, including rape, were equally distressing in both captivity settings, possibly reflecting the cultural connotations of such events. Witnessing torture was also unrelated to the context of captivity. As noted earlier, the psychological impact of witnessing torture might reflect an evolutionarily determined preparedness to react with distress to fear in conspecifics.

Associations between sense of control and distress during torture

The association between loss of control and intensity of distress during various torture events was examined in 343 cases (excluding 89 Turkish survivors on whom the control ratings were not available) by computing the Pearson correlation coefficient between control and distress ratings with respect to each reported stressor event. The correlations in relation to all but two stressor events (forced extraction of teeth, excrement in food) were significant with a p value < 0.001 for 41 of the 45 stressor events. These findings lend further support to the role of uncontrollability of stressors in anxiety or fear responses.

Associations between resilience and sense of control during torture

Greater resilience significantly correlated with less loss of control during 31 of the 45 stressor events (p < 0.001 for 26 events). However, it did not relate to some events involving physical pain or discomfort (Palestinian hanging, electrical torture, burning parts of the body, forced extraction of teeth, stretching of extremities, needles under toenails or fingernails, rope bondage, forced standing with weight on, exposure to bright light, loud music, or cold showers), threats of rape, and solitary confinement. These findings point to the uncontrollable nature of these stressor events in the context in which they were experienced. We should emphasize here that these correlations do not reflect only the impact of a particular torture method independent of other stressor events. Stressor events occur in clusters and they potentiate the effects of each other (see below). For example, being beaten while naked and blindfolded involves three concurrent stressor events, each of which magnifies the distress associated with the others. Such stressor interactions

---

[1] It is important to note that these findings imply nothing about the effectiveness of various forms of torture in resilient individuals. We know from interviews with political activists that an experience of severe physical torture implies neither a psychological breakdown nor submission to torturers. Evidence (Başoğlu, 2009) from the same studies suggests that physical torture is not even associated with long-term psychological damage in survivors. This reflects the ability of highly resilient political activists to tolerate severe pain, utilize various coping strategies, and maintain a sense of control over the situation.

define the context of the torture setting. The control and distress ratings thus reflect the relative impact of a particular stressor event experienced together with other stressor events.

Contextual factors in captivity – stressor interactions

In a previous report (Başoğlu, 2009) the contextual characteristics of the torture setting was examined by a principal components analysis of the distress ratings associated with the torture events listed in the *Exposure to Torture Scale*. The analysis yielded 12 components, which explained 59% of the total variance. The first three components that showed high loadings on more than two items were interpreted. The first component showed high loadings on (in descending order from 0.68 to 0.34) food deprivation, sleep deprivation, prevention of hygiene, water deprivation, pulling by hair, forced standing, beating over the ears, denial of privacy, infested surroundings, restriction of movement, threats of torture and death, rope bondage, prevention of urination / defecation, deprivation of medical care, witnessing torture, exposure to extreme hot / cold, humiliating treatment, stripping naked, beating, fluctuations of interrogators' attitude, cold showers, exposure to bright light, sham executions, throwing feces to detainee, solitary confinement, verbal abuse, forced standing with weight on, asphyxiation / suffocation, threats against family, and exposure to loud music. The second component, on the other hand, showed high loadings on severe forms of physical torture such as electrical torture, hanging by the hands, Palestinian hanging, falaqa, stretching of extremities, and needles under toenails or fingernails. Thus, Component 1 represented what is often referred to as cruel, inhuman, and degrading treatment (CIDT), whereas Component 2 represented physical torture. The third component represented sexual torture with high loadings on sexual advances, rape, fondling of genitals, and threats of rape. As the distress ratings of events not experienced by the survivors were coded as 0, these components represented interactions among the distressing effects of stressor events that were administered concurrently or sequentially. The survivors from former Yugoslavia scored higher on Component 1, whereas the survivors from Turkey scored higher on Component 2. Mean Distress Scores correlated positively with the CIDT component ($r = 0.58$, $p < 0.001$) and negatively with the physical

torture component ($r = -0.39$, $p < 0.001$), showing that CIDT accounted for perceived overall severity of torture. These components revealed various contextual characteristics of the captivity setting in the two study sites. Potentially life-threatening (e.g. deprivation of basic needs), fear-inducing treatments (e.g. threats of harm to self and close ones, sham executions, asphyxiation), and humiliating treatments were the major determinants of perceived severity of the torture experience. Such appraisal of threat appeared to be more characteristic of the overall context of war captivity setting in former Yugoslavia, consistent with our earlier formulation of war captivity involving greater perceived threat to safety.

Orthogonal rotation of the components yielded fairly distinct stressor clusters. Rotated Component 1 represented distress associated with deprivation of basic needs and the adverse circumstances of the captivity environment. Component 2 showed high loadings on beating, pulling by the hair, threats of torture and death, forced standing, rope bondage, humiliating treatment, verbal abuse, beating over the ears, and witnessing torture. Component 3 was characterized by electrical torture, falaqa, hanging by the hands, Palestinian hanging, blindfolding, humiliating treatment, verbal abuse, and cold showers. Component 4 represented sexual torture, whereas distress associated with extreme temperatures, isolation, forced stress positions, and being stripped naked characterized Component 5. These stressor clusters provided clues regarding the intent in combined use of particular torture methods, that is, to maximize psychological impact by enhancing the unpredictability and uncontrollability of stressors. Some likely examples include: (a) deprivation of multiple basic needs (rotated Component 1); (b) threats of torture / death during beating or exposure to forced stress positions to maximize fear, restriction of movement during beating to remove behavioral control, humiliating treatment to induce helplessness through inability to act on anger (rotated Component 2); (c) removing visual control over physical torture events and thus making them more unpredictable by blindfolding or removing behavioral control over electrical torture by combining it with hanging by the hands (rotated Component 3); and (d) exposure to cold temperatures / showers, stress positions, or isolation while naked (rotated Component 5). The clustering of these stressors also reflected their mutually enhancing effects. These findings are generally consistent with our review of survivors' accounts of elements of unpredictability and uncontrollability of various torture events.

Resilience and context of captivity as predictors of PTSD

The contribution of resilience and captivity context to PTSD was examined by a multiple regression analysis. Captivity context was represented by two types of variables: (1) a study site variable (Turkey vs. Former Yugoslavia) that contrasted two different socio-political contexts of captivity, i.e. detention / imprisonment for political reasons during a repressive regime versus war-related captivity or prisoner-of-war (POW) experience, and (2) study participants' scores on the three unrotated *Exposure to Torture Scale* components (CIDT, physical torture, and sexual torture) that represented appraisal of threat arising from the overall contextual characteristics of the captivity setting. The number of PTSD symptoms (based on Structured Clinical Interview for DSM-IV assessment) occurring at some stage after the torture was used as the dependent variable in this analysis, as this was the only measure of PTSD common to both studies. Age, sex, education, marital status, time since last torture, and level of resilience were entered into the regression equation at step 1 and the captivity context variables at step 2. The overall regression model was significant ($R^2 = 0.24$, $F_{10,410} = 12.4$, $p < 0.001$). The pre-trauma variables explained 9% of the variance in PTSD severity, while captivity context variables explained a further 15% of the variance. The resilience variable showed significant prediction at step 1 ($\beta = 0.14$, $p < 0.01$) but this prediction just failed to reach significance at step 2 ($\beta = 0.09$, $p = 0.06$). In the full regression model PTSD severity significantly related to CIDT ($\beta = 0.32$, $p < 0.001$), lower education ($\beta = 0.15$, $p < 0.001$), war-related captivity / POW experience ($\beta = 0.18$, $p < 0.05$), and sexual torture ($\beta = 0.12$, $p < 0.05$). Physical torture showed no significant prediction ($\beta = 0.08$, $p = 0.22$). Thus, PTSD severity most strongly related to the contextual characteristics of the captivity setting. It is worth noting that when the distress ratings in relation to torture events were entered into the regression equation, no single torture event showed a significant prediction. This suggests that it was the context of torture setting defined by stressor clusters rather than individual stressors *per se* that accounted for traumatic stress.

Fear and helplessness effects of torture and their association with PTSD

The fear and helplessness effects of torture were assessed using a 12-item *Fear and Loss of Control Scale*, which is part of the *Emotions and Beliefs after War* (EBAW) questionnaire (Başoğlu et al., 2005). Each item was rated on a 0–8 scale (0 = not at all true, 4 = moderately true, 8 = very true). Table 2.2 shows the item endorsement rates in 343 survivors (excluding 89 Turkish survivors on whom EBAW data were not available).

These findings suggest that fear and helplessness responses are quite common among torture survivors. It is worth noting that at assessment the mean time since torture was 39 months in Turkish survivors and 95 months in survivors from former Yugoslavia countries. The Turkish survivors had somewhat more intense anticipatory fear, whereas the survivors from former Yugoslavia had more severe helplessness responses, possibly reflecting the contextual differences in post-captivity settings. At the time of assessment the war in former Yugoslavia was over, whereas some of the Turkish study participants still faced some realistic threat of arrest and torture after release from captivity. Nevertheless, regardless of the trauma context, these findings point to the chronic and generalized nature of fear and helplessness responses in

Table 2.2 Endorsement rates of Fear and Loss of Control Scale items (N = 343)[a]

	%
Fear responses	
I fear for my life.	47
I feel I am in danger.	38
I feel my loved ones are in danger.	43
I sometimes feel I am being followed.	42
I feel fearful in crowded places.	40
I have developed some fears that I did not have before.	58
I am afraid of coming across the torturers some day.	53
I cannot lead my normal life for fear of the same events happening again.	50
I am frightened when I see someone who might be from the other side.	52[b]
Helplessness responses	
I feel I have lost control over my life.	42
My life is largely controlled by others.	34
I think I cannot change anything in my life.	56

[a] Endorsement defined as a rating 4 (moderately true) or higher.
[b] Item used only in Former Yugoslavia sample.

torture survivors long after their trauma. In this respect torture survivors closely resemble earthquake survivors (see Chapter 1, Table 1.3).

To examine the association between post-trauma fear and helplessness and PTSD, a multiple regression analysis was conducted using total Clinician-Administered PTSD Scale (CAPS; Blake et al. 1990) scores as the dependent variable and entering age, sex, education, marital status, time since last torture, and level of resilience into the regression equation at step 1, the captivity context variables at step 2, and *Fear and Loss of Control Scale* score at step 3. The pre-trauma variables explained 5% of the variance in PTSD severity, while captivity context variables and *Fear and Loss of Control Scale* explained a further 16% and 24% of the variance, respectively. Thus, post-trauma fear and helplessness was the strongest predictor of PTSD, even when the effects of all other variables were controlled for. In the full regression model significant predictors were post-trauma fear and helplessness ($\beta = 0.53$, $p < 0.001$) and CIDT ($\beta = 0.21$, $p < 0.001$).

Evidence from a study of war survivors

In this section we examine similar evidence from our study (Başoğlu et al., 2005) of war survivors in former Yugoslavia countries pointing to the role of helplessness in war-related traumatic stress. This study included 1079 war survivors with no torture experience (see Table 1 in Introduction). War experiences were assessed using a 54-item *Exposure to War Stressors Scale* (EWSS), which is part of the *Structured Interview for Survivors of War* (Başoğlu et al., 2005). Each war stressor was assessed for loss of control and perceived distress during the event using the same control and distress scales described earlier for torture survivors. As in torture survivors, the control ratings were based on a detailed assessment of various coping strategies employed during the stressor events. In addition, global ratings of distress (0 = no distress, 4 = extreme distress) and loss of control (0 = completely in control, 4 = not at all in control / entirely helpless) associated with war experiences were also obtained. The latter scales measured the cumulative impact of all trauma experiences during the war.

Sample characteristics

Of the 1079 study participants, 18% were recruited from Sarajevo, Bosnia and Herzegovina, 23% from Banja Luka, Republica of Srpska, 20% from Rijeka, Croatia, and 39% from Belgrade, Serbia. Ethnic status was Bosniak in 17%, Croat in 18%, Serb in 58%, and mixed or other in 7%. The mean age was 37 (SD = 12) and 48% of the study participants were male and 54% were married. Eleven percent of the participants were rated as fairly to very well prepared for trauma. The survivors reported experience of a mean of 10 (SD = 6) stressor events during the war. Time since the last trauma event was 77 (SD = 36) months. Twenty-three percent of the survivors had a diagnosis of lifetime PTSD, while 13% had current PTSD and 7% had current Major Depressive Episode.

Associations among resilience, loss of control, and distress

Table 2.3 shows the endorsement rates of war-related events and mean control and distress ratings. Various findings are consistent with those pertaining to torture survivors. Detention camp experience was among the most distressing war events, even though it did not involve torture. This lends further support to earlier findings pointing to the highly distressing nature of captivity *per se*. Events that led to witnessing of pain, suffering, or death in others were also associated with high levels of distress. The resilience variable correlated significantly with global rating of loss of control ($r = 0.30$, $p < 0.001$) and distress ($r = 0.22$, $p < 0.001$). Thus, survivors with greater resilience experienced less loss of control and distress in relation to their overall war experience. The control and distress ratings with respect to all but three war stressors were highly intercorrelated (p's < 0.001 for 40 stressor events).

Fear and helplessness effects of war trauma

Table 2.4 shows the endorsement rates of the *Fear and Loss of Control Scale* items. The rates of fear and helplessness responses were similar in war survivors but generally lower than those in torture survivors. This suggests that torture has greater fear- and helplessness-inducing effects than other war-related stressor events. Nevertheless, these findings suggest that different types of war stressors lead to the same psychological

Table 2.3 Distress and control ratings associated with war-related stressors (N = 1079)

	n	Distress[a]	Control[b]
Rape	2	4.0 (0.0)	3.0 (1.4)
Witnessing torture of close ones	8	3.8 (0.5)	3.0 (0.9)
Identifying bodies of close ones (mass graves)	49	3.4 (0.7)	2.1 (1.3)
Detention / concentration camp experience	13	3.3 (0.6)	2.7 (1.1)
Stepping on a landmine during the war	23	3.3 (0.7)	1.6 (1.1)
Witnessing violent death of close ones	80	3.3 (0.8)	2.1 (1.2)
Learning about violent death of close ones	452	3.3 (0.7)	2.1 (1.2)
Learning about the torture of close one(s)	271	3.1 (0.7)	2.0 (1.2)
Learning about rape of close ones	31	3.1 (0.9)	2.3 (1.0)
Detention / imprisonment of close one(s)	229	3.1 (0.8)	2.0 (1.2)
Witnessing acts of atrocities	20	3.1 (1.1)	1.8 (1.4)
Close ones missing in action	100	3.1 (0.8)	1.8 (1.2)
Witnessing serious injury to close one(s)	127	3.0 (0.9)	1.7 (1.2)
Living in enemy-controlled territory	179	3.0 (0.8)	1.9 (1.1)
Forced labor	6	3.0 (0.6)	1.2 (0.8)
Witnessing violent death of others	278	3.0 (0.9)	1.7 (1.1)
Forced displacement	429	3.0 (1.0)	1.8 (1.2)
Threat of death by suffocation	55	3.0 (0.8)	1.8 (1.2)
Learning about serious injury to close one(s)	371	3.0 (0.8)	1.7 (1.1)
Being ambushed	140	2.9 (0.9)	1.5 (1.0)
Serious injury to self	134	2.9 (1.2)	1.8 (1.3)
Prisoner-of-war experience / imprisonment	7	2.9 (1.1)	1.6 (1.0)
Witnessing others being seriously injured	391	2.9 (0.9)	1.6 (1.2)
Disappearance of close ones	115	2.8 (0.8)	1.9 (1.1)
Exposure to shelling	755	2.8 (0.9)	1.7 (1.1)
Dealing with mutilated bodies	168	2.8 (0.9)	1.3 (0.9)
Total destruction of home (e.g. by shelling)	246	2.8 (1.1)	1.6 (1.3)
Being targeted by sniper fire	353	2.8 (1.0)	1.6 (1.2)
Witnessing torture of others	39	2.7 (1.1)	1.9 (1.2)
Exposure to random fire	604	2.7 (0.9)	1.5 (1.0)
Loss of property	621	2.7 (1.0)	1.5 (1.1)
Refugee experience	437	2.7 (1.0)	1.4 (1.0)
Witnessing dead bodies in mass graves	33	2.7 (1.1)	1.3 (1.1)
Aerial bombardment	614	2.7 (1.1)	1.5 (1.1)
Loss of social status or occupation	385	2.6 (1.0)	1.4 (1.1)
Dealing with severely injured people	294	2.6 (0.9)	1.1 (0.9)
Severe damage to home (e.g. by shelling)	223	2.5 (1.1)	1.5 (1.1)
Other explosions	236	2.5 (1.0)	1.5 (1.1)
Combat experience of close one(s)	814	2.4 (1.1)	1.2 (1.0)

Table 2.3 (cont.)

	n	Distress[a]	Control[b]
Defection of close one to enemy side	67	2.3 (1.2)	1.0 (1.1)
Deprivation of vital needs (e.g. food, water)	365	2.3 (1.1)	1.3 (1.1)
Combat experience	358	2.3 (0.9)	1.1 (0.9)
Responsibility for others' lives (in the military)	167	2.2 (1.1)	0.7 (0.8)
Learning about others committing suicide	339	2.2 (1.1)	1.1 (1.0)
Sudden disappearance of close one without notice	125	2.1 (1.1)	1.1 (1.1)
Participation in 'territory cleaning missions'	139	2.1 (1.1)	0.9 (0.9)
Killing enemy in one to one combat	49	1.9 (1.4)	1.0 (1.1)

Note: items endorsed by less than 1% of the sample are not included (i.e. Witnessing rape of close ones / others, Rape with consequent pregnancy, Captivity/multiple rape/forced pregnancy, Experience of suffocation, Stepping on a landmine after the war).
[a] = not at all distressing, 4= extremely distressing.
[b] = completely in control, 1= slight loss of control, 2= moderate loss of control, 3= marked loss of control, 4= not at all in control / entirely helpless.

Table 2.4 Endorsement rates of Fear and Loss of Control Scale items in war survivors (N = 1079)[1]

	%
Fear responses	
I fear for my life.	20
I feel I am in danger.	10
I feel my loved ones are in danger.	14
I sometimes feel I am being followed.	9
I feel fearful in crowded places.	20
I have developed some fears that I did not have before.	32
I am afraid of coming across the perpetrators some day.	20
I cannot lead my normal life for fear of the same events happening again.	22
Helplessness responses	
I feel I have lost control over my life.	18
My life is largely controlled by others.	19
I think I cannot change anything in my life.	40

[1] Endorsement defined as a rating 4 (moderately true) or higher.

outcomes. Considering that this assessment was conducted a mean of 77 months after the trauma and several years after the cessation of the war, fear and helplessness responses seem to run a chronic course, even in conditions of relative safety. This might reflect in part the conditioned nature of fears induced by war events.

Role of helplessness in war-related PTSD

A multiple regression analysis examined the role of fear and helplessness in PTSD, using the total CAPS score as the dependent variable. Age, sex, education, marital status, time since the trauma, and psychological preparedness for trauma were entered at step 1, while the trauma exposure variables (total number of war stressors reported and global ratings of loss of control and perceived distress during war events) were entered at step 2 and the *Fear and Loss of Control Scale* score at step 3. The variance explained in PTSD symptoms at each step was 10%, 19%, and 19%, respectively. In the full regression model severity of PTSD related to post-trauma fear and helplessness ($\beta = 0.50$, $p < 0.001$), number of war events ($\beta = 0.21$, $p < 0.001$), loss of control during the trauma ($\beta = 0.12$, $p < 0.001$), older age ($\beta = 0.10$, $p < 0.001$), male gender ($\beta = 0.09$, $p < 0.001$), lower education ($\beta = 0.08$, $p < 0.001$), and shorter time since trauma ($\beta = 0.06$, $p < 0.05$). Thus, post-trauma fear and helplessness was the strongest predictor of PTSD severity.

Also worth mentioning is an additional finding relating to detention camp or POW experience, which was reported by 19 survivors. Compared with others who had no detention camp experience, these survivors had higher scores on CAPS (mean = 27, SD = 22 vs. mean = 15, SD = 22, $p < 0.01$) and *Fear and Loss of Control Scale* (mean = 31, SD = 24 vs. mean = 18, SD = 18, $p < 0.05$). Nine of these survivors (47%) developed PTSD at some stage after the trauma, compared with 23% of those without detention camp or POW experience (χ^2 with continuity correction = 5.1,

$p < 0.05$). The association between detention camp experience and PTSD was also confirmed by a regression analysis involving individual war events as independent variables. These findings are consistent with the Table 2.3 data, which show detention camp experience among the war stressors with the highest distress and loss of control ratings.

Role of cognitive factors in war and torture trauma

Cognitive theories maintain that traumatic stress responses may be mediated by inability to find an acceptable explanation for the trauma (Lifton and Olson, 1976; Ursano et al., 1992; Winje, 1998) and violation of beliefs that the world is a just and orderly place (Janoff-Bulman, 1989; Janoff-Bulman, 1992; Lerner and Miller, 1978). Furthermore, lack of redress for trauma, such as investigation of human rights violations, uncovering of truth, punishment of those responsible for human rights violations, and commemoration and compensation, is believed to aggravate social and psychological problems and impede healing processes in survivors (Carmichael et al., 1996; Gordon, 1994; Lagos, 1994). We examined the role of such cognitive processes in a pooled sample of 1079 war and 230 torture survivors in former Yugoslavia countries.

The assessment instruments were detailed in the main study report (Başoğlu et al., 2005). To summarize, the impact of trauma on beliefs was assessed by a 48-item *Emotions and Beliefs after War* (EBAW) questionnaire. A comparison of war survivors with matched controls at two study sites (Banja Luka and Rijeka) demonstrated that EBAW items measured the impact of trauma on beliefs. A factor analysis of the questionnaire yielded seven factors, which explained 55% of the total variance. The factors were orthogonally rotated. The items that defined each factor (i.e. with loadings over 0.32; Tabachnick and Fidell, 2001) and the item endorsement rates are shown in Table 2.5.

Factor 1 included all the items of the *Fear and Loss of Control Scale* presented earlier in this chapter and represented fear and associated helplessness responses. Factor 2 reflected various emotions associated with perceived impunity for those held responsible for trauma, including demoralization, distress, anger, helplessness, pessimism, sense of injustice, and loss of faith in people. This finding lends further support

to our statement earlier in this chapter that humans respond with anger, hostility, and aggression to threats to physical and psychological well-being (Averill, 1982; Baron, 1977) and that not being able to act on such emotions generates feelings of helplessness. Compared with non-tortured survivors, tortured survivors had significantly higher scores on Factor 1 (mean = -0.15, SD = 0.86 vs. mean = 0.69, SD = 0.98, $p < 0.001$) and Factor 2 (mean = -0.08, SD = 0.96 vs. mean = 0.35, SD = 0.77, $p < 0.001$). This finding suggests that torture has stronger fear and helplessness effects than other war traumas.

Factor 3 represented fatalistic thinking and increased faith in God and religion, while Factor 4 represented loss of meaning in war cause. The latter factor also seemed to reflect feelings of helplessness and hopelessness arising from a sense of defeat, loss of war cause, and loss of hope for the future of the country. In view of the between-site differences on the mean scores of this factor (Belgrade mean = 0.24, SD = 0.94, Banja Luka mean = -0.12, SD = 0.87, Sarajevo mean = -0.04, SD = 0.86, Rijeka mean = -0.29, SD = 0.88, F = 22.5, $p < 0.001$), this factor seemed to reflect a sense of defeat in the Serbian war survivors. The other factors represented belief in the benevolence of people and justice in the world, desire for vengeance, and loss of faith in God and religion. A desire for vengeance and beliefs in God, religion and benevolence of people might also be regarded as reflecting to some extent cognitive efforts to regain sense of control over uncontrollable stressor events. Fatalistic thinking as a form of coping response was discussed in Chapter 1.

This study also included an 18-item assessor-rated *Redress for Trauma Survivors Questionnaire* (RTSQ), which obtained information about the survivor's appraisal of redress for trauma. The items related to telling of trauma story to authorities or NGOs, retributive justice (investigation, trial, and punishment of those held responsible for trauma), compensation for trauma, activities in remembrance of past events, community responses to survivors (recognition of past suffering, contribution to war effort, people's attitudes towards survivors), meaning attributed to trauma (Was past suffering worthwhile, given the present circumstances of the country?), social and political responses to human rights violations (community protests, international protests, international media coverage, efforts by foreign governments to stop human rights violations, efforts by NGOs to stop

Table 2.5 Emotions and Beliefs after War factors and item endorsement rates (N = 1309)

	%[a]	Factor loadings
Factor 1: Fear and loss of control over life (13.4%)		
I feel I am in danger.	13	0.80
I feel my loved ones are in danger.	17	0.72
I sometimes feel I am being followed.	13	0.69
I have lost control over my life.	22	0.68
I cannot lead my normal life for fear of the same events happening again.	27	0.67
I am frightened when I see someone who might be from the other side.	25	0.66
I feel fearful in crowded places.	24	0.64
I fear for my life.	24	0.63
I developed certain fears that I never had before.	38	0.61
I am afraid of coming across the perpetrators some day.	26	0.57
My life is largely controlled by others.	22	0.56
There is nothing I can change in my life.	44	0.45
Factor 2: Emotional responses to impunity (13.4%)		
I feel demoralized when I see the perpetrators getting away with what they did.	61	0.75
I feel rage at the thought of perpetrators getting away with their deeds.	59	0.74
I feel distressed by the thought of the perpetrators of such atrocities getting away with what they did.	78	0.74
There is nothing I want more in life than seeing the perpetrators punished.	58	0.74
Everything in life loses meaning when I see the perpetrators getting away with what they have done.	59	0.73
Seeing atrocities go unpunished makes me feel helpless.	57	0.67
The perpetrators getting away with their deeds makes me pessimistic about the future.	58	0.64
I feel angry when I think of what they did to me and to my loved ones.	82	0.64
It is great injustice that the perpetrators get away with what they did.	92	0.62
So many atrocities going unpunished made me lose my faith in humanity.	60	0.56
The international community's indifference to and lack of awareness in what happened annoy me.	73	0.54
Factor 3: Fatalistic thinking / Increased faith in God and religion (8.6%)		
Suffering for what is right is God's will.	43	0.79
What happened to me was God's test of my faith.	34	0.77
If a person suffers for what is right they will be rewarded in the afterlife.	40	0.77
What happened to me was God's will.	43	0.74
I have stronger faith in God.	58	0.72
Faith in God is of great help in difficult times.	79	0.70
God is on the side of the poor and the oppressed.	57	0.66
Factor 4: Loss of meaning in the war cause (8.5%)		
The struggle for my country and people lost its meaning for me.	48	0.77
I believe our cause is lost.	51	0.77
My struggle for this country has been in vain.	56	0.73
I feel hopeless when I consider what we have achieved so far in our struggle.	54	0.64
I feel nothing will ever change in the world.	55	0.57
I believe the current situation of my country is not likely to improve.	54	0.45
I have no trust in the State.	74	0.42
My comrades have disappointed me.	42	0.41
Factor 5: Belief in the benevolence of people and justice in the world (4.7%)		
I believe good will always prevail over evil.	80	0.77
I have faith in justice.	75	0.72
Sooner or later, people find punishment for their bad deeds.	79	0.68
I believe in essence people are good.	76	0.52
Factor 6: Desire for vengeance (3.5%)		
Sometimes I daydream that I take revenge on the perpetrators.	19	0.75
In my dreams I commit acts of revenge against the perpetrators.	20	0.70
If I had the chance, I would punish the perpetrators with my own hands.	38	0.52

Table 2.5 (cont.)

	%[a]	Factor loadings
Factor 7: Loss of faith in God and religion (2.7%)		
I have less faith in religion.	23	0.70
I have lost faith in God.	25	0.64
I do not believe in God's justice.	40	0.37

[a] Endorsement defined as a rating 4 (moderately true) or higher.

human rights violations), and global rating of sense of justice ("Considering what you and/or your close ones went through, do you think justice has been served in your case? How satisfied are you with this outcome?" 1 = very dissatisfied, 4 = no effect /don't know, 7 = very satisfied). The same satisfaction rating was also obtained for each redress event. According to the global rating of sense of injustice, 79% of the study participants were dissatisfied with justice, while 15% were satisfied.

A principal components analysis of the EWSS in the pooled sample yielded 12 components representing captivity and torture events, exposure to shelling and random enemy fire, active combat experiences, displacement and refugee experiences, trauma events (torture, death, disappearance, imprisonment) of close ones, witnessing injury and violent death of close ones, defection of close ones to enemy side, exposure to mass graves and mutilated bodies, rape / witnessing rape of others, stepping on a landmine, sudden destruction of home / exposure to explosions, and combat experience of close ones.

A multiple regression analysis was conducted, including CAPS total scores as the dependent variable. Age, sex, marital status, education, time since trauma, and preparedness for trauma were entered into the equation at step 1, global rating of loss of control during the trauma at step 2, the 12 EWSS component scores at step 3, the 18 RTSQ items at step 4, the scores on all EBAW factors, except the Fear and Loss of Control factor at step 5, and the scores on the latter factor at step 6. The Fear and Loss of Control factor scores were entered after the other EBAW factors to examine the percentage of variance explained by fear-induced helplessness over and above the variance explained by the other EBAW factors. Table 2.6 shows the percentage of variance explained at each step and significant predictors in the full regression model.

Several findings are worth noting. First, the helplessness variables together explained as much variance (19%) as all trauma exposure variables combined, even when the Fear and Loss of Control factor was entered at the last step. When the latter variable was entered at the second step (not shown in Table 2.6) with the global rating of loss of control during the trauma, together they explained 28% of the variance, while the trauma exposure variables explained 10% of the variance. This suggests that fear and helplessness during and after the trauma is a stronger predictor of PTSD than the distress experienced during the war events. Second, appraisal of redress explained the smallest percentage of variance (2%). Third, among the EBAW factors, Fear and Loss of Control explained 10% of the variance as opposed to 4% explained by all other factors combined. Thus, helplessness associated with appraisal of ongoing threat to safety was a much stronger predictor of PTSD than helplessness related to perceived impunity for those held responsible for trauma and sense of defeat and loss of belief in war cause. Fourth, the resilience variable showed significant prediction at the first step ($\beta = 0.06$, $p < 0.05$), although it was no longer a significant predictor at subsequent steps when the effect of loss of control during the trauma was controlled for. This reflected shared variance between the two variables. Finally, the strongest predictors in the full regression model were post-trauma fear and helplessness, captivity and torture experiences, and exposure to enemy fire and casualties.

Concluding remarks

Survivor accounts of torture experience reveal striking parallels between inescapable shock experiments in animals and human responses to unpredictable and uncontrollable torture stressors. Psychological responses to torture appear to be primarily geared towards maintaining control over torture stressors through cognitive,

Table 2.6 Multiple regression analysis of factors associated with PTSD in war and torture survivors (n = 1309)

	R^2	Change statistics
Step 1	0.15	$F_{6,1222} = 36.7$, $p < 0.001$
Step 2	0.09	$F_{1,1221} = 150.4$, $p < 0.001$
Step 3	0.19	$F_{12,1209} = 32.8$, $p < 0.001$
Step 4	0.02	$F_{18,1191} = 2.7$, $p < 0.001$
Step 5	0.04	$F_{6,1185} = 14.9$, $p < 0.001$
Step 6	0.10	$F_{1,1184} = 286.1$, $p < 0.001$
Overall model	0.59	$F_{44,1228} = 38.9$, $p < 0.001$
	β	p
Older age	0.08	0.001
Lower education	0.07	0.001
Loss of control during trauma	0.10	0.001
Captivity- and torture-related stressors	0.22	0.001
Exposure to enemy fire and casualties	0.19	0.001
Combat experience involving acts of killing	0.12	0.001
Loss of resources / Refugee experience	0.05	0.03
Learning about trauma experiences of close ones	0.04	0.04
Exposure to mass graves and mutilated bodies	0.05	0.01
Combat experience of close ones	−0.07	0.001
Community's recognition for past suffering	0.06	0.04
Emotional responses to impunity	0.13	0.001
Loss of meaning in the war cause	0.12	0.001
Less belief in the benevolence of people and justice in the world	0.12	0.001
Desire for vengeance	0.13	0.001
Fear and helplessness	0.37	0.001

behavioral, emotional, and psychophysiological processes. Both anecdotal data from interviews with torture survivors and empirical evidence from our studies strongly suggest that unpredictability and uncontrollability of torture stressors play an important role in acute and chronic post-traumatic stress. Evidence also suggests that immunization against traumatic stressors is possible in humans. Resilience processes not only afford some protection from traumatic stress but also appear to play an important role in natural recovery from torture trauma.

The association between fear-induced helplessness and PTSD is consistent with findings pertaining to earthquake trauma reviewed in Chapter 1. Similar findings from studies of survivors of rape (Regehr et al., 1999), fire (Maes et al., 2001), physical or sexual assault (Kushner et al., 1993; O'Neill and Kerig, 2000), childhood sexual abuse (Bolstad and Zinbarg, 1997), and nuclear accident (Davidson et al., 1982) suggest that different types of traumas, whether of human design or due to natural causes, share the same mechanisms of traumatic stress. These findings imply that traumatic stress reactions can be reversed by interventions designed to enhance sense of control over fear, as will be detailed in Part 2. The relatively small role of beliefs about justice and trust in PTSD suggests that interventions that focus on fear may be sufficient in recovery from traumatic stress.

Our findings also have important implications on definition of torture. Since the 9/11 events there has been much debate on what constitutes torture. After reports (Amnesty International, 2005) of human rights abuses by the US military in Guantanamo Bay, Iraq, and Afghanistan, a US Defense Department working group report (US Defense Department, April 4, 2003) on detainee interrogations and a US Justice Department memorandum (US Justice Department, December 30, 2004) on US torture policy argued for a fairly narrow definition of torture that excludes mental pain and suffering caused by various acts that do not cause severe physical pain. According to this definition, various interrogation and detention procedures, such as blindfolding, hooding, forced nudity, isolation, forced standing, rope bondage, deprivation (of sleep, light, water, food, or medical care), and psychological manipulations designed to break a person's resistance (e.g., humiliating treatment or other acts designed to create fear, terror, or helplessness in the detainee), do not constitute torture. The implications of our findings for an evidence-based definition of torture were reviewed in two recent articles (Başoğlu et al., 2007; Başoğlu, 2009). Although this issue is beyond the scope of this chapter, it is worth briefly summarizing the main points of these articles in the light of additional information provided in this chapter. Most importantly, Table 2.1 data show that various stressor events that are said not to involve intense physical pain (e.g. forced stress positions, asphyxiation, sham executions, sexual torture, threats of rape, death, torture, or harm against family, witnessing torture, blindfolding, humiliating treatment, solitary confinement, sleep deprivation, and prevention of urination / defecation) can be as distressing as physical torture. Table 2.3 data suggest that stressor events involving witnessing death, injury, torture, or suffering of close ones and other people are also among the most distressing events experienced by war survivors outside a captivity setting. Thus, it is difficult to make a distinction between CIDT and physical torture events in terms of associated distress. Furthermore, evidence shows that it is fear and helplessness associated with CIDT rather than physical torture that account for chronic psychological damage in survivors. Second, our findings suggest that contextual factors need attention in any consideration of what constitutes torture. These procedures, even when they do not involve physical violence, are inherently coercive and potentially traumatic. This is supported by the fact that 47% of the war survivors who had detention or POW experience in our study in former Yugoslavia developed PTSD, even though they were not tortured. Finally, the severity of acute or chronic traumatic stress does not appear to be a reliable criterion in defining torture, considering that resilient survivors responded to many stressor events with relatively less distress and many did not develop PTSD, despite severe torture. Furthermore, not all stressors perceived as most distressing (including physical torture) related to PTSD. Yet, it makes neither logical nor moral sense to disqualify such events as torture on these grounds, as many of them constitute torture by any definition.

References

Abramson, L., Metalsky, G. and Alloy, L. (1989). Hopelessness depression: A theory-based subtype of depression. *Psychological Review*, **96**, 358–372.

Alloy, L., Kelly, K., Mineka, S. and Clements, C. (1990). Comorbidity in anxiety and depressive disorders: A helplessness/hopelessness perspective. In *Comorbidity of Mood and Anxiety Disorders*, ed. J. D. Maser and C. R. Cloninger. Washington: American Psychiatric Press, 499–543.

Amnesty International. (2005). *Amnesty International Report 2005*. Accessed on April 30, 2010 at http://www.amnesty.org/en/library/info/POL10/001/2005.

Averill, J. R. (1982). *Anger and Aggression: An Essay on Emotion*. New York: Springer-Verlag.

Baron, R. A. (1977). *Human Aggression*. New York: Plenum Press.

Başoğlu, M. (2009). A multivariate contextual analysis of torture and cruel, inhuman, and degrading treatments: Implications for an evidence-based definition of torture. *American Journal of Orthopsychiatry*, **79**, 135–145.

Başoğlu, M., Livanou, M. and Crnobarić, C. (2007). Torture vs other cruel, inhuman, and degrading treatment: Is the distinction real or apparent? *Archives of General Psychiatry*, **64**, 277–285.

Başoğlu, M., Livanou, M., Crnobarić, C., Franćišković, T., Suljić, E., Đurić, D. and Vranešić, M. (2005). Psychiatric and cognitive effects of war in former Yugoslavia: Association of lack of redress for trauma and posttraumatic stress reactions. *Journal of the American Medical Association*, **294**, 580–590.

Başoğlu, M., Mineka, S., Paker, M., Aker, T., Livanou, M. and Gök, S. (1997). Psychological preparedness for trauma as a protective factor in survivors of torture. *Psychological Medicine*, **27**, 1421–1433.

Başoğlu, M., Paker, M., Özmen, E., Taşdemir, O. and Şahin, D. (1994a). Factors related to long-term traumatic stress responses in survivors of torture in Turkey. *Journal of the American Medical Association*, **272**, 357–363.

Başoğlu, M., Paker, M., Özmen, E., Taşdemir, O., Şahin, D., Ceyhanlı, A. and İncesu, C. (1996). Appraisal of self, social environment, and state authority as a possible mediator of posttraumatic stress disorder in tortured political activists. *Journal of Abnormal Psychology*, **105**, 232–236.

Başoğlu, M., Paker, M., Paker, O., Özmen, E., Marks, I., İncesu, C., Şahin, D. and Sarımurat, N. (1994b). Psychological effects of torture: A comparison of tortured with nontortured political activists in Turkey. *American Journal of Psychiatry*, **151**, 76–81.

Beck, A. T., Kovacs, M. and Weissman, A. (1975). Hopelessness and suicidal behavior: An overview. *Journal of the American Medical Association*, **234**, 1146–1149.

Bersh, P., Schoenfeld, W. and Notterman, J. (1953). The effect upon heart rate conditioning of randomly varying the interval between conditioned and unconditioned stimuli. *Proceedings of the National Academy of Sciences*, **39**, 563–570.

Blake, D. D., Weathers, F. W., Nagy, L. M., Kaloupek, D. G., Charney, D. S. and Keane, T. M. (1990). Clinician-Administered PTSD Scale (CAPS) – Current and Lifetime Diagnostic Version. Boston: National Center for Posttraumatic Stress Disorder, Behavioral Science Division.

Bolstad, B. R. and Zinbarg, R. E. (1997). Sexual victimization, generalized perception of control, and posttraumatic stress disorder symptom severity. *Journal of Anxiety Disorders*, **11**, 523–540.

Carmichael, K., Mckay, F. and Dishington, W. (1996). The need for REDRESS: Why seek a remedy – Reparation as rehabilitation. *Torture*, **6**, 7–9.

Davidson, L. M., Baum, A. and Collins, D. L. (1982). Stress and control-related problems at Three Mile Island. *Journal of Applied Social Psychology*, **12**, 349–359.

Fleshner, M., Laudenslager, M. L., Simons, L. and Maier, S. (1989). Reduced serum antibodies associated with social defeat in rats. *Physiology and Behavior*, **45**, 1183–1187.

Gordon, N. (1994). Compensation suits as an instrument in the rehabilitation of tortured persons. *Torture*, **4**, 111–114.

Gudjonsson, G. H. (1991). The application of interrogative suggestibility to police interviewing. In *Human Suggestibility: Advances in Theory, Research, and Application*, ed. J. F. Schumaker. New York: Routledge, 279–288.

Gudjonsson, G. H. (2003). *The Psychology of Interrogations and Confessions: A Handbook*. Chichester: John Wiley and Sons.

Gudjonsson, G. H. and Clark, N. (1986). Suggestibility in police interrogation: A social psychological model. *Social Behaviour*, **1**, 83–104.

Gudjonsson, G. H. and Mackeith, J. A. C. (1982). False confessions: Psychological effects of interrogation. A discussion paper. In *Reconstructing the Past: The role of Psychologists in Criminal Trials*, ed. A. Trankell. Deveneter, The Netherlands: Kluwer, 253–269.

Guile, M. (1987). Differential gastric ulceration in rats receiving shocks on either fixed-time or variable time schedules. *Behavioral Neurosciences*, **101**, 139–140.

Hayes, L. and Rowan, J. (1988). *National Study of Jail Suicides: 7 Years Later*. Alexandria, VA: National Center on Institutions and Alternatives. Accessed on April 4, 2010 at http://www.nicic.org/pubs/pre/006540.pdf.

Jackson, R., Alexander, J. and Maier, S. (1980). Learned helplessness, inactivity and associative deficits: Effects of inescapable shock on response choice escape learning. *Journal of Experimental Psychology: Animal Behavior Processes*, **6**, 1–20.

Janoff-Bulman, R. (1989). Assumptive worlds and the stress of traumatic events: Applications of the schema construct. *Social Cognition*, 113–136.

Janoff-Bulman, R. (1992). *Shattered Assumptions: Towards a New Psychology of Trauma*. New York: Free Press.

Kushner, M. G., Riggs, D. S., Foa, E. B. and Miller, S. M. (1993). Perceived controllability and the development of posttraumatic stress disorder (PTSD) in crime victims. *Behaviour Research and Therapy*, **31**, 105–110.

Lagos, D. (1994). Argentina: Psycho-social and clinical consequences of political repression and impunity in the medium term. *Torture*, **4**, 13–15.

Lee, R. and Maier, S. (1988). Inescapable shock and attention to internal versus external cues in a water discrimination escape task. *Journal of Experimental Psychology: Animal Behavior Processes*, **14**, 302–310.

Lerner, M. J. and Miller, D. T. (1978). Just world research and the attribution process: Looking back and ahead. *Psychological Bulletin*, **85**, 1030–1051.

Lifton, R. J. and Olson, E. (1976). The human meaning of total disaster: The Buffalo Creek experience. *Psychiatry*, **39**, 1–18.

Lunde, I. and Ortmann, J. (1992). Sexual torture and the treatment of its consequences. In *Torture and its Consequences: Current Treatment Approaches*, ed. M. Başoğlu. London: Cambridge University Press, 310–329.

Maes, M., Delmeire, L., Mylle, J. and Altamura, C. (2001). Risk and preventive factors of post-traumatic stress disorder (PTSD): Alcohol consumption and intoxication prior to a traumatic event diminishes the relative risk to develop PTSD in response to that trauma. *Journal of Affective Disorders*, **63**, 113–121.

Maier, S., Drugan, R. C., Grau, J., Hyson, R., Maclennan, A. J., Moye, T., Madden, J. and Barchas, J. D. (1983a). Learned helplessness, pain inhibition, and the endogenous opiates. In *Advances in the Analysis of Behavior: Vol 3. Biological Factors in Learning*, ed. M. D. Zeiler and P. Harzem. New York: Wiley, 275–323.

Maier, S., Jackson, R. and Tomie, A. (1987). Potentiation overshadowing, and prior exposure to inescapable shock. *Journal of Experimental Psychology: Animal Behavior Processes*, **13**, 260–270.

Maier, S., Sherman, J. J., Lewis, J., Terman, G. and Liebeskind, J. (1983b). The opioid / nonopioid nature of stress induced analgesia and learned helplessness. *Journal of Experimental Psychology: Animal Behavior Processes*, **9**, 80–90.

Maier, S. F., Drugan, R. C. and Grau, J. W. (1982). Controllability, coping behavior, and stress-induced analgesia in the rat. *Pain*, **12**, 47–56.

McCleery, R. (1961). Authoritarianism and the belief system of the incorrigibles. In *The Prison*, ed. D. Cressey. New York: Holt, Rinehart and Winston, 260–306.

Mineka, S. (1987). A primate model of phobic fears. In *Theoretical Foundations of Behavior Therapy*, ed. H. Eysenck and I. Martin. New York: Plenum Press, 81–111.

Mineka, S. and Hendersen, R. W. (1985). Controllability and predictability in acquired motivation. *Annual Review of Psychology*, **36**, 495–529.

Mineka, S. and Kihlstrom, J. F. (1978). Unpredictable and uncontrollable events: New perspective on experimental neurosis. *Journal of Abnormal Psychology*, **87**, 256–271.

Mineka, S. and Öhman, A. (2002). Phobias and preparedness: The selective, automatic, and encapsulated nature of fear. *Biological Psychiatry*, **52**, 927–937.

Mineka, S., Watson, D. and Clark, L. A. (1998). Comorbidity of anxiety and unipolar mood disorders. *Annual Review of Psychology*, **49**, 377–412.

Minor, T., Jackson, R. and Maier, S. (1984). Effects of task irrelevant cues and reinforcement delay on choice escape learning following inescapable shock: Evidence for a deficit in selective attention. *Journal of Experimental Psychology: Animal Behavior Processes*, **10**, 543–556.

O'Neill, M. L. and Kerig, P. K. (2000). Attributions of self-blame and perceived control as moderators of adjustment in battered women. *Journal of Interpersonal Violence*, **15**, 1036–1049.

Overmier, J. B. (1985). Toward a reanalysis of the causal structure of the learned helplessness syndrome. In *Conditioning and Cognition: Essays on the Determinants of Behavior*, ed. F. R. Brush and J. B. Overmier. Hillsdale, NJ: Lawrence Erlbaum, 211–228.

Overmier, J. B. and Murison, R. (1989). Poststress effects of danger and safety signals on gastric ulceration in rats. *Behavioral Neurosciences*, **103**, 1296–1301.

Regehr, C., Cadell, S. and Jansen, K. (1999). Perceptions of control and long-term recovery from rape. *American Journal of Orthopsychiatry*, **69**, 110–115.

Royal College of Psychiatrists (2002). *Suicide in Prisons* (Council Report CR99). London: Royal College of Psychiatrists.

Seligman, M. E. P. and Maier, S. F. (1967). Failure to escape traumatic shock. *Journal of Experimental Psychology: Animal Behavior Processes*, **74**, 1–9.

Shalev, S. (2008). *A Sourcebook on Solitary Confinement*. London: Mannheim Centre for Criminology, London School of Economics and Political Science. Accessed on April 28, 2010 at http://www.solitaryconfinement.org/sourcebook.

Sherwood, E. (1986). The power relationship between captor and captive. *Psychiatric Annals*, **16**, 653–655.

Skylv, G. (1992). The physical sequelae of torture. In *Torture and its Consequences: Current Treatment Approaches*, ed. M. Başoğlu. London: Cambridge University Press, 38–55.

Spiegel, D. and Fink, R. (1979). Hysterical psychosis and hypnotizability. *American Journal of Psychiatry*, **136**, 377–381.

Stuart, H. (2003). Suicide behind bars. *Current Opinion in Psychiatry*, **16**, 559–564.

Suedfeld, P. (1990). Torture: A Brief Overview. In *Psychology and Torture*, ed. P. Suedfeld. New York: Hemisphere Publishing Corporation.

Tabachnick, B. G. and Fidell, L. S. (2001). *Using Multivariate Statistics*. Boston: Allyn and Bacon.

Toch, H. (1992). *Mosaic of Despair: Human Breakdown in Prison*. Washington DC: American Psychological Association.

US Defense Department (April 4, 2003). Working Group Report on Detainee Interrogations in the Global War on Terrorism: Assessment of Legal, Historical, Policy and Operational Considerations. In *The Torture Papers*, ed. K. J. Greenberg and J. L. Dratel. Cambridge: Cambridge University Press, 286–359.

US Justice Department (December 30, 2004). *Memorandum for James B. Comey Deputy Attorney General Re: Legal standards applicable under 18 U.S.C. §§ 2340–2340A*. Accessed on April 30, 2010 at http://www.justice.gov/olc/18usc23402340a2.htm.

Ursano, R., Tzu-Cheg, K. and Fullerton, C. S. (1992). Posttraumatic stress disorder and meaning: Structuring human chaos. *Journal of Nervous and Mental Disease*, **180**, 756–759.

Weiss, J. (1971). Effects of punishing the coping response (conflict) on stress pathology in rats. *Journal of Comparative and Physiological Psychology*, **77**, 14–21.

Weiss, J. (1977). Psychological and behavioral influences on gastrointestinal lesions in animal models. In *Psychopathology: Experimental Models*, ed. J. Maser and M. E. P. Seligman. San Francisco: Freeman, 232–269.

Weiss, J., Glazer, H. and Poherecky, L. (1976). Coping behavior and neurochemical changes in rats: an alternative explanation for the original 'learned helplessness' experiments. In *Animal Models in Human Psychobiology*, ed. G. Serban and A. Kling. New York: Plenum Press, 141–173.

Williams, J. and Maier, S. (1977). Transsituational immunisation and therapy of learned helplessness in the rat. *Journal of Experimental Psychology: Animal Behavior Processes*, **3**, 240–252.

Winje, D. (1998). Cognitive coping: The psychological significance of knowing what happened in the traumatic event. *Journal of Traumatic Stress*, **11**, 627–643.

Chapter 3

Assessment

In this chapter we review assessment instruments that we have developed in the course of our work with earthquake, war, and torture survivors for various purposes. An understanding of what assessment involves is helpful in understanding the basic principles of Control-Focused Behavioral Treatment (CFBT) described in Chapter 4. Gaining some familiarity with these instruments at this stage is also useful, because some of them are also used as part of treatment procedures. The assessment tools are reviewed in two sections. We first review various self-rated screening instruments that can be used for quick and cost-effective assessment of survivors' treatment needs, as well as evaluation of intervention outcomes. Some general guidelines as to how the data they generate can be interpreted and used in planning treatment services are also provided. These instruments are an indispensable component of outreach treatment delivery programs targeting large survivor populations but can also be useful in primary healthcare or outpatient settings in quick assessment of incoming referrals. In the second section we briefly review some additional instruments designed for research purposes. Psychometric information on some of the instruments reviewed in this chapter is available in our published studies. Available psychometric data on as yet unpublished instruments are provided for readers who may want to use these tools in their work.

The instruments used in screening and assessment of treatment outcome are all designed in accordance with the learning theory formulation of traumatic stress detailed in Part 1. Hence, the primary focus in assessment is traumatic stress reactions, including fear and avoidance responses, PTSD, depression, and associated functional impairment. As assessment of prolonged grief may also be needed in the aftermath of mass trauma events causing widespread casualties, we developed two instruments for this purpose, which are reviewed in Chapter 5.

Screening of earthquake survivors

Screening tools for earthquake survivors include the self-rated *Screening Instrument for Traumatic Stress in Earthquake Survivors, Fear and Avoidance Questionnaire*, and *Depression Rating Scale*.

Screening Instrument for Traumatic Stress in Earthquake Survivors (SITSES)

The SITSES (Appendix A) was originally developed for screening of large survivor groups. It was validated in a sample of 130 earthquake survivors (Başoğlu et al., 2001) and re-validated in a second study of 387 survivors. The scale, originally developed in Turkish, has been translated into English, Greek, Urdu, and Chinese. It consists of three parts: *Survivor Information Form, Traumatic Stress Symptom Checklist*, and *Severity of Disability Scale*. The titles of scale components below include the letter E at the end to distinguish them from their war trauma versions.

Survivor Information Form (SIF-E)

The SIF-E is a 21-item questionnaire that elicits information about demographic characteristics and various risk factors for traumatic stress. It has recently been revised by omitting the redundant items and adding two new ones (item #20 relating to anticipatory fear of future earthquakes and item #21 relating to sense of control over life) that proved to be the most important predictors of traumatic stress in later work.

Traumatic stress symptom checklist (TSSC-E)

The TSSC-E is a screening instrument designed to assess PTSD symptoms and depression that frequently accompany PTSD. It consists of 17 PTSD and 6 depression symptoms, each rated on a 0–3 scale (0 = not at all bothered, 3 = very much bothered). It has sensitivity and specificity of 0.81 when the diagnosis of PTSD is based on a cut-off point of 25 in the total scores of the

17 PTSD items (overall correct classification rate 81%). Similarly, a diagnosis of major depression based on a cut-off of 38 in the total scores of 23 TSSC-E items yields a sensitivity of 0.83 and specificity of 0.73 (overall correct classification rate 77%). It is worth noting that the scale underestimates depression rates when PTSD symptoms are relatively mild or absent, because the total score used in predicting depression includes the PTSD item scores, thus making it difficult for any case to reach the threshold for depression (based on 17 PTSD + 6 depression items) without reaching the threshold for PTSD (based on 17 PTSD items). Thus, although the scale is useful in assessing rates of depression comorbid with PTSD, it does not reliably estimate rates of depression in the absence of PTSD. To overcome this problem we developed a separate questionnaire to assess depression, which is presented later in this chapter. The total TSSC-E score can also be used in estimating PTSD diagnosis. A score of 33 appears to be the optimal cut-off, yielding sensitivity of 0.80 and specificity of 0.79 (correct classification rate 80%). However, any cut-off between 25 and 40 might be useful, depending on whether one opts for greater sensitivity or specificity in predicting PTSD.

Although the TSSC-E was originally designed to assess the symptoms in the last week, another validation study (involving 289 earthquake survivors) showed that a last-month version of the scale performs just as well as the last-week version (unpublished data). Thus, the scale can be used to assess symptoms in the last month (by simply replacing the words 'last week' by 'last month' in the instructions), if the need arises. However, the two versions are unlikely to yield substantially different results, because survivors often tend to overlook the time frame for symptoms indicated in the instruction.

Severity of Disability Scale (SDS)

The SDS includes three items, each of which is rated in relation to the traumatic stress problems elicited by the TSSC-E. The first item assesses the severity of overall distress associated with traumatic stress symptoms on a 0–3 scale (0 = not at all, 3 = extremely). This item correlated highly with the Clinician-Administered PTSD Scale (CAPS; Aker et al., 1999; Blake et al., 1990) item of subjective distress (r = 0.60, p < 0.001; Başoğlu et al., 2001) and the TSSC-E scores (r = 0.74, p < 0.001) in a pooled sample of 4332 earthquake survivors from five surveys (Başoğlu et al., 2002; Başoğlu et al., 2004; Livanou et al., 2002; Şalcıoğlu

et al., 2003; Şalcıoğlu et al., 2007; see Table 2 in Introduction for methodological details).

The second item assesses the extent of associated functional impairment in work, social life, and family relationships on a 0–3 scale (0 = no impairment / I can lead my daily life, 1 = slight impairment / I can lead my daily life with a little effort, 2 = marked impairment / there is marked disruption in my daily life, 3 = severe impairment / I cannot do most of the things in my daily life). This item correlates significantly with CAPS ratings of social (r = 0.52, p < 0.001) and occupational (r = 0.54, p < 0.001) disability (Başoğlu et al., 2001). It was also highly correlated with the TSSC-E score (r = 0.71, p < 0.001) in the pooled sample of five surveys. These findings demonstrate that PTSD symptoms are closely associated with overall distress and functional impairment.

The third SDS item (*Would you like to have help from a psychiatrist or psychologist for your problems?*) assesses the survivor's perceived need for help and likely response to a treatment offer. This item is included in the scale, because PTSD or depression scores may not always reflect survivors' likely response to a help offer, as we will see later. In addition to 'yes' and 'no' responses, this item also allows a 'don't know / not sure' response to identify those who are reluctant to accept help for various reasons. Such cases often need some information about the nature of their problems and how treatment can be useful in dealing with them before they agree to treatment.

Screening Instrument for Traumatic Stress in Earthquake Survivors – Child Version (SITSES-C)

Children respond to earthquakes in much the same way as adults do. Generalized fear and associated stress symptoms, such as hypervigilance, startle, sleeping difficulty, memory / concentration problems, and avoidance behaviors are fairly common. Other commonly encountered problems in children include decline in school performance, bed wetting, and clinging behaviors. Accordingly, we developed a modified version of the SITSES for children (Appendix A). It also consists of a *Survivor Information Form*, *Traumatic Stress Symptom Checklist – Child Version*, and a *Severity of Disability Scale*.

Although we did not have a chance to validate the instrument against assessor-ratings of PTSD, depression, and functional impairment, we examined its psychometric properties in a sample of 322 children

(54% male; mean age 12) assessed as part of an epidemiological study of earthquake survivors (Başoğlu et al., 2004). We found it quite useful in assessing treatment needs of children aged 6 to 15, as well as their response to treatment. The scale is easy to administer, as children often find the items' wordings fairly easy to understand.

Survivor Information Form – Child Version (SIF-C)

The SIF-C is a briefer version of the SIF-E. It includes 15 items. The last two items tap the intensity of fear during the earthquake and anticipatory fear in relation to aftershocks. Unlike its adult version, it does not include an item tapping sense of control over life due to the difficulties in assessing this construct in children. This construct is assessed indirectly by using the fear items. The predictive validity of the scale items was examined by a multiple regression analysis, including demographic, personal history, and trauma characteristics as independent variables and child version of the *Traumatic Stress Symptom Checklist* scores as the dependent variable. The regression model explained 27% of the variance in severity of PTSD symptoms. The strongest predictor was fear during the earthquake ($\beta = 0.41$, $p < 0.001$), consistent with similar findings from other studies of child (Giannopoulou et al., 2006; Roussos et al., 2005) and adult (Başoğlu et al., 2004; Başoğlu et al., 2002; Bergiannaki et al., 2003; Kılıç et al., 2006; Kılıç and Ulusoy, 2003; Livanou et al., 2002; Livanou et al., 2005; Şalcıoğlu et al., 2003; Şalcıoğlu et al., 2007) earthquake survivors. Past trauma experience ($\beta = 0.14$, $p < 0.01$) and closer proximity to the epicenter ($\beta = 0.13$, $p < 0.05$), although significant, were relatively weak predictors. These findings lend further support to the learning theory model of traumatic stress reviewed in Part 1.

Traumatic Stress Symptom Checklist – Child Version (TSSC-C)

The TSSC-C includes 18 items relating to PTSD symptoms and six items relating to depression symptoms. The scale differs from its adult version in certain ways. The items are worded as questions rather than as statements, because children find it easier to respond to the former. In addition, the scale includes two items relating to behavioral avoidance, one item tapping avoidance of distressing trauma reminders and the other item measuring avoidance related to anticipatory fear of future earthquakes. The items are rated on a 0–3 scale, the anchor points of which are defined in a simple fashion (*no, a little, fairly, very much*) to make rating easier for children.

A reliability analysis (model alpha) of the scale items yielded a Cronbach's alpha of 0.90 with item-total score correlations ranging from 0.30 to 0.62 and inter-item correlations ranging from 0.06 to 0.50. A factor analysis of the scale items yielded a general factor (40% of the total variance) with high positive item loadings ranging between 0.31 and 68. The scale total scores correlated significantly with *Fear and Avoidance Questionnaire* scores ($r = 0.65$, $p < 0.001$). These findings support the internal consistency and construct and concurrent validity of the scale.

Severity of Disability Scale – Child Version (SDS-C)

The SDS-C consists of two items measuring the severity of overall distress associated with traumatic stress reactions (0 = not bothered at all, 3 = very much bothered) and impairment in daily activities, such as going to school, attending classes, doing homework, helping with housework, playing or meeting with friends (0 = I can do everything as usual, 4 = I cannot do any of the things I used to do). These items were highly correlated with TSSC-C ($r = 0.64$ and $r = 0.56$, respectively; p's < 0.001).

Fear and Avoidance Questionnaire (FAQ)

A detailed assessment of avoidance behaviors in survivors is of critical importance in delivering treatment, considering that CFBT primarily focuses on avoidance behaviors when they are present. The FAQ (Appendix A) includes 35 items relating to activities or situations most commonly avoided by earthquake survivors. Each item measures the extent of difficulty associated with each activity or situation on a 0–3 scale (0 = no difficulty / can do it easily, 3 = extreme difficulty / cannot do it at all). Psychometric properties of the FAQ were examined in a study (Şalcıoğlu, 2002) of 551 earthquake survivors conducted at mean 20 months after the disaster. Reliability analysis of its items yielded a Cronbach's α value of 0.97. A factor analysis yielded five meaningful factors, representing avoidance behaviors relating to concrete buildings, earthquake reminders, outdoor activities, media news about earthquakes, and sleep. The scale score highly correlated with the TSSC-E item relating to avoidance of trauma reminders ($r = 0.67$) and TSSC-E score ($r = 0.75$) (all p's < 0.001). The scale was also sensitive to clinical improvement in our treatment studies (Başoğlu et al., 2003a; Başoğlu et al., 2003b; Başoğlu et al., 2005b; Başoğlu et al., 2007; Başoğlu et al., 2009).

In a pooled sample of 2238 survivors from three surveys (Başoğlu et al., 2004; Şalcıoğlu et al., 2003; Şalcıoğlu et al., 2007), where the FAQ was used, the total FAQ score correlated highly with the SDS items relating to overall perceived distress ($r = 0.65$, $p < 0.001$) and functional impairment ($r = 0.61$, $p < 0.001$). Functional impairment scores from 0 to 3 respectively corresponded to mean 3 ($SD = 5$), 9 ($SD = 8$), 17 ($SD = 9$), and 21 ($SD = 8$) markedly or extremely severe avoidance behaviors endorsed in the FAQ. This finding demonstrates the close association between avoidance behaviors and perceived functional impairment in earthquake survivors.

The FAQ can be useful in several ways. It provides useful information regarding the extent and severity of avoidance behaviors. Higher FAQ scores often indicate a strong fear component in the clinical picture and thus signal likely good response to CFBT. Second, because the FAQ highlights the extent of functional impairment caused by fear, it is helpful in explaining the treatment rationale to survivors and making a convincing case for their need for treatment. This can be most useful when they are reluctant to agree to the idea of confronting their fears. In such cases, the FAQ ratings can be useful in demonstrating to survivors the kind of 'price' they pay for surrendering to their fear. In many cases we observed that the mere act of filling in the questionnaire helps survivors gain awareness of the nature and extent of their problem. It helps them to recognize the connection between fear and their presenting complaints and see their stress symptoms as a treatable condition. Third, the FAQ serves as a particularly useful measure of treatment outcome, considering the treatment focus on avoidance behaviors. Early treatment response in FAQ scores is often a good prognostic sign for post-treatment outcome. As such, the scale score provides the therapist with useful feedback on treatment progress. Fourth, it serves as an item pool for avoidance behaviors, from which treatment (exposure) tasks can be selected. This is particularly useful when the treatment is delivered in a single session without subsequent monitoring of progress. The avoidance profile provided by the scale serves as the framework for treatment, defines treatment targets, and guides the survivors throughout their self-administered exposure practices. Finally, when rated regularly (e.g. weekly), it also provides an opportunity for self-monitoring of progress. Declining scores may act as rewarding feedback for the survivor, thereby reinforcing motivation for further progress.

As the FAQ was originally prepared for use in Turkey, some of its items may not be applicable in other post-disaster settings. Items like entering multi-storey buildings, elevators, going near the seaside, watching TV, or reading newspapers may not reflect the realities of certain third world country settings. The scale nevertheless provides useful examples of the kind of avoidance behaviors one needs to search for in assessment. It can be easily modified by omitting irrelevant items and adding new ones that reflect common avoidance behaviors in a particular post-disaster setting.

Depression Rating Scale (DRS)

For reasons noted earlier, the TSSC-E is not sufficiently reliable in assessing depression in the absence of PTSD. We also needed a more comprehensive depression scale as an outcome measure in treatment studies and currently available depression scales, such as the Beck Depression Inventory (BDI; Beck et al., 1979; Hisli, 1987), posed various problems in administration, particularly with survivors of lower socio-educational status. Hence, we developed a stand-alone depression scale that was easier to administer. This scale is provided in Appendix A for readers who might prefer a simple screening tool for depression validated in a developing country setting.

The DRS consists of 19 items, 14 of which assess the Major Depressive Episode symptoms as defined in DSM-IV. Five items tap irritability, hopelessness, crying spells, somatisation, and decreased libido commonly observed in depressed patients. The psychometric properties of the DRS were examined in a study of 205 earthquake survivors (unpublished data). A reliability analysis yielded a Cronbach's alpha of 0.94. Item-total correlations ranged from 0.41 to 0.82 and inter-item correlations ranged from 0.19 to 0.82. A factor analysis of the scale items yielded a general depression factor (56% of the total variance) with high positive item loadings, ranging from 0.42 to 0.85. These findings support the internal consistency and construct validity of the scale.

Table 3.1 shows sensitivity and specificity of 14 DRS items with respect to the corresponding item ratings of the Major Depressive Episode module of the Structured Clinical Interview for DSM-IV (SCID; First et al., 1996). A cut-off of 2 in item scores yielded optimum sensitivity and specificity values, correctly classifying 67% to 91% of the cases. The agreement between the two scales was moderate to good on 11 items and fair on 3 items. To identify a cut-off

Table 3.1 Concordance of Depression Rating Scale items with assessor-rated depression symptoms

	SE	SP	% CC	κ
Depressed mood	88	69	77	54
Loss of pleasure	75	76	75	51
Weight change	67	78	74	43
Appetite change	68	80	76	48
Sleep problems	80	80	80	60
Agitation	75	67	69	38
Retardation	56	80	72	36
Fatigue	91	75	83	65
Loss of energy	67	91	79	58
Feelings of guilt	51	88	80	40
Feelings of worthlessness	60	84	79	41
Concentration difficulty	74	84	78	56
Indecisiveness	55	85	67	37
Suicidal thoughts	80	92	91	48

SE = Sensitivity, SP = Specificity, % CC = Percent correctly classified.
All κ's < 0.001.

that best predicted diagnosis of depression, scale scores of 15 to 35 were checked against SCID diagnosis of current Major Depressive Episode. A score of 28 yielded optimum sensitivity (0.85), specificity (0.86), correct classification rate (85%), and concordance rate ($\kappa = 0.69$, $p < 0.001$). It also yielded a depression rate of 41% in the study sample, compared with 38% based on the SCID (McNemar test not significant). The scale showed excellent concurrent validity with the BDI ($r = 0.86$) and correlated highly with General Health Questionnaire-28 (GHQ; Goldberg and Hillier, 1979; Kılıç, 1996; $r = 0.75$), TSSC-E ($r = 0.75$), CAPS ($r = 0.66$), and FAQ ($r = 61$)(all p's < 0.001). These findings support the validity of the scale.

Screening of war and torture survivors

Screening instruments for war and torture survivors include the *Screening Instrument for Traumatic Stress in Survivors of War*, *Depression Rating Scale*, and two measures of prolonged grief (reviewed in Chapter 5). A war and torture trauma version of the FAQ has not yet been developed.

Screening Instrument for Traumatic Stress in Survivors of War (SITSOW)

The SITSOW (Appendix A) is a modified version of SITSES and consists of *Survivor Information Form*, *Traumatic Stress Symptom Checklist*, and *Social Disability Scale*. The psychometric properties of the scale were examined in a study involving 948 survivors of war trauma in the countries of former Yugoslavia (Serbia, Croatia, Bosnia-Herzegovina, Republica Srpska), including combat, torture, internal displacement, refugee experience, and aerial bombardment (Başoğlu et al., 2005a). The titles of scale components below include the letter W at the end to distinguish them from their earthquake trauma versions.

Survivor Information Form (SIF-W)

The SIF-W consists of 17 items relating to demographic, personal history, and trauma characteristics. It has recently been revised by omitting the redundant items and adding some new ones that proved to be important predictors of post-traumatic stress. The latter includes two items relating to anticipatory fear of further threat to safety and sense of control over life.

Traumatic Stress Symptom Checklist (TSSC-W)

TSSC-W includes 17 items tapping PTSD symptoms as defined by DSM-IV. Unlike the earthquake version, it does not include depression items. The scale was found to have excellent internal consistency with a Cronbach's alpha of 0.96 (range of item-total correlations 0.70 to 0.83; range of inter-item correlations 0.50 to 0.78). A factor analysis of the scale items yielded a single factor (62% of the total variance) with item loadings ranging from 0.71 to 0.85. These findings supported the internal consistency and construct validity of the scale. The criterion validity of the TSSC-W items was established using the CAPS ratings of PTSD symptoms. A cut-off of 2 yielded optimum sensitivity and specificity and correctly classified 70% to 86% of the survivors. Agreement between the self- and clinician-rated PTSD symptoms was good in 2 (kappa > 0.61), moderate in 12 (kappa values 0.43 to 0.53), and fair in 3 items (kappa values 0.23 to 0.33).

A cut-off of 25 in the scale scores yielded optimum sensitivity (0.86), specificity (0.84), correct classification rate (84%), and concordance value ($\kappa = 0.61$, p < 0.001). Based on this cut-off score the rate of PTSD in the sample was 32%, compared with 22% based on the CAPS (McNemar test < 0.001). Thus, the scale overestimated PTSD diagnosis by 10%. This does not pose a problem in fieldwork, given that higher scale sensitivity reduces the likelihood of missing cases in need of treatment. The scale score correlated highly with CAPS, BDI, and GHQ total scores (r range = 0.74 to 0.80, all p's < 0.001), indicating satisfactory concurrent validity. It also showed meaningful correlations with various SIF-W items, a finding that supports the validity of both scales.

Severity of Disability Scale

The SDS is the same scale as its counterpart in the SITSES. It is rated in relation to the traumatic stress problems elicited by the TSSC-W. The validity of its items was assessed in relation to the corresponding CAPS items measuring subjective distress and disability. High correlations were found between the SDS and CAPS item of distress (r = 0.66) and between the SDS functional impairment item and CAPS items relating to social (r = 0.61) and occupational (r = 0.58) disability (all p's < 0.001). SDS distress and functional impairment items also correlated highly with TSSC-W (r = 0.83 and r = 0.79, p's < 0.001).

Depression Rating Scale (DRS)

The psychometric properties of the DRS, originally developed with earthquake survivors, were re-examined in our study of 948 war survivors. A reliability analysis yielded a Cronbach's alpha of 0.96; item-total correlations ranged from 0.58 to 0.85 and inter-item correlations ranged from 0.35 to 0.76. A factor analysis of the DRS items yielded a single factor (58% of the total variance) with item loadings ranging from 0.58 to 0.87. Thus, the scale showed satisfactory internal consistency and construct validity. As in earthquake survivors, a cut-off score of 28 yielded optimum sensitivity (0.80), specificity (0.83), correct classification rate (83%), and concordance value ($\kappa = 0.40$, p <0.001) in relation to the SCID diagnosis of Major Depressive Episode. Relative to the latter, this cut-off score overestimated the diagnosis of depression by 13%. The scale showed excellent concurrent validity with the BDI (r = 0.90) and also correlated highly with GHQ (r = 0.83), TSSC-W (r = 0.87), and CAPS (r = 0.74) (all p's < 0.001).

Identifying survivors in need of treatment

Several lines of information provided by the scales reviewed so far are useful in assessing treatment needs in survivors. These include the risk factors for traumatic stress, total TSSC, DRS, and FAQ scores, severity of functional impairment, and response to treatment offer. The relative importance of these data in determining treatment need depends on the setting in which the screening tools are used. We used it most commonly for screening of survivors in shelters, camps, schools, factories, and communities most severely affected by mass trauma events. At times the targeted population included several thousand people. Incoming data were regularly computerized and analyzed to identify survivors in need. Once they were identified, they were classified according to the estimated urgency of their problem. As the SITSES and SITSOW are most likely to be used for similar purposes in such settings, it might be useful to examine how the data can be used in advance planning of care services for a large survivor population.

Association between post-traumatic stress and perceived need for help

The TSSC score is a useful indicator of problem severity but may not always reflect survivors' need for help. It should therefore be evaluated together with survivors' responses to help offer. Some data showing how these two variables are inter-related might be helpful in this regard. We examined this issue in both earthquake and war survivors. Table 3.2 shows mean TSSC scores in cases with *yes*, *no*, and *don't know* responses to the treatment offer in both survivor groups. The sample of earthquake survivors included 3267 non-treatment-seeking cases screened during an outreach program (Başoğlu et al., 2002; Başoğlu et al., 2004; Şalcıoğlu et al., 2003; Şalcıoğlu et al., 2007) and 1027 cases that sought treatment from our community center in the disaster region (Livanou et al., 2002). Also shown are the rates of non-PTSD (or sub-threshold PTSD), probable PTSD, and probable depression diagnoses within each response category to allow an impression of how they relate to perceived need for help. Note that the TSSC-E and TSSC-W scores are not directly comparable because of their different item count.

Table 3.2 Mean TSSC scores and rates of PTSD and depression diagnoses in relation to perceived need for help

Perceived need for help	n	Mean TSSC score	Sub-threshold PTSD[1]	Probable PTSD[2]	Probable depression[3]
Earthquake survivors					
Community sample	3267	25 (17)	64%	36%	25%
Yes	840	37 (15)	35%	65%	51%
No	1617	16 (13)	86%	14%	8%
Not sure	810	30 (14)	52%	48%	32%
Clinical sample	1027	37 (15)	35%	65%	51%
War survivors					
Community sample	946	18 (14)	68%	32%	23%
Yes	230	31 (12)	28%	72%	58%
No	437	9 (9)	94%	6%	3%
Not sure	279	21 (12)	61%	39%	25%

TSSC = Traumatic Stress Symptom Checklist.
[1] TSSC-E PTSD sub-scale score (sum of 17 PTSD items) < 25, TSSC-W score < 25.
[2] TSSC-E PTSD sub-scale score > 24, TSSC-W score > 24.
[3] TSSC-E total score > 37 for earthquake survivors, DRS score > 27 for war survivors.

Several findings in Table 3.2 are of interest. In earthquake survivors, the TSSC-E scores were higher in the clinical than in the community sample; treatment-seeking survivors were twice as likely to have probable PTSD and depression as the community sample survivors. On the other hand, the presence of only sub-threshold PTSD in 35% of the treatment-seekers shows that help-seeking survivors do not always have symptoms severe enough to meet the diagnosis of PTSD. Help-seeking behavior in such cases is often prompted by the distressing and disabling effects of fear-related traumatic stress symptoms (e.g. hypervigilance, avoidance of trauma reminders, startle) that often predominate the clinical picture or depression symptoms secondary to PTSD symptoms. This is further supported by the fact that 35% of the community sample survivors who perceived a need for help also had sub-threshold PTSD.

Among the 'no' responders in the community sample, 86% did not have probable PTSD (mean TSSC-E score = 12, SD = 8). This shows that absence of PTSD is a fairly reliable predictor of lack of perceived need for help. On the other hand, 14% of these cases had probable PTSD with a mean TSSC-E score of 39 (SD = 9) above the cut-off for probable depression. This meant that about 1 in 7 survivors in the community with probable PTSD did not perceive a need for help, even when they were depressed.

In the community sample the survivors with a 'don't know' response were more similar to the 'yes' responders in their TSSC scores than to the 'no' responders. Such survivors can thus be regarded as potentially in need of treatment. Possible reasons for their uncertain response (detailed later in this chapter) often include misconceptions about their psychological problems or treatment issues, which can be easily overcome by providing them with sufficient information on these issues. Thus, when possible, it may be worthwhile to find out the reasons for uncertain responses and deal with them.

The data for war survivors show largely similar results. The fact that 72% of the survivors with 'yes' responses to treatment offer had probable PTSD lends further support to an association between PTSD and perceived need for help. On the other hand, 28% of the war survivors who perceived a need for help had only sub-threshold PTSD. Among the 'no' responders, 94% did not meet the diagnosis of probable PTSD, once again pointing to absence of PTSD as a fairly reliable predictor of lack of perceived need for help. On the other hand, 6% of these cases (1 in 16) with probable PTSD (and a mean TSSC-W score of 32, SD = 6) did not perceive a need for help. It is also worth noting that 39% of the war survivors with a 'don't know' response had probable PTSD.

The relationship between the TSSC score and perceived need for help can be better appreciated when the responses to the treatment offer are plotted against the entire TSSC score range. Figure 3.1 shows how the rates of yes, no, and not sure responses to treatment

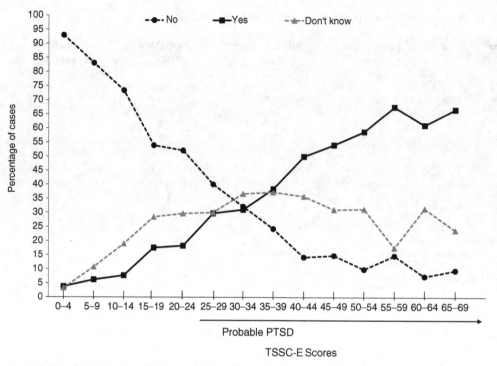

Figure 3.1 Association between TSSC scores and responses to treatment offer in earthquake survivors. TSSC-E = Traumatic Stress Symptom Checklist – Earthquake version.

offer differ across the TSSC scores (shown as 5-point intervals) in the community sample.

Figure 3.1 clearly demonstrates a strong linear association between the TSSC-E scores and treatment acceptance or rejection. Treatment acceptance steadily rises as the TSSC-E score increases, reaching a maximum at the 55–59 score interval. In contrast, treatment rejection rates show a steady decline and reach a low point at the TSSC-E score interval of 40–44 and tend to stabilize thereafter. Thus, it appears that resistance against the idea treatment reaches its lowest point as the TSSC-E score goes over the cut-off point of 38 for depression. This is indeed the breaking point for many survivors, where they can no longer cope with the crippling effects of traumatic stress symptoms. On the other hand, uncertainty about the need for treatment reaches a peak within a TSSC-E score range of 30 to 40 and begins to decline as the TSSC-E score goes over 40, reflecting a steadily increasing perceived need for help beyond this point.

It is also worth noting that the rate of 'no' responses does not fall below 10%, when the TSSC-E score goes over 40, which indicates PTSD and comorbid depression. In contrast, perceived need for help steadily rises

even within the score range of 0–29, which is below the threshold of 33 for PTSD diagnosis. This apparent contradiction, consistent with Table 3.2 data, points to other factors that might influence perceived need for help. Indeed, in a regression analysis personal history of psychiatric illness requiring treatment and female gender were associated with treatment acceptance, independent of the TSSC-E score.

Figure 3.2 shows the same analysis for war survivors. A strong linear association between the TSSC-W scores and treatment acceptance or rejection is again evident. Treatment rejection rates show a steady decline and reach a low point at the score interval of 30–34 and tend to stabilize thereafter. On the other hand, uncertainty about the need for treatment reaches a peak within a score range of 15–19, stabilizes until a score range of 35–39, and begins to decline as the score goes over 40. However, as in earthquake survivors, the rate of uncertain or 'no' responses does not fall to 0 within the score range of 30 to 49, while perceived need for help steadily rises even within the score range of 0–24, which is below the cut-off of 25 for PTSD diagnosis.

The high rates of depression in both earthquake and war survivors who perceived a need for help might

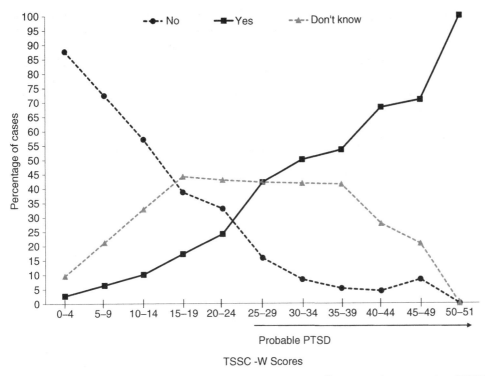

Figure 3.2 Association between TSSC scores and responses to treatment offer in war and torture survivors. TSSC-W = Traumatic Stress Symptom Checklist –War version.

raise the question whether it was PTSD or depression that explained help-seeking behavior in our studies. It is worth recalling from Part 1 that depression in our studies of earthquake and war survivors was largely secondary to PTSD, while only 15% of earthquake survivors and 3% of war survivors without PTSD had depression. We examined the relative contributions of PTSD and depression in a multinomial logistic regression analysis involving responses to treatment offer as the dependent variable in war survivors. In view of the comorbidity between PTSD and depression, we created three independent measures, including diagnoses of (a) PTSD comorbid with depression, (b) PTSD alone without depression, and (c) depression alone without PTSD, based on TSSC-W scores. Controlling for demographic and personal history variables, PTSD comorbid with depression emerged as the strongest predictor of 'yes' responses (OR = 104.9), followed by PTSD alone (OR = 11.8) and depression alone (OR = 9.8). Thus, while PTSD and depression both independently contributed to perceived need for help, increasing the likelihood of treatment acceptance by about 10 times, their combination made perceived need for help 105 times more likely.

In a similar analysis with earthquake survivors, PTSD comorbid with depression was also the strongest predictor of 'yes' responses (OR = 12.8), followed by PTSD alone (OR = 4.8). Diagnosis of depression was not used in this analysis because of too few cases with depression alone (n = 6). The same analysis including diagnosis of depression was conducted in a separate sample of 387 earthquake survivors (Şalcıoğlu, 2004) where PTSD and depression were assessed independently using assessor-rated instruments. In this analysis, PTSD comorbid with depression was again the strongest predictor (OR = 43.4), followed by depression alone (OR = 10.1) and PTSD alone (OR = 8.3).

These findings suggest that both PTSD and depression contribute to perceived need for treatment in war and earthquake survivors but their combination increases the likelihood of the latter by 3- to 10-fold. Considering that PTSD is the primary process leading to depression in most earthquake and war survivors, PTSD could be regarded as the underlying causal factor in treatment-seeking behavior. The implications of these findings for mental healthcare policies are reviewed in Chapter 8.

Determining priorities in treatment planning

The above findings suggest that priorities in treatment planning can be based on TSSC-E scores in earthquake survivors and TSSC-W and DRS scores in war survivors. The SIF items relating to fear of trauma recurrence and loss of control over life can also be useful in identifying cases at high risk for PTSD and depression. The FAQ score and SDS items provide useful additional information about the extent of avoidance behaviors and functional impairment. Survivors with high scores on these measures are most likely to need priority attention in treatment planning.

In cases with uncertain or negative response to treatment offer, it is helpful to bear in mind that the problem in a non-negligible proportion of these cases may be serious enough to warrant help. In our work with earthquake survivors, we explored the reasons for uncertain or negative responses in cases with scores over 20, whenever possible (e.g. during home visits). Some of these reasons deserve attention. Because post-traumatic stress problems are quite prevalent in a disaster-struck community, many survivors may not recognize them as a problem requiring treatment. This is particularly true for avoidance behaviors, which many survivors see as a justifiable precautionary measure against future occurrence of trauma events (Başoğlu et al., 2002; Şalcıoğlu et al., 2008), even when such avoidance relates to conditioned fears of an irrational nature. Negative responses may reflect hopelessness effects of depression or grief in some survivors. Some survivors may not see the connection between their trauma and symptoms, particularly when psychosomatic symptoms (e.g. pain in parts of the body) predominate the clinical picture. There may also be cultural factors that determine response to help offer. Men may be more reluctant to accept treatment, regarding it as a sign of weakness. Survivors with no previous experience with psychiatric treatments may be more reluctant to accept treatment offer. This might be due to concerns about being prescribed drugs. Indeed, in our fieldwork we observed that many survivors were concerned about taking 'brain numbing' drugs. There may also be concerns about stigma associated with receiving mental healthcare. In some cases reluctance to accept treatment may reflect a negative experience with interventions delivered by other psychosocial aid groups. We observed, for example, that many earthquake survivors were quite unhappy about their previous experience with psychological debriefing. All these factors need to be taken into account in interpreting responses to treatment offer. In our fieldwork we were able to overcome many survivors' initial reluctance to the idea of treatment with an explanation of the nature of their problems and effective ways of overcoming them.

Assessment of intervention outcomes

Outreach treatment delivery programs targeting relatively large survivor populations require self-rated instruments to assess intervention outcomes. The TSSC-E, DRS, FAQ, and Global Improvement Scale (GIS; Appendix A) are often sufficient in assessing treatment outcome in earthquake survivors. We have not yet used TSSC-W, DRS, and GIS in assessing treatment outcome in war survivors but we expect them to be also useful with these survivors. The TSSC-E and FAQ are sensitive to clinical change and their change scores correlate highly with change in CAPS scores. DRS is also sensitive to clinical change and its pre-post-treatment change scores correlate significantly ($r = 0.67$, $p < 0.001$) with change scores in BDI.

The GIS, which was developed and used in a recent treatment study (Başoğlu et al., 2007), measures overall improvement on a 0–4 scale (0 = no change, 1 = slightly improved / less than 20%, 2 = moderately improved / 20–60%, 3 = much improved / 60–80%, 4 = very much improved / more than 80%). It has a self- and assessor-rated version. In our treatment study the 0–4 ratings of the GIS-Self respectively corresponded to mean 0%, 9%, 28%, 53%, and 79% reduction in PTSD symptoms (measured by the CAPS) at post-treatment. The respective figures for GIS-Assessor were mean 0%, 12%, 40%, 59%, and 78%. Thus, the calibration of the scales appeared to be reasonably realistic. The two scales showed high correlations with each other and pre- to post-treatment change in TSSC-E, FAQ, and BDI.

To assess functional impairment related to post-traumatic stress in our treatment studies, we used a Work and Social Adjustment (WSA) scale (Appendix A) in addition to the SDS of the SITSES, because the SDS did not appear to be sufficiently sensitive to clinical change. The WSA scale is an extensively modified version of the original scale developed by Mundt et al. (2002). As this scale was modified recently, its psychometric properties are not yet examined.

Research instruments

In this section we briefly review various research instruments that we used with earthquake, war, and torture survivors in examining mechanisms of traumatic stress, intervention outcomes, and mechanisms of change during treatment. We developed most of these instruments with a view to testing various hypotheses generated by the learning theory formulation of traumatic stress. These instruments are not provided in this book because of space constraints.

Structured Interview for Survivors of Torture (SIST)

The SIST (Başoğlu et al., 1997) is designed for the assessment of torture survivors. It consists of two parts. Part 1 contains 51 items tapping demographic and personal history characteristics, psychological preparedness for torture, and post-trauma social support and adjustment. Part 2 consists of an *Exposure to Torture Scale*, which includes 46 items relating to captivity and torture experiences and perceived distress and uncontrollability ratings in relation to each experience. It also includes a *Global Distress Rating* and a *Global Sense of Control Rating* to assess the survivors' overall perceived distress or loss of control during torture.

Structured Interview for Survivors of War (SISOW)

The SISOW (Başoğlu et al., 2005a) was modified from the SIST for assessment of war survivors. In addition to demographic and personal history characteristics, it includes an *Exposure to War Stressors Scale* that elicits information on 54 war-related stressor events and perceived distress and uncontrollability associated with each event. It also includes the *Exposure to Torture Scale* of the SIST. *Global Distress* and *Global Sense of Control Ratings* assess the survivors' overall perceived distress or loss of control associated with war and torture trauma.

Structured Interview for Survivors of Earthquake (SISE)

The SISE (Şalcıoğlu, 2004), modified from the SIST and SISOW, was originally designed to examine pre- and post-earthquake risk factors for traumatic stress in detail. Indeed, much of the data on mechanisms of traumatic stress in earthquake survivors reviewed in

Chapter 1 were based on this instrument. It consists of four parts, altogether involving 39 items. Part 1 includes information about demographic characteristics and personal history of psychiatric illness and trauma. Part 2 includes an *Exposure to Earthquake Stressors Scale* that consists of 44 items tapping earthquake experiences and perceived distress in relation to each experience. Part 3 elicits information about economic and social resource loss. Part 4 elicits information on severity of anticipatory fear of earthquakes, loss of control over life in general, and perceived need for help.

Structured assessment of PTSD and depression

Treatment research may require structured assessment of PTSD and depression in addition to self-rated measures of these conditions. Various structured interviews for psychiatric disorders, such as the SCID (First et al., 1996) among others, may be available to mental health professionals in developing countries, though they may require validation if they have not been previously validated for use in a particular country. Among measures of PTSD, we found the CAPS (Blake et al., 1990) most useful, because it provides ratings of symptom frequency and intensity and a total score that can be used as a measure of severity of traumatic stress.

Assessment of sense of control in treatment – Sense of Control Scale

Assessment of sense of control in treatment research might be useful, not only in studies of CFBT but also in other intervention outcome research. The learning theory model of traumatic stress reviewed in Part 1 suggests that interventions are effective to the extent that they enhance sense of control over fear or stressor events. Thus, the impact of a particular intervention on sense of control assessed early in treatment is likely to be a useful indicator of good outcome. We developed a *Sense of Control Scale* (SCS) for this purpose (Appendix A). The SCS was first used in assessing the impact of Earthquake Simulation Treatment on sense of control (Başoğlu et al., 2007) and shown to have satisfactory psychometric properties. Its five items tap reduction in fear or distress, sense of control, courage, self-confidence, and expectations of coping in relation to feared situations. It has good internal consistency with Cronbach's alpha values ranging from 0.91 to 0.94 at different post-treatment assessment points. The total SCS score correlates highly with reduction in PTSD, depression, and functional impairment scores. It is most useful when administered early in treatment (e.g. after the delivery of self-exposure instructions or the first self-administered or therapist-aided exposure session) to assess the early impact of treatment.

Assessment of cognitive effects of trauma

In our studies of the phenomenology of earthquake (Şalcıoğlu, 2004), and war and torture trauma (Başoğlu et al., 2005a) we used two questionnaires to measure cognitive effects of trauma. The *Redress for Trauma Survivors Questionnaire* (RTSQ) elicits information about attributions of responsibility for trauma, implementation of civil sanctions for those held responsible, sense of injustice associated with perceived impunity for those held responsible for trauma, compensation of survivors, commemoration, and other socio-political events with a symbolic redress value for survivors. This measure did not have any predictive value with respect to post-trauma psychological outcomes in war, torture, and earthquake survivors.

The *Emotions and Beliefs after Trauma* (EBAT) is a self-rated questionnaire measuring (a) appraisal of impunity for those held responsible for trauma and associated emotions, (b) fear associated with perceived threat to safety and loss of control over life, and (c) loss of faith in people and beliefs about justice in the world and benevolence of people. The war trauma version of the EBAT (*Emotions and Beliefs after War – EBAW*) includes two additional sub-scales, one assessing change in appraisal of war / political cause and expectations about the future of the country and the other relating to beliefs about God and religion. Among its subscales, the *Fear and Loss of Control Scale* was the strongest predictor of traumatic stress reactions in survivors of war (Başoğlu et al., 2005a) and earthquake (Şalcıoğlu, 2004) (see also Part 1).

A misconception about assessment

In closing this chapter a common misconception about assessment deserves brief attention. Some believe that assessment of trauma survivors using questionnaires or even screening instruments may further traumatize them. There is no convincing literature evidence in support of this view. Furthermore, we observed that questionnaire assessment often has a therapeutic effect on survivors by helping them recognize their problems, particularly their fear and avoidance, as symptoms and develop a sense of control over these problems. In some cases this may even lead to self-instigated exposure to feared situations and complete recovery. Indeed, such beneficial effects of assessment in our treatment studies (Başoğlu et al., 2005b; Başoğlu et al., 2007) led to 10% to 20% improvement in PTSD symptoms in waitlist control subjects. Similar levels of improvement allocated to a repeated assessment condition have also been reported in other treatment studies (Ehlers et al., 2005; Foa et al., 1999; Foa et al., 2005). It was indeed such findings that led us to make use of screening instruments as therapy tools in delivering CFBT. Their use in treatment is described in Chapter 4.

References

Aker, A. T., Özeren, M., Başoğlu, M., Kaptanoğlu, C., Erol, A. and Buran, B. (1999). The Turkish version of Clinician-administered PTSD Scale for DSM-IV: A study of its reliability and validity. *Turkish Journal of Psychiatry*, **10**, 286–293.

Başoğlu, M., Kılıç, C., Şalcıoğlu, E. and Livanou, M. (2004). Prevalence of posttraumatic stress disorder and comorbid depression in earthquake survivors in Turkey: An epidemiological study. *Journal of Traumatic Stress*, **17**, 133–141.

Başoğlu, M., Livanou, M., Crnobarić, C., Frančišković, T., Suljić, E., Đurić, D. and Vranešić, M. (2005a). Psychiatric and cognitive effects of war in former Yugoslavia: Association of lack of redress for trauma and posttraumatic stress reactions. *Journal of the American Medical Association*, **294**, 580–590.

Başoğlu, M., Livanou, M. and Şalcıoğlu, E. (2003a). A single session with an earthquake simulator for traumatic stress in earthquake survivors. *American Journal of Psychiatry*, **160**, 788–790.

Başoğlu, M., Livanou, M., Şalcıoğlu, E. and Kalender, D. (2003b). A brief behavioural treatment of chronic post-traumatic stress disorder in earthquake survivors: Results from an open clinical trial. *Psychological Medicine*, **33**, 647–654.

Başoğlu, M., Mineka, S., Paker, M., Aker, T., Livanou, M. and Gök, S. (1997). Psychological preparedness for trauma as a protective factor in survivors of torture. *Psychological Medicine*, **27**, 1421–1433.

Başoğlu, M., Şalcıoğlu, E. and Livanou, M. (2002). Traumatic stress responses in earthquake survivors in Turkey. *Journal of Traumatic Stress*, **15**, 269–276.

Başoğlu, M., Şalcıoğlu, E. and Livanou, M. (2007). A randomized controlled study of single-session behavioural treatment of earthquake-related post-traumatic stress disorder using an earthquake simulator. *Psychological Medicine*, **37**, 203–213.

Başoğlu, M., Şalcıoğlu, E. and Livanou, M. (2009). Single-case experimental studies of a self-help manual for traumatic stress in earthquake survivors. *Journal of Behavior Therapy and Experimental Psychiatry* **40**, 50–58.

Başoğlu, M., Şalcıoğlu, E., Livanou, M., Kalender, D. and Acar, G. (2005b). Single-session behavioral treatment of earthquake-related posttraumatic stress disorder: A randomized waiting list controlled trial. *Journal of Traumatic Stress*, **18**, 1–11.

Başoğlu, M., Şalcıoğlu, E., Livanou, M., Özeren, M., Aker, T., Kılıç, C. and Mestçioğlu, Ö. (2001). A study of the validity of a Screening Instrument for Traumatic Stress in Earthquake Survivors in Turkey. *Journal of Traumatic Stress*, **14**, 491–509.

Beck, A. T., Rush, A. J., Shaw, B. F. and Emery, G. (1979). *Cognitive Therapy of Depression*. New York: Guilford Press.

Bergiannaki, J. D., Psarros, C., Varsou, E., Paparrigopoulos, T. and Soldatos, C. R. (2003). Protracted acute stress reaction following an earthquake. *Acta Psychiatrica Scandinavica*, **107**, 18–24.

Blake, D. D., Weathers, F. W., Nagy, L. M., Kaloupek, D. G., Charney, D. S. and Keane, T. M. (1990). *Clinician-Administered PTSD Scale (CAPS) – Current and Lifetime Diagnostic Version*. Boston: National Center for Posttraumatic Stress Disorder, Behavioral Science Division.

Ehlers, A., Clark, D. M., Hackmann, A., Mcmanus, F. and Fennell, M. (2005). Cognitive therapy for post-traumatic stress disorder: Development and evaluation. *Behaviour Research and Therapy*, **43**, 413–431.

First, M. B., Spitzer, R. L., Gibbon, M. and Williams, J. B. W. (1996). *Structured Clinical Interview for DSM-IV Axis I Disorders – Non-patient Edition (SCID-I/NP, Version 2)*. New York: Biometrics Research Department, New York State Psychiatric Institute.

Foa, E. B., Dancu, C. V., Hembree, E. A., Jaycox, L. H., Meadows, E. A. and Street, G. P. (1999). A comparison of exposure therapy, stress inoculation training, and their combination for reducing posttraumatic stress disorder in female assault victims. *Journal of Consulting and Clinical Psychology*, **67**, 194–200.

Foa, E. B., Hembree, E. A., Cahill, S. P., Rauch, S. A. M., Riggs, D. S., Feeny, N. C. and Yadin, E. (2005). Randomized trial of prolonged exposure for posttraumatic stress disorder with and without cognitive restructuring: Outcome at academic and community clinics. *Journal of Consulting and Clinical Psychology*, **73**, 953–964.

Giannopoulou, I., Strouthos, M., Smith, P., Dikaiakou, A., Galanopoulou, V. and Yule, W. (2006). Post-traumatic stress reactions of children and adolescents exposed to the Athens 1999 earthquake. *European Psychiatry*, **21**, 160–166.

Goldberg, D. and Hillier, V. F. (1979). A scaled version of the General Health Questionnaire. *Psychological Medicine*, **9**, 139–145.

Hisli, N. (1987). A study on the validity of Beck Depression Inventory. *Turkish Journal of Psychology*, **6**, 118–122.

Kılıç, C. (1996). General Health Questionnaire: A study of its validity and reliability. *Turkish Journal of Psychiatry*, **7**, 3–10.

Kılıç, C., Aydın, I., Taşkıntuna, N., Özçürümez, G., Kurt, G., Eren, E., Lale, T., Özel, S. and Zileli, L. (2006). Predictors of psychological distress in survivors of the 1999 earthquakes in Turkey: Effects of relocation after the disaster. *Acta Psychiatrica Scandinavica*, **114**, 194–202.

Kılıç, C. and Ulusoy, M. (2003). Psychological effects of the November 1999 earthquake in Turkey: An epidemiological study. *Acta Psychiatrica Scandinavica*, **108**, 232–238.

Livanou, M., Başoğlu, M., Şalcıoğlu, E. and Kalender, D. (2002). Traumatic stress responses in treatment: Seeking earthquake survivors in Turkey. *Journal of Nervous and Mental Disease*, **190**, 816–823.

Livanou, M., Kasvikis, Y., Başoğlu, M., Mytskidou, P., Sotiropoulou, V., Spanea, E., Mitsopoulou, T. and Voutsa, N. (2005). Earthquake-related psychological distress and associated factors 4 years after the Parnitha earthquake in Greece. *European Psychiatry*, **20**, 137–144.

Mundt, J. C., Marks, I. M., Shear, M. K. and Greist, J. H. (2002). The Work and Social Adjustment Scale: A simple measure of impairment in functioning. *British Journal of Psychiatry*, **180**, 461–464.

Roussos, A., Goenjian, A. K., Steinberg, A. M., Sotiropoulou, C., Kakaki, M., Kabakos, C., Karagianni, S. and Manouras, V. (2005). Posttraumatic stress and depressive reactions among children and adolescents after the 1999 earthquake in Ano Liosia, Greece. *American Journal of Psychiatry*, **162**, 530–537.

Şalcıoğlu, E. (2002). *Long-term psychological consequences of 1999 Kocaeli earthquake*. MA Thesis. Institute of Social Sciences, Boğaziçi University, Istanbul.

Şalcıoğlu, E. (2004). *The effect of beliefs, attribution of responsibility, redress and compensation on posttraumatic stress disorder in earthquake survivors in Turkey.* PhD Dissertation. Institute of Psychiatry, King's College London, London.

Şalcıoğlu, E., Başoğlu, M. and Livanou, M. (2003). Long-term psychological outcome for non-treatment-seeking earthquake survivors in Turkey. *Journal of Nervous and Mental Disease,* **191**, 154–160.

Şalcıoğlu, E., Başoğlu, M. and Livanou, M. (2007). Post-traumatic stress disorder and comorbid depression among survivors of the 1999 earthquake in Turkey. *Disasters,* **31**, 115–129.

Şalcıoğlu, E., Başoğlu, M. and Livanou, M. (2008). Psychosocial determinants of relocation in survivors of the 1999 earthquake in Turkey. *Journal of Nervous and Mental Disease,* **196**, 55–61.

Chapter 4

Control-focused behavioral treatment

In Part 1 we reviewed the evidence pointing to the role of helplessness in traumatic stress reactions. We also discussed the possible evolutionary basis of 'risk-taking' behaviors to overcome fear and how such behaviors facilitate natural recovery from trauma. Control-Focused Behavioral Treatment (CFBT) was designed as an intervention to facilitate natural recovery processes by restoring sense of control over anxiety, fear, or distress. Its underlying principle is to reduce helplessness responses by encouraging behaviors that are likely to enhance sense of control over stressor events and life in general. Although it primarily relies on exposure in achieving this aim, in view of the fact that a wide range of stressful life events associated with anxiety and depression may interact with the impact of trauma and contribute to helplessness, it may also include other interventions (e.g. problem-solving, behavioral activation, training in various skills needed to overcome life problems, etc.) likely to have an impact on sense of control over life. As such, CFBT is an empowerment strategy that can be used in dealing with other psychological problems that arise from helplessness and /or hopelessness responses to stressful life events (e.g. generalized anxiety, depression) or those that may benefit from increased control over the problem behaviors (e.g. anxiety disorders, addictions, eating disorders, habit disorders, etc.). In this chapter we describe its applications in facilitating recovery from trauma in earthquake, war, and torture survivors.

In view of the evidence pointing to the close association between helplessness and anxiety, fear, and avoidance in trauma survivors, CFBT focuses primarily on trauma cues or reminders that evoke the latter responses. Its primary aim is to reverse traumatic stress processes by increasing anxiety or distress tolerance. A treatment focus on trauma cues is feasible in most cases, considering trauma cues evoke anxiety / distress in the overwhelming majority of trauma survivors and often lead to avoidance behaviors. Indeed, in our studies (Başoğlu et al., 2005; Şalcıoğlu, 2004) we were able to identify distressing trauma reminders in 96% of earthquake survivors and 92% of war survivors with PTSD. Avoidance behaviors were present in 97% of earthquake and 90% of war survivors with PTSD. It is worth clarifying at this point what we mean by avoidance behaviors. While DSM-IV criteria for PTSD (American Psychiatric Association, 1994) makes a distinction between behavioral and cognitive avoidance (defined as avoidance of thoughts, feelings, or conversations associated with the trauma), such a distinction is rather ambiguous and arbitrary because most forms of avoidance have a behavioral as well as a cognitive component. For example, avoidance of talking about the trauma may have a cognitive component in involving avoidance of thoughts / feelings but it is also behavioral in nature because it involves avoidance of talking behavior. Furthermore, thoughts and feelings could also be conceptualized as behaviors in the broad sense of the term. We therefore use the term avoidance behaviors to refer to both cognitive and behavioral avoidance.

In this chapter we provide a detailed description of CFBT accompanied by case vignettes and a discussion of various treatment procedures. A review of various issues pertaining to treatment of problem cases is also provided. Later in the chapter we describe various applications of CFBT in earthquake survivors, including single-session CFBT, delivery of treatment in groups, and Earthquake Simulation Treatment.

Pre-treatment assessment

An initial assessment immediately before the first session using the screening instruments reviewed in Chapter 3 (*Screening Instrument for Traumatic Stress in Earthquake Survivors – SITSES, Screening Instrument for Traumatic Stress in War Survivors – SITSOW, Fear and Avoidance Questionnaire – FAQ,* and *Depression Rating Scale – DRS*) is most helpful during treatment for several reasons. These scales provide useful information on severity of trauma exposure and traumatic stress reactions and the extent of associated functional impairment. In earthquake survivors the FAQ provides useful information for assessment of avoidance behaviors. In survivors who have lost close ones during the traumatic events, the assessment tools for grief reviewed in Chapter 5 may be useful in identifying possible prolonged grief reactions. Second, the scales can be used to provide the survivor with valuable feedback regarding the nature and severity of their problems and their need for treatment. They are also useful in explaining the treatment and its rationale. Furthermore, this initial assessment serves as a baseline for the survivor's psychological condition against which progress in treatment can be evaluated. Subsequent assessments during treatment can provide useful feedback for both the therapist and the survivor. Declining scores may act as rewarding feedback for the survivor, thereby reinforcing motivation for further progress.

First session

Step 1: identifying trauma cues and avoidance behaviors

At the outset of the session it is helpful to ask about the survivor's main presenting complaints and explore further to establish their connection with particular trauma events. If the trauma is recent (e.g. as in the aftermath of mass trauma events), it is fairly easy to establish this connection, as most survivors report distress caused by re-experiencing symptoms, anticipatory fear of similar events in the future, and hyperarousal symptoms. If depression is present, the presenting complaints may concern symptoms that cause severe interference with daily activities (e.g. loss of interest, lack of energy, loss of pleasure). Somatic complaints (e.g. pain in parts of the body) may also be observed in mass trauma survivors from developing countries, particularly those with lower socio-educational status. Once the presence of traumatic stress problems is ascertained, the following step helps to bring the session to focus on these problems:

> *Let us now have a closer look at your problems. I understand from the questionnaires you filled in that you are having quite a few stress-related problems. I can see that you have marked problems like …*
>
> (Read some of the endorsed Traumatic Stress Symptom Checklist – TSSC – and DRS items)

There is usually no need to probe into trauma experiences at any stage of the treatment but the initial inquiry about presenting complaints sometimes prompts the survivor to relate their trauma experiences. While we have observed that earthquake survivors often engage in a detailed account of their trauma story (e.g. where they were and what they did during the earthquake, etc.), survivors of war or torture trauma may not find it easy to relate their story in detail. If the survivor volunteers the trauma story, this could be used as an opportunity to gain an understanding of their trauma experiences. As wars, armed conflicts, and torture occur in a wide range of different settings and contexts, it may be helpful to gain some understanding of the geographical, historical, social, and political context of the traumatic events experienced by the survivor. Did the trauma occur in the context of political persecution by a repressive regime, conflict between rival groups or warring ethnic groups in a country, a larger scale regional war, or other circumstances? It is also useful to understand the nature and extent of the survivor's involvement in the political processes in their country of origin. Is the survivor a political activist committed to a political group or cause or an ordinary civilian who got caught up in the conflict in their country of origin? The latter survivors often develop more severe traumatic stress than experienced political activists (Başoğlu et al., 1997).

Assessment of trauma cues and associated avoidance behaviors in earthquake survivors is a fairly straightforward procedure, because such assessment can be conducted using the FAQ. This questionnaire provides all the information necessary for treatment, so a detailed assessment of trauma cues is usually not necessary in earthquake survivors. As a similar questionnaire is not yet available for war and torture survivors, such information needs to be elicited during the first session.

Assessment of avoidance behaviors in earthquake survivors

Once avoidance behaviors are elicited using the FAQ, it is helpful to identify the ones that cause most impairment in daily functioning. For example, avoidance of concrete buildings might have led the entire family to seek refuge in a survivor camp solely out of fear, even when their house may have sustained no damage during the earthquake. It might also have made it difficult for the survivor to visit friends or relatives, thereby causing disruption in social life. Some survivors even quit their job because of fear of buildings. Avoidance of distressing sights of devastated buildings might have made it impossible to undertake daily activities. Avoidance of sexual intercourse might have severely strained a marital relationship. Note that the FAQ does not include an exhaustive list of possible avoidance behaviors. To make sure that important avoidance behaviors are not missed, it might be helpful to ask questions like *Is there anything else you have difficulty doing now because of your fear of earthquakes?*" In most cases it is possible to identify at least several avoidance behaviors with significant impact on daily activities.

Assessment of avoidance behaviors in war and torture survivors

Distressing trauma cues can be internal (e.g. intrusive thoughts or memories of trauma events), or external, involving situations or activities that act as reminders of the trauma by way of their resemblance to various aspects of the trauma events. For example, medical investigations involving electrodes attached to the body (as in electrocardiography) may act as a trauma cue in torture survivors with an experience of electrical torture. Undressing for a medical examination may evoke distress or fear in survivors with an experience of being stripped naked during torture. Swimming in pools or sea may be avoided in cases with suffocation experience resulting from submersion under water (or 'waterboarding'). A woman with a history of rape may avoid sexual activity or physical contact with their partners or men in general. A job interview by an authority figure may evoke memories of brutal interrogations.

Trauma cues may also reflect secondary fear conditioning effects of the trauma. Various aspects of the original trauma setting, objects, sights, smells, sounds, tastes, or tactile sensations present at the time of the trauma may become associated with the trauma and act as reminders in other contexts or settings. We have seen a torture survivor, for example, who could not wear white socks, because their color acted as a reminder of the blank sheet of paper that she was forced to sign as confession to a crime she had not committed; her 'confession' was later typed on the paper. Trauma cues may also evoke fear by signaling further threat to safety. For example, a torture survivor may avoid crowded places for fear of coming across police officers, even when there is no realistic risk of re-arrest and further torture. The following questions are often helpful in identifying trauma cues and associated avoidance behaviors:

1. *Do thoughts or memories of these events enter your mind against your will and make you feel so distressed that you have to make an effort to push them out of your mind?*
2. *Are there any situations or activities in your daily life that remind you of past events and make you feel distressed, anxious, or fearful?*
3. *Do you go out of your way to avoid any of these situations or activities either because they remind you of past events or because you think there is a danger of reliving the same events?*

The first question is aimed at identifying intrusive trauma memories associated with distress and avoidance. The second question elicits information about anxiety cues associated with past trauma and the third one clarifies which of these cues are associated with avoidance behaviors. It is helpful to elicit information on as many trauma cues as possible and make a list of them. Various situations or events that trigger flashbacks could also reveal useful information about distressing trauma cues. It is useful to bear in mind that stimulus generalization in the process of fear conditioning may lead to highly idiosyncratic examples of trauma cues in some cases (e.g. the torture survivor with avoidance of white socks). Hearing people speak English acted as a distressing trauma cue in an ex-Guantanamo detainee (who eventually decided to overcome such distress by taking English courses). Some survivors develop overt avoidances of various trauma cues, which are fairly easy to identify. However, more subtle and elaborate forms of avoidance may be more difficult to detect. Some survivors may have changed their life routines in subtle ways to avoid trauma cues. Others may divert their attention from distressing thoughts by occupying themselves with other activities. When trying to sleep, they may keep the TV on or listen to music just to interrupt the flow of thoughts into their mind. Some survivors rely on safety signals in executing certain activities. In cases with high levels of distress or fear, some form of avoidance is highly likely and further probing (e.g. *"Is there anything you have difficulty doing now because of your fears or distress that you could easily do before the trauma events?"*) might help identify them.

We should note here an assessment of trauma cues and associated avoidance behaviors may indirectly elicit information about the nature of trauma experiences. For example, avoidance of men in female survivors may point to an experience of sexual abuse or rape. Avoidance of electrical appliances may suggest an experience of electrical torture. If the survivor does not relate such experiences in detail, there is no need to probe into them. Some survivors find it easier to talk about their trauma as they recover from its effects later in treatment. As the trauma story unravels in treatment, it may reveal additional trauma cues that were not elicited in the first session. Thus, assessment of trauma cues is not limited to the first session. It is a process that continues throughout treatment. Two case vignettes are provided below from case studies (Başoğlu & Aker, 1996; Başoğlu et al., 2004a) to illustrate the nature of trauma cues and associated avoidance behaviors in survivors of torture.

Case vignette #1

A 23-year-old, single, female survivor was detained by the police and tortured for 20 days in the early 1990s. The purpose of the torture was to obtain information about political activist relatives and a confession incriminating various people. Torture involved verbal abuse, blindfolding, beating, stripping naked, hanging, electrical shocks to fingers and nipples, cold showers, sexual advances, several incidents of rape, insertion of a baton into the anus, submersion into water, forced ingestion of salty water, being led to believe she was going up a flight of stairs when blindfolded, threats of torture and death to family, exposure to bright light, and threats of further torture. On psychiatric examination she had full-blown PTSD. She was anxious, dysphoric, but not depressed. She avoided a wide range of situations or activities that either reminded her of her torture experience or evoked intense fear because of perceived threat of re-arrest and torture. These included the following:

1. *Avoidance behaviors associated with generalized conditioned fears:*
   - staying home alone
   - sleeping in the dark
   - going out alone
   - going to public places, such as a post office or a coffee house
   - meeting friends, going to social meetings
   - getting in a car on her own
   - going up a flight of stairs alone (a reminder of the occasion when she was led to believe she was going up a flight of stairs when she was blindfolded)
   - walking near the street (she was picked up by a police car when walking on the street side of the pavement)

   - walking by a police station
   - going near police officers on the street or tall men with a moustache (thus resembling the police officers who conducted her torture)
   - going near white Ford cars (resembling the police car that picked her up on the street)
   - talking and making appointments on the phone (for fear of police surveillance of telephone conversations)
   - carrying someone else's telephone number on her (for fear of getting that person into trouble with the police in case of re-arrest)

2. *Avoidance behaviors associated with distressing trauma reminders:*
   - watching certain movies
   - drinking tea (she was offered a cup of tea during interrogation)
   - reading newspapers, talking about sex (reminder of her rape)
   - talking about her torture experience, signing a paper (reminder of the confession she signed)
   - sound of a police wireless radio

This case is fairly characteristic of torture survivors who continue to live in their home country in an environment of continued threat of arrest and torture. Generalized fear and avoidance relate to a wide range of situations and activities and in some cases may reflect in part a certain degree of realistic risk of re-arrest and torture. Nevertheless, the nature and extent of generalized fears and avoidance often go well beyond reasonable self-protective behaviors. Although there was some risk of re-arrest and torture in this case, a realistic evaluation of her circumstances (e.g. she was not a militant political activist sought by the authorities) did not justify fear and avoidance to an extent that crippled her daily functioning and made her almost housebound. As detailed in Part 1, fear conditioning leads to a wide range of avoidance behaviors, many of which have little self-protective value. Such fear and avoidance may even persist in a safe environment, as illustrated by the second case vignette.

Case vignette #2

A 22-year-old, male, single asylum-seeker, who had arrived in Sweden in 1997, had been detained and tortured on eight separate occasions between 1994 and 1997 in his home country and spent 18 months in prison on one occasion. He reported an experience of more than 20 different forms of torture, including forced stress positions, severe beatings, electric torture, being hanged by the arms, near-suffocation, and sham executions. He left his country after this last detention. In psychiatric examination he had full-blown PTSD with additional complaints of fatigue, headaches, and pains in the chest. He also complained of feeling that he was still at risk of re-arrest and torture, despite the fact that he knew he was perfectly safe in Sweden. He avoided social interactions and had difficulty in forming close relationships. His social avoidance and concentration difficulties made it difficult to attend language courses and learn Swedish. He avoided sleeping because of fear of nightmares. He had difficulty socializing because he felt anxious with people and also feared that he might lose control and assault someone. He avoided travelling on buses because this triggered flashbacks of a past incident when the police had boarded a bus he was on and arrested some people. He did not watch TV and movies because certain news or scenes of violence reminded him of his torture experience. He avoided dealings with the Swedish immigration office and his lawyer because this meant having to talk about his torture experience.

This case also shows that avoidance behaviors can develop in relation to various traumatic stress symptoms. The intensity of fear associated with perceived threat to safety can have a profound impact on the person's daily functioning. We have seen an Iraqi refugee, for example, who fled his country in the 1990s to settle in London. His fear of recapture by Iraqi agents was so intense and pervasive that he avoided going home every night, spending all night travelling on London busses and going home at daybreak when he was completely exhausted. His fear of recapture and further persecution by the Iraqi authorities did not appear realistic, because he was not a high-profile political activist or someone holding a high position in any political organization in his country. An exhaustive list of all possible avoidance behaviors is not possible, given that such behaviors may take highly idiosyncratic forms.

Trauma cues in war survivors also vary considerably according to the nature of the war events experienced. As in torture survivors, assessment needs to focus on situations or activities that act as distressing reminders of past trauma or that are perceived as posing further threat to safety. Traumatized survivors often tend to avoid situations where they think similar

events are likely to occur. For example, visits to a territory previously held by the enemy may be avoided, even when the war is over and such a visit involves no realistic threat. Depending on the nature of the particular trauma event, other war trauma cues include airplane or helicopter sounds, military personnel or other people in uniform, sights of devastation, sudden loud sounds (e.g. explosions), crowded places, movies involving violence, people with physical injury, ambulances, sirens, hospital settings, and media news or TV pictures of any form of violence or disaster. Two additional case vignettes presented in Chapter 9 illustrate further the nature of trauma cues in asylum-seekers exposed to various forms of war trauma, including torture.

Step 2: explaining treatment and its rationale

Once the trauma cues and associated traumatic stress responses are identified, the next step is to help the survivor understand why they need treatment for traumatic stress problems and what treatment involves and how it works. Some survivors may not be fully aware of how their traumatic stress problems affect their life functioning or they may simply not perceive traumatic stress reactions as a treatable problem. It is therefore useful practice to ensure that the survivor fully understands the impact of traumatic stress on their life and their need for treatment.

Clarifying the need for treatment

In explaining the need for treatment, it is best to get the survivor to draw their own conclusions about the impact of traumatic stress on their life, rather than presenting such analysis in the form of an argument. For example:

So far we established that you have considerable distress in relation to the trauma events you experienced. Various situations or activities that remind you of these events make you feel so distressed that you avoid many of them. Let us examine more closely how fear, avoidance, and related stress problems affect your life. Tell me how the symptoms you marked in this questionnaire [read endorsed TSSC items] affect your functioning at home / work / school or your social life. Tell me more about important chores / duties / responsibilities that you need to take care of everyday but cannot because of these problems.

This introduction is followed by a more detailed discussion of how specific traumatic stress symptoms lead to impaired functioning in important areas of the survivor's life. For example, avoidance behaviors may seriously hinder their occupational and social functioning or even making it difficult to maintain their job. Memory / concentration problems caused by intrusive trauma-related thoughts, heightened levels of anxiety / distress evoked by frequent encounters with a wide range of trauma reminders, and hypervigilance may cause serious impairment in their learning capacity and school, work, and social performance. Chronic fatigue caused by reduced sleep (associated with generalized anxiety and / or frequent nightmares) may further hamper their performance in everyday tasks. Irritability and problems of anger control may impair their relationships with family, friends, and colleagues at work. They may have various somatic complaints as a manifestation of chronic anxiety. The latter may have also led to depression and other complications, such as drug and alcohol abuse, thereby further aggravating the problems.

Explaining the treatment and its rationale

Once the survivor fully understands how traumatic stress affects their life, they are ready for an explanation of the treatment and its rationale.

OK, now that we have clarified how your problems affect your life, let us consider what can be done about them. Fear is your worst enemy here, considering how it affects your life. Instead of fighting and defeating the enemy, you have so far chosen to surrender to fear by avoiding it. Avoidance means you are letting fear take control of your life. [In non-tortured war survivors: By doing this, you are also surrendering to those responsible for what you have been through. Is this not exactly how they wanted to see you – terrified and helpless? In torture survivors: Think about your torture experience. They tried to break your will in every way possible and make you totally helpless, so that you would surrender and comply with their demands. Given your current state, would you not say they have so far succeeded in achieving their aims?] Considering that avoiding distress / fear maintains stress problems, the logical thing to do here is to overcome your fears by not avoiding them. You need to do this in a systematic fashion until you learn to tolerate and control your anxiety. This means you will have to make an effort not to avoid situations or activities that make you anxious. You stand a good chance of recovery with this treatment. I will tell you more about what you need to do in treatment later. At this point you need to decide whether you want to fight your anxiety and take control over your life or surrender to your fear and live your life in fear and helplessness. This is entirely your choice and you will need to take the responsibility for it. Which one will it be?

Note that this discourse highlights the primary role of distress / fear and associated avoidance / helplessness in traumatic stress. Presenting a choice between chronic illness and recovery and placing responsibility for this choice squarely on the survivor counters the victim role by urging the survivor to take action against the problem. Informing the survivor that the chances of recovery with treatment are high instills hope and alleviates feelings of helplessness and hopelessness (e.g. *I will never get better*).

Presenting fear as the *enemy*, avoidance as *surrendering* to the enemy, and not avoiding fear as *fighting* and *defeating* the enemy serves to enhance sense of control over fear and encourages survivors to relinquish the victim role by taking action against their problem. Survivors of mass trauma events of human design, such as war, torture, atrocities, and acts of terrorism can easily relate to such discourse, because these terms are not merely allegories relating to fear; they relate to real people perceived as the enemy or perpetrators of human rights abuses. Note that such discourse is similar to the one often used in military training of soldiers or in training of political activists. Indeed, using a similar discourse many leaders in history have been able to mobilize masses against a designated enemy and lead them to armed conflicts or wars. Among other examples of this phenomenon are the Kamikaze pilots in World War II, militant political activists, and suicide bombers of today. Such discourse appears to facilitate cognitive control over natural fear of dying and avoidance associated with life-threatening situations. Combat-related allegories are also helpful in natural disaster survivors, even when used only in reference to fear. This is because people have a natural tendency to personify fear as an adversary and think in terms of fighting, beating, overcoming, defeating, conquering, or winning a victory over fear. Most languages probably have similar expressions, which reflect such a natural tendency in people. In Turkish, for example, *being enslaved by fear* is one of the many expressions that describe inability to control fear.

Presenting fear, avoidance, and helplessness as a form of surrender to the 'enemy' makes much sense to war survivors, given that much of war violence and gross human rights violations are often designed to terrorize people and force them into total submission and surrender. Such discourse may be particularly helpful in survivors of torture, rape, physical assaults, or other forms of direct victimization, who often have strong feelings of injustice, anger, and desire for vengeance against the perpetrators. These emotions can be channeled into a desire to recover from trauma by helping the survivor see recovery as an act of retribution against or victory over the perpetrators. Survivors of torture, particularly political activists, often relate very well to such suggestions, because they often attribute similar meanings to successful coping with the torture (e.g. not breaking down or submitting to the torturers in any way) and surviving the event in relatively good health. They tend to regard this as their victory over the torturers, as the following case illustrates.

> A female political activist in her early 30s was detained by the police and subjected to various forms of torture, including insertion of a baton into her vagina. During the latter event she was mockingly told by the torturers that she would never be able to have children. After her release she experienced various post-traumatic stress problems but her main problem related to intrusive thoughts of not being able to have children. Despite repeated medical examinations and assurances from doctors that she sustained no damage in her reproductive organs, she was continually distressed by these thoughts. She knew that her fear made no sense but she could not control it. A few years later, she fell pregnant with her first child but she nevertheless continued to feel anxious throughout her pregnancy, thinking that the baby might turn out to be abnormal in some way. When she finally gave birth to a perfectly normal and healthy baby, her first remark was *"The victory is mine."* Following this event she substantially recovered from the trauma.

When confronted with a choice between recovery and illness, most survivors state that they want to get better and that they are prepared to make an effort for it. Political activists often relate very well to the treatment rationale, because it is consonant with the norms and values of political activist groups, which often promote commitment to cause, self-sacrifice, courage, and resilience in their members. If the treatment is taking place in an environment where there is ongoing threat to safety (e.g. the survivor's home country), some survivors may raise the question as to whether it is not normal to fear and avoid situations that pose a realistic

threat to safety. The question could be answered by pointing to the survivor's irrational nature of conditioned fears. For example, the following explanation would be useful for the survivor in case vignette #1.

> *Fear and avoidance are normal to the extent that they serve to protect you from real danger. Traumatic events cause many irrational fears that serve no such purpose. Let us consider which of your fears are rational. For example, you avoid watching certain movies, reading newspapers, signing papers, going up a flight of stairs on your own, and drinking tea, because these situations remind you of the distressing events you experienced during your detention. Does avoiding such activities make you any safer? Consider your avoidance of staying alone at home, sleeping in the dark, going out alone, going to public places, meeting friends, men with moustaches, and white Ford cars. Are these really reasonable precautions that protect you from being detained again, given that the police know where you live? Such fears are not normal, not only because they do not actually protect you from danger but also because they make it impossible for you to lead a reasonably normal life. Surely, there is some risk of similar events happening to you but you need to learn to live with such risks in life. You may die in a car accident any time but you do not stop going out or using transport for this reason. You do not avoid going out simply because you might be killed by a flowerpot falling on your head on the street. There are many real dangers in everyday life but we do not make an effort to avoid them. We learn to live with such risks, because otherwise it would be impossible to lead a normal life.*

Similar challenging questions might also be raised by earthquake survivors, particularly during the early months of the disaster when aftershocks are most frequent. While not directly challenging the treatment rationale, some may try to justify their fear by asking whether it is not normal to be afraid of earthquakes, given that they cause so many deaths. Again, this issue could be tackled by highlighting the irrational nature of conditioned fears after earthquake trauma. The following account illustrates the similarities in the irrational nature of conditioned fears in earthquake and torture trauma.

> *You have to make a distinction here between normal fear of earthquakes and irrational fears that serve no purpose. Fear is normal to the extent that it makes you take reasonable precautions to protect yourself against earthquakes. Earthquakes cause a lot of*

irrational fears in people. Let us just consider which of your fears serve a useful purpose. For example, you no longer sleep in the room where you experienced the earthquake. You do this because being in that room brings back your fear. Other than perhaps making you feel a bit better, does sleeping in another room make you any safer during an earthquake? Similarly, you do not take a shower alone at home, go to bed with clothes on, and sleep with lights on. Are these really reasonable precautions that make you any safer during an earthquake? Such fears are not rational, because they do not actually protect you from earthquakes. Moreover, they make it impossible for you to lead a normal life. You might perhaps think that your avoidance of buildings is realistic because being in a building during an earthquake poses some danger. While this is true to a certain extent, you cannot continue to avoid all buildings forever and expect to lead a normal life. You will eventually have to re-settle in a building. The most you can do is to take reasonable precautions against injury during an earthquake and learn to live with the risk. Bear also in mind that there are many other hazards in the world, besides earthquakes, that can cause loss of life. For example, the chances of dying in a car accident are probably higher than dying in an earthquake. Yet you do not stop going out or using transport thinking that there might be an accident. Certain domestic chores, such as ironing or cooking may lead to fires in the house. Yet, you do not give up these activities because they involve a risk to life. Because we are not aware of these dangers in our everyday lives, we do not make an effort to avoid them. We learn to live with such risks, because otherwise it would be impossible to lead a normal life.

Less commonly, some earthquake survivors object to the idea of taking calculated risks as unacceptable and display an unreasonably argumentative attitude towards the therapist, trying to justify their avoidance as a reasonable means of minimizing the probability of harm during an earthquake. It is best to avoid engaging in lengthy discussions with such cases and to display a firm attitude regarding the treatment rationale. It is also worth telling them that treatment need not involve realistically dangerous situations (e.g. entering a building known to be structurally severely damaged) and that not avoiding feared situations that entail no real danger (including undamaged buildings) is sufficient. If this does not help, simply remind the survivor that whether or not they want to get better is entirely up to them.

Explaining how treatment works

A good understanding of how the treatment works on the part of both the therapist and the survivor is essential for success in therapy. To illustrate how CFBT works, it is worth briefly reviewing the processes of change during exposure to fear cues. Figure 4.1 compares the change processes in anxiety and sense of control during exposure that ends with escape from the situation (avoidance) with those that occur during continued exposure where control over fear is exercised (non-avoidance).

It is helpful to recall our discussion in Part 1 as to how repeated exposures to uncontrollable stressors induce a state of helplessness, reducing pre-trauma sense of control over stressors to a level where the person no longer has expectations of control over the outcomes of future stressor events. The dotted line labeled as pre-session baseline sense of control represents this reduced level of sense of control before an encounter with a stressor event. Such low sense of control facilitates actual loss of cognitive, behavioral, and emotional control when a trauma cue is encountered. As sense of control drops to a maximum low, anxiety rapidly rises, reaching a peak. Heightened loss of control and anxiety triggers avoidance or escape behavior, which in turn leads to a reduction in loss of control and anxiety. If the person manages to stay in the situation and continues to experience heightened anxiety, they eventually learn to tolerate and control it. It is important to note here that anxiety may not reduce substantially in some cases (dotted arrow in Figure 4.1), even when sense of control increases. This does not pose a problem for therapy, as the purpose of exposure is to enhance tolerance and control of anxiety, rather than reduce it. Accordingly, the treatment aim needs to be presented in such a way that the person makes an effort to invite, challenge, tolerate, and control fear / distress rather than try to reduce it. In a post-earthquake situation, challenging fear means, for example, entering an undamaged building and doing things to maintain anxiety for as long as possible, such as seeking and focusing on additional fear cues (e.g. examining supporting columns for signs of damage, looking at cracks on the wall plaster, standing in a place where ground vibrations caused by passing trucks can be felt, etc.), tackling more frightening aspects of the situation (e.g. going to the upper floors), and inviting anxiety-evoking thoughts (e.g. 'an earthquake might happen now'). In the example of the survivor in case vignette #1,

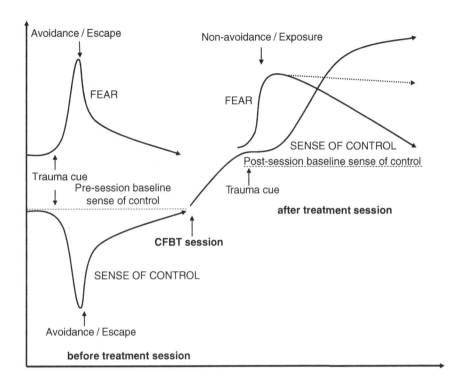

Figure 4.1 Processes of change in fear and sense of control during exposure to trauma cues before and after first treatment session.

challenging fear means not only going out alone but also doing things to invite fear, such as going to crowded places, going near police officers or men with a moustache on the street, approaching white Ford cars, walking close to the street, etc. It is such newly acquired ability to challenge fear and not mere reduction in anxiety that accounts for perceived improvement in treatment. Such experience often signifies a major *victory* or *liberation* from fear, particularly in survivors with a long history of pervasive fear, avoidance, and feelings of helplessness. Fear reduction is not a requirement for a sense of well-being, as the latter is more closely related to increased sense of control (see Chapter 6 for more discussion of this issue). Accordingly, the treatment rationale makes no explicit reference to anxiety reduction in treatment. Although anxiety often diminishes as the treatment progresses, setting anxiety reduction as the treatment goal is not consistent with the expressed aim of the therapy. It may be counterproductive in survivors who may not experience reduction in their anxiety or who experience a return in anxiety at some stage during treatment, leading them into thinking that the treatment is not working or that they are a treatment failure.

The context-dependent nature of fear reduction is a well-known problem in traditional exposure treatment that accounts for return of fear in situations different in their contextual characteristics from the one in which fear reduction took place (Bouton, 1988; Hermans et al., 2005; Mineka et al., 1999; Mystkowski et al., 2002; Rodriguez et al., 1999; Rowe & Craske, 1998). Accordingly, some authors (Craske et al., 2008; Vansteenwegen et al., 2005; Vansteenwegen et al., 2007) recommend that exposure treatment is conducted in multiple contexts so that treatment effects are generalized and the likelihood of relapse is reduced. This is not a requirement in CFBT, simply because it does not aim at reducing anxiety in any context. In CFBT each fear-evoking situation is regarded as an opportunity to build up anxiety tolerance or resilience. Generalized improvement can occur in both fear and related traumatic stress reactions with one session of CFBT (e.g. as in Earthquake Simulation Treatment described later in this chapter; see also Chapter 6), suggesting that increased sense of control, unlike anxiety reduction, can generalize to other contexts. The remarkably low rate of relapse in our treatment studies with earthquake survivors (evidence reviewed in Chapter 6), despite ongoing aftershocks (i.e. unconditioned stimuli), is further evidence of generalized treatment effects.

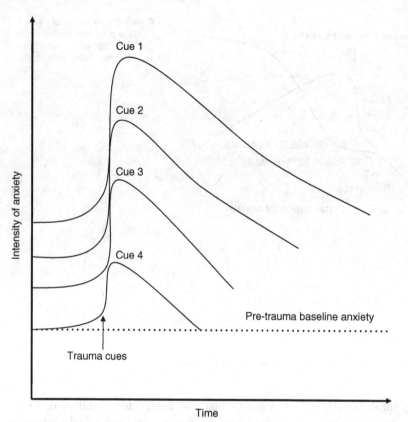

Figure 4.2 Pattern of anxiety reduction with repeated exposures to trauma cues.

Once the first encounter with a feared situation is managed successfully, the increase in sense of control makes subsequent encounters with the same or similar situations easier to tackle. At each subsequent exposure peak anxiety (highest anxiety level reached during the encounter) tends to be lower in intensity and increase in sense of control and decrease in anxiety occurs faster. Such improvement process can also be observed within the same exposure session when fear cues of increasing intensity are presented in succession.[1] Figure 4.2 shows the pattern of change

in anxiety with repeated encounters with anxiety cues as treatment progresses.

Note that the baseline anxiety level before an encounter with a trauma cue is higher than the pre-trauma baseline anxiety level (dotted line), because of anticipatory anxiety or hypervigilance associated with expectations of further threat to safety. An increase in sense of control after each exposure reduces anticipatory anxiety, resulting in lower baseline anxiety before the next encounter with another trauma cue. Enhanced sense of control also leads to lower peak anxiety during the next exposure and faster return to pre-exposure baseline anxiety level. Thus, as peak anxiety declines with repeated exposures to different anxiety cues, so does baseline anxiety, which may eventually return to pre-trauma level. This is often

---

[1] For example, in our study (Başoğlu et al., 2007) of Earthquake Simulation Treatment in earthquake survivors, the magnitude of simulated tremors ranged from 1 (corresponding to a 3- to 4-strong earthquake on the Richter scale) to 5 (magnitude of about 7 on the Richter scale). We obtained within-session anxiety ratings throughout the session based on a 0–8 scale to examine the process of change. At each tremor magnitude level sufficient time was allowed for substantial increase in sense of control to occur before moving to the next level up. At each higher level anxiety surged to a peak and then started to decline. Peak anxiety was highest (mean 6.5, SD = 1.7) at level 1, steadily declining as higher levels were achieved,

reaching its lowest point (mean 1.0, SD = 0.9) at level 5 (unpublished data). In addition, the time required for a substantial increase in sense of control and reduction in anxiety was much longer at the lower tremor magnitude levels, decreasing as the session progressed to higher levels. In fact, 80% of the session time was spent at the lowest levels.

accompanied by a substantial reduction in traumatic stress and depression symptoms (evidence reviewed in Chapter 6).

While such a detailed account using visual illustrations of change processes in treatment may be helpful in some survivors with higher socio-educational status, a brief explanation as follows is sufficient in most cases.

When you come across situations that make you distressed or anxious, you feel an urge to get away from them and you often surrender to this urge. When you get away, your anxiety diminishes and you feel relieved. This is obviously not an effective strategy, given that it has not helped you with your fear and stress problems. Instead, try confronting your anxiety by not avoiding distressing situations every time you come across one. This will give you an opportunity to learn how to tolerate and control anxiety. Once you manage to do this, your confidence in yourself will grow and you will find it easier to tackle other anxiety-evoking situations. As your resilience against anxiety increases, you will feel less helpless and this will lead to an improvement in your stress problems. To use an analogy, building up your resilience by allowing yourself to experience anxiety is like getting vaccinated against a virus. You need a small dose of the virus in your system so that your body can build up its defense against the virus. This is also like practicing weight-lifting. The more you do it, the stronger you get and the more weight you can lift.

Note that the emphasis in this account is on *tolerance* and *control* of fear or distress, rather than a reduction of these emotions. Although it is acceptable practice to inform the survivor that anxiety is likely to reduce during as well as between encounters with feared situations, this should not be set as *the* treatment goal or emphasized. Anxiety needs to be presented, not as an undesirable phenomenon that needs to be reduced or eradicated at all costs, but rather as an opportunity to test, reinforce, and enhance one's capacity to tolerate and control it. As discussed in detail in Part 1, this is the process that leads to resilience. Such resilience-building processes, often referred to as a 'toughening' (Dienstbier, 1989) or 'steeling' effect in psychiatric literature (Bleuler, 1974; Rutter, 1985), are also widely utilized in training of soldiers, special forces, commandos, and militant political activists. It is also worth noting that a good understanding of this process on the part of the survivor is one of the most important predictors of good outcome with CFBT. Survivors who quickly grasp the treatment rationale and actively seek opportunities to challenge their fear recover much faster and to a greater extent than others.

Step 3: defining treatment tasks and giving self-exposure instructions

Once the survivor is prepared to go along with treatment, the next step is to describe the course of action required to achieve the treatment aim. Such action involves (a) normalizing life routines by not avoiding anxiety-evoking situations as they are encountered in daily life and (b) focused exposure exercises in relation to specific anxiety-evoking situations.

Anti-avoidance instructions for earthquake survivors

Anti-avoidance instructions relate to both anticipatory fear of recurrence of trauma and distressing reminders of the trauma experiences. The following instructions relate to fear of future earthquakes.

Overcoming fear of earthquakes

There are things that you can do to overcome your fear of earthquakes in your daily life at home. For example,

- *Take a bath as usual, making sure that you do not cut short your time in the bathroom for fear of earthquakes. If you have stopped taking a bath when you are alone at home, make an effort and do it.*
- *At night get undressed before going to bed, turn the light off, close the bedroom door, and do not keep the TV or radio on until you sleep.*
- *Do not avoid sleeping in the dark or when you are alone at home.*
- *Do not keep someone in the family awake at night in case an earthquake happens.*
- *If you are afraid of sleeping alone in the house, make a point of sleeping alone whenever you need to.*
- *If you have stopped sleeping in the room where you experienced the earthquake, make a point of sleeping in that room.*
- *Do not seek the company of someone in the house because it makes you feel safer. Make sure you can stay in the house all by yourself. Do not go out of your way to visit friends, relatives, or neighbors when you are in fear. Take every opportunity to overcome your fear of being alone in the house.*
- *Stop trying to avoid earthquakes by watching out for signs of an impending earthquake. For example, do not repeatedly check the ceiling lights*

or keep a glass of water on the table to detect signs of any movement. Do not keep listening to sounds of dogs or birds or keep watching the sky or the sea for any signs of an impending earthquake. Stop watching TV or listening to the radio all the time in the hope that you may hear something about future earthquakes. Do not keep checking with your friends to see if they have heard any rumors about an earthquake in the near future.

- *If you have fear of various other situations that you did not have before the earthquake, make a point of not avoiding them. For example, confront and overcome any fear of confined spaces, heights, lifts, going out alone, swimming, or travelling in public transport. There may be many other things that you can do to overcome your fears. Just ask yourself "What is it that I do in the belief that it will protect me in case of an earthquake?" Make a list of them. Then examine each action carefully to see if it realistically makes you any safer. Bear in mind that feeling safe and actually being safe are not necessarily the same thing. Remember also that it is impossible to avoid earthquakes by being alert all the time or trying to detect early signs. The best you can do is to take some realistic precautions and learn to live with the reality of earthquakes.*

Note that some of these instructions are designed to help the survivor challenge fear, while others are aimed at blocking behaviors or cues that have a safety signal value. As described in detail in Chapter 1, many survivors resort to such safety signals in reducing their anxiety, so it is important to make the survivor aware of the anti-therapeutic effects of such dependency on safety signals.

Below are examples of anti-avoidance instructions relating to trauma reminders:

Overcoming trauma-related distress

Some of the avoidance behaviors you marked in the Fear and Avoidance Questionnaire may relate to distressing reminders of your earthquake experiences. Every time you come across these reminders, take it as an opportunity to build up your resilience by not avoiding them. For example:

- *Do not avoid sights of devastation or destroyed buildings. If you need to pass by such locations in your everyday life, make sure that you do not take a different route. Look closely at these sights, examine them, and do not try to avoid any memories of the earthquake that may come to your mind. If necessary, make a point of going to*

these locations and stay there until you have complete control over your distress.
- *Do not avoid talking about things you experienced during the earthquake with friends, acquaintances, or others.*
- *Take every opportunity to participate in conversations or discussions about earthquakes.*
- *Do not avoid earthquake-related news in the media. On the contrary, challenge your distress and listen to such news on TV or radio or read about them in the newspapers.*
- *Do not avoid any other reminders of the earthquake. If necessary, make a point of looking at pictures of acquaintances that died in the earthquake, seeing particular people or visiting particular locations in the region that bring back your memories, and attending community meetings, ceremonies for the dead, anniversaries of the disaster, and so on.*
- *Whenever something reminds you of your earthquake experiences, do not try to avoid memories, thoughts, or images about your experiences by pushing them away from your mind. Do not try to divert your attention from these thoughts or prevent them from entering your mind by occupying yourself with other activities, such as keeping the radio on, reading something, or doing housework. Instead, focus your attention on these thoughts and go through the earthquake events as they happened over and over again until you no longer feel the need to avoid them in your mind. You will see that when you do not try to avoid such thoughts, they will come to your mind less frequently.*

Because the FAQ provides a detailed list of most common avoidance behaviors that interfere with daily functioning, it may serve as a useful guide in normalizing life routines. Thus, it may be helpful to give the survivor a copy of their own ratings and ask them to give priority to avoidance behaviors that they consider as causing most problems in daily life. Generally, avoidances that impair work, family, and social functioning are deemed as most troublesome by most people but there may also be individual variations in this respect.

Anti-avoidance instructions for war and torture survivors

Many of the instructions listed above would also apply to war and torture survivors, given that life-threatening traumatic events lead to similar avoidance behaviors in survivors. The following example in relation to the survivor in case vignette #1 illustrates this point.

Overcoming torture-induced fear and distress

Think about how you used to go about your daily life before your detention experiences. Make an effort to resume your normal daily life routines by not avoiding anxiety-evoking situations. Stay alone at home whenever necessary. Turn off the lights when you go to bed. Whenever the need arises, go out of your home alone to public places, take a taxi, attend social meetings, and meet with friends. Challenge your fear by walking near the streets and walking by police stations, going near white Ford cars, police officers, or men with moustaches on the street. Drink tea, watch TV, and read newspapers, as you did before. Do not avoid any conversations with friends that remind you of your detention experiences. Take every opportunity to engage in such conversations. If you feel the need to talk to a close friend about your detention experiences, do not avoid it simply because you would feel distressed by doing so. Do not avoid any other reminders of the event. Make a point of doing things that you know will bring back your memories. Whenever something reminds you of your torture, do not try to avoid distressing thoughts or images by pushing them away from your mind. Do not try to divert your attention from these thoughts or prevent them from entering your mind by occupying yourself with other activities, such as listening to the radio, reading something, or doing housework. Instead, focus your attention on these thoughts and go through the events as they happened over and over again until you no longer feel the need to avoid them in your mind. You will see that when you do not try to avoid such thoughts, they will come to your mind less frequently.

Some survivors who are well aware of the disabling effects of fear on their life and desperately looking for a way out of the problem are quick to act on anti-avoidance instructions and make systematic efforts to stop avoiding anxiety-evoking situations. They eventually resume their normal life without having to conduct systematic exposure homework exercises (therapist- or self-administered) in relation to specific situations. However, as some survivors may not be able to stop avoiding certain situations because of high levels of anxiety, it is best to prescribe a few focused exposure exercises in relation to most troublesome feared situations and a more detailed description of how they need to go about conducting these exercises.

Focused self-exposure exercises

Survivors often find it more difficult to tackle situations that not only evoke distressing memories of past trauma but also signal further threat to safety. Locations where the original trauma was experienced often involve both distress and fear cues and thus are often among the situations that pose most difficulty for survivors. Staying alone at home, for example, might pose the greatest difficulty in people who experienced the traumatic event while at home (e.g. as in many earthquake survivors or people who were captured at home during a raid by security forces, enemy soldiers, paramilitaries, etc.). Entering buildings poses a major problem for earthquake survivors, while torture survivors often find it difficult to go into situations they associate with risk of being detained and tortured again. Focused self-exposure exercises in relation to such situations serve several purposes. They help survivors understand how they can deal with their anxiety in situations associated with high levels of distress or fear. Successful completion of such an exposure task enhances their sense of control over anxiety, which often generalizes to other situations, making subsequent tasks easier to tackle. Furthermore, they may help survivors overcome certain avoidance behaviors associated with severe functional impairment (e.g. avoidance of buildings in displaced earthquake survivors) and thereby facilitate a more rapid return to normal life functioning.

Most survivors, particularly those with high motivation for treatment, often do not pose problems in complying with self-exposure instructions. In some cases, however, exposure tasks may need to be broken into easier steps. For example, in a displaced earthquake survivor who wants to overcome fear of resettling at home, this task could be broken into more manageable steps as follows:

Step 1: Go near the building and stand near the door.
Step 2: Go into the building, have a look around and then leave.
Step 3: Go into your home, have a cup of coffee and then leave.
Step 4: Go back home, tidy up the place and then leave.
Step 5: Spend the whole day at home and leave in the evening.
Step 6: Spend the day and the evening at home and leave late at night.
Step 7: Start spending the nights at home.

It is important to negotiate each step with the survivor and reach an agreement. They can make each step as easy or difficult as they like. Once an agreement on the course of action is reached, the survivor will need to know how to go about conducting the exercise.

> *As you begin your exercise, you may experience anxiety symptoms, such as sweating, shaking, rapid heartbeat, dizziness, or feeling faint. These symptoms are unpleasant but essentially harmless. You may feel a strong urge to leave the building. Try to control this urge by not giving into it. Tell yourself 'I am going to beat this fear once and for all.' Do not be afraid of feeling anxious. Remember the vaccination example. You need such anxiety to build up your endurance against it. Always remember: This is a battle with fear. Either you will conquer your fear or it will conquer you.*
>
> *As you begin to tolerate anxiety better and better, you will notice an increase in your self-confidence. When this happens, challenge your fear by inviting it. This means doing things to increase your fear. For example, you may be standing near the door and therefore not feeling too anxious. You know that if you go further inside, you will be more anxious, thinking that it will not be easy to get out in case of an earthquake. Muster your courage and go into your home. If you know that going into the room where you experienced the earthquake will increase your fear, go into that room to challenge your fear. The cracks on the wall plaster might make you more anxious. Instead of turning your eyes away from them, go around looking for cracks and examining them. At every step of the way, think as follows: 'What can I do now to invite my fear?' For example, if going up to the upper floors of the building makes you more anxious, do it. If thinking about your experiences during the earthquake makes you more anxious, think about them. Tell yourself 'An earthquake might happen right now'. Sometimes heavy vehicles passing by cause vibrations in buildings. If such vibrations scare you, go and stand at a location where they are most strongly felt. These are just some examples of how you can challenge fear and you may be able to find many other ways of doing it. Once you have learned how to do this, you can consider the battle won. This is an early sign that shows you will be successful in this treatment.*
>
> *At each step terminate the exercise only when you feel that you can leave the building at your own will and not because of your fear. This will mean that you have achieved total control over your fear and are no longer helpless against it. You can congratulate yourself for this achievement! You will be feeling great about yourself. The next time you go back, you are likely to be less anxious than you were the first time. This is because you have greater control*

over your anxiety. Each further step will seem easier to you as you progress through treatment. Therefore, do things to invite your fear while you are there.

If your anxiety gets too intense, stay where you are and find somewhere to sit. Focus your mind on symptoms of anxiety. Tell yourself 'I will not give in to this fear. I will not let it take control over me.' Do NOT try to divert your attention elsewhere. Do not, for example, start reading something, talking to someone or examining something. Otherwise, you would be defeating the purpose of the exercise. If at some point you give in to your fear and leave the building, do not worry. This does not mean failure yet. Have a short break and wait outside. Try to muster more courage and go back inside. If you fail again, do not worry; you can always give it another try some other day. Keep trying and you will eventually succeed. Once you successfully complete the step, move on to the next step and then to the next one until you complete the whole exercise.

Once the survivor achieves this task and resettles at home, they may find it easier to deal with their fear of other buildings. A single focused exposure exercise might be sufficient in some cases in helping them resume their normal life activities. Others, however, may need additional exercises in relation to other buildings, such as homes of friends or relatives, schools, shopping places, banks, hospitals, schools, government offices, cinemas, and so on. Note that a potential problem in exposure exercises is avoidance of anxiety by distracting attention from anxiety cues (e.g. by occupying oneself with another activity). It is thus important to warn the survivor against such avoidance.

The treatment procedure described above also applies to war and torture survivors. To illustrate how an exposure exercise can be structured in relation to a difficult task, let us again consider the survivor in case vignette #1.

Step 1: Go out of your home alone and walk to a nearby public place (e.g. local shops) where you are less likely to come across police officers.

Step 2: Meet with a friend or a close one in a public place where you are less likely to come across many police officers. Walk close to the street. Talk to a few men with a moustache, asking for directions. Approach white Ford cars as much as possible, whenever you see one.

Step 3: Meet with a friend or a close one in a busy public place where there are many police

*officers around. Try to get closer to them (e.g.
by walking past them). If possible, talk to a
police officer asking for directions.*

Step 4: *Repeat Step 2 and Step 3 on your own.*

Similar graduated exposure exercises can be defined in
relation to all other feared situations that the survivor
finds difficult to tackle. In the above case, for example,
the exposure task relating to staying alone at home
might involve staying alone at home during daytime at
the first step, then during the early hours of the evening, and finally during the whole night.

As live exposure sessions involve a strong element
of exposure to trauma memories, additional imaginal
exposure to trauma memories is not necessary.
Exposure to trauma memories in a live exposure context often has greater therapeutic impact than any
form of imaginal exposure taking place in a clinical
setting (see Chapter 6 for more discussion of this
issue). Simply advising the survivor not to try to
avoid intrusive trauma thoughts as they occur is likely
to be useful in many cases. More resistant cases can be
helped by asking them to invite and challenge intrusive
thoughts each time they occur by mentally focusing on
the most distressing trauma memories and images
until they are no longer intolerable. They can also be
encouraged to talk about their trauma to others and
engage in conversations about trauma events.

Survivors with no avoidance of distressing trauma
cues are quite rare. Indeed, we did not have to treat any
such cases in our practice with survivors of earthquake, war, or torture. Theoretically, however, exposure to distressing trauma cues, even when there is no
avoidance, is likely to have similar tolerance-building
effects in such cases. Their treatment might be even
easier, considering that lack of avoidance, despite sufficiently severe trauma-induced distress to warrant
treatment, suggests that the person is already capable
of maintaining control over the problem. This issue,
however, needs to be explored by further research.

Closing the session

As compliance with self-exposure instructions is the
single most important predictor of treatment success,
it is often useful to emphasize the importance of this
issue to the survivor before closing the session. CFBT
is largely a self-help intervention in its heavy reliance
on anti-avoidance or self-exposure exercises, particularly when therapist involvement in conduct of these
exercises is minimal. Treatment success thus depends

entirely on the survivor's compliance with treatment
instructions. The responsibility for success or failure
in treatment needs to be placed squarely on the survivor, because this is the only way of helping them break
the cycle of helplessness or overcome their victim role.
The following explanation might be useful in this
regard:

*Now that we have clarified and agreed on what you
need to do to get better, you need to understand
clearly that success or failure in treatment depends
entirely on you and that you will have to take the
responsibility for the outcome. If you make sufficient
efforts to overcome your problems, your chances of
recovery are very high. Almost all people who fail in
treatment do so because they do not carry out their
treatment exercises. You may experience some setbacks along the way but you need not worry about
them as long as you keep making an effort. I will
guide you through this process and may even help
you with some exposure exercises you may find difficult to tackle, but I will also expect sufficient progress
each time I see you. You also need to bear in mind
that you do not have unlimited time in treatment.
Most people improve after 10 sessions. People who
are most likely to recover with this treatment usually
show signs of improvement within the first few
weeks. This means I will have an idea about your
chances of recovery quite early in treatment. If you
are not making sufficient progress, this will most
likely mean you are not complying with treatment,
in which case I may have to consider terminating the
treatment.*

Setting a time frame for treatment and making con-
tinuation of treatment conditional on progress not
only enhances treatment compliance but also avoids
waste of valuable therapist time in non-compliant
cases. This is a particularly important issue in post-
disaster settings where large numbers of survivors may
be awaiting urgent care. It is also useful to advise the
survivor to involve close ones in treatment, whose
support and help might be valuable in successful execution of difficult exposure tasks. Sharing progress
with close ones (e.g. arranging some kind of family
celebration for major achievement in treatment) could
have strong motivation enhancing effects. Using what
they learned in treatment, they could also try and help
their close ones who may have been exposed to the
same or similar trauma events. We observed on many
occasions that treated earthquake survivors were able
to help their family members, friends, or relatives by
encouraging them to administer the same treatment.

Such efforts to help others might also help enhance their sense of control.

In situations where weekly sessions are not feasible or where treatment attendance is likely to be irregular (e.g. every 2 or 3 weeks), it is worth giving the survivor copies of the TSSC, DRS, and FAQ (for earthquake survivors), and Global Improvement Scale-Self for weekly self-administration until the next session. Declining scale scores might act as a reward and reinforce treatment compliance. It is worth noting in this connection that weekly ratings of progress also provide valuable outcome evaluation data for operational research.

Subsequent sessions

Subsequent sessions involve essentially the same procedures, so they are not described separately here. They involve monitoring of progress to ensure compliance with treatment instructions, provide verbal praise for progress achieved, and deal with problems encountered in treatment. The self-ratings administered before each session are helpful in assessing progress. At the first monitoring session the most important task is to understand the impact of the first session on the survivor's sense of control over distress or fear. Increased sense of control often manifests itself as reduced avoidance.[2] Evidence (Şalcıoğlu et al., 2007a) shows that reduced behavioral avoidance is the earliest sign of improvement in treatment, followed by a reduction in other traumatic stress symptoms in subsequent weeks. Thus, reduced avoidance at the first monitoring session may not be accompanied by marked improvement in other symptoms. Nevertheless, reduced behavioral avoidance is the single most important predictor of successful treatment outcome, so it is important to assess the extent of such change. In earthquake survivors the FAQ ratings are often useful for quick assessment of overall reduction in behavioral avoidance.

---

[2] We examined this issue in 10 earthquake survivors, for example, by giving them a single session of exposure to earthquake tremors in an earthquake simulator to increase their sense of control over fear and then assessed their progress for 6 months to examine the impact of the session on their avoidance behaviors. Although we refrained from giving them explicit self-exposure instructions after the session (to avoid their confounding effects), we observed substantial reduction in behavioral avoidance and improvement in PTSD at 3-month follow-up in eight survivors.

As noted earlier, some survivors, particularly those who relate well to the treatment rationale and show strong motivation for change, make rapid progress in treatment. A few successful attempts at confronting distressing situations often enhance their sense of control further, which in turn makes more difficult situations easier to handle. Such initial progress at the outset often means a great deal to survivors, because they see it as confirmation of their ability to overcome their problem. In such cases focused exposure exercises in relation to particular situations may not be necessary; simple encouragement for further progress may suffice.

Some survivors may not be able to make such progress, either because of generalized feelings of helplessness (e.g. '*I can't do it*') or high levels of anxiety during encounters with avoided situations or both. In such cases one needs to find out whether they attempted focused exposure exercises prescribed in relation to particular situations. They may have had difficulty in initiating these exercises or made failed attempts at them. Such problems often occur when survivors do not plan and execute exposure exercises in a graduated fashion, despite instructions to this effect in the first session. In such cases, a graduated exposure plan needs to be worked out together with the survivor, breaking difficult tasks into more manageable steps, as described earlier. Note also that the survivor does not have to complete the whole task in 1 week. If necessary, a single task may be executed step by step over the course of several weeks. In some cases getting a close friend or a family member to participate in this process and oversee exposure exercises may be helpful. With close monitoring of progress over a few more sessions and strong support and encouragement, most survivors are able to complete their exercises. Once they overcome this initial obstacle, they often find subsequent exposure tasks easier to handle. In a few cases, however, therapist-administered exposure sessions may be needed to overcome this problem. Although several therapist-administered exposure sessions are likely to be sufficient in most cases, more may be needed in very severe cases.

Therapist-administered live exposure

A therapist-administered exposure session might be considered at the very first session, when an anxious survivor rejects the idea of self-exposure or expresses strong reluctance about it. In some cases the need for this intervention may arise later in treatment, if a survivor turns out to be unable to initiate even graduated self-exposure exercises, despite all the support and encouragement from the therapist. It may also be considered in survivors who can initiate self-exposure but try to reduce their anxiety by distracting their attention away from distress cues or by relying on some safety signals (e.g. the presence of someone during the exercise). Although the latter problem could also be overcome with proper monitoring, guidance, and encouragement, a therapist-administered session might save considerable therapist time and effort in treatment.

In deciding on the exposure setting, it is best to consider a task that the survivor finds most difficult to tackle on their own, so that the session has maximum impact on their sense of control. This task can be identified by simply asking the survivor if there is any task they find so difficult to tackle that, if they managed to do it just once, they would feel confident enough to tackle other tasks on their own. For most survivors such tasks involve situations that evoke fear. To illustrate how the exposure session can be conducted, let us assume that the task involves going to a street café located in a busy part of the town. Note that this example is selected to make the session description relevant to different trauma experiences. For example, the reason for avoiding this place might be fear of earthquakes in an earthquake survivor, fear of re-arrest by police in a torture survivor, fear of bombs in a person who survived a bomb explosion on the street during a war or terror attack, or fear of some other trauma event previously experienced in that café or other similar public places. Before conducting an exposure session it is helpful to understand first how the survivor feels about your presence in the feared situation. In some cases the therapist's presence acts as a safety signal and reduces anxiety during exposure. If the survivor feels more anxious about the idea of going into the café alone, it is best to let them tackle the exercise alone, while you wait outside. If your presence does not make any difference to the survivor, you can then accompany them into the café. The survivor's anxiety is likely to be most intense when they arrive at the café. If they feel a strong urge to quit the session, they can be told that they are free to leave whenever they want but this would only mean surrendering to their problem. Repeating the treatment rationale using the same discourse as in the first sessions might be helpful. If this is of no help, it is best to consider

graduated exposure. Depending on the most fear-evoking aspects of the situation for a particular survivor, this can be organized in different ways. With earthquake survivors, for example, the therapist may take a seat outside the café in the first instance. As the survivor gains more self-confidence, the therapist can lead them into the café and take a seat close to the door. As the final step, the survivor can be asked to move to a seat as far away from the door as possible. This whole process may need to be done in reverse order with a torture survivor who is afraid of being seen by police officers passing by the café or with someone who is afraid of a bomb explosion on the street. Whenever the survivor's anxiety increases, care needs to be taken to ensure that they do not avoid fear cues by distracting their attention away from the situation (e.g. thinking about something else, observing someone closely, reading, looking at posters or pictures on the wall, etc.). They may be asked to challenge their fear by focusing on fear-evoking thoughts (e.g. an earthquake / bomb explosion might happen any time / police may raid the café, etc.). If, at any stage, the survivor feels too distressed to take the next step, the following explanation might be helpful:

In the beginning you thought even getting near the café was difficult enough for you. Yet, here you are now inside the café, feeling more in control. If I asked you to go out now and come back in again, would you be able to do that? [The answer is often yes.] Well, this is what I meant when I said you would be feeling more confident in facing your fear if you stayed in the situation. Would you have ever imagined you would be able to do even this much? [The answer is often no.] Well, this is how it happens. The next step might seem too difficult to you now but when you do it you will be telling me the same thing. You can quit anytime you like but why not complete the whole task now so that you can celebrate your success with your close friends by inviting them to this café!

Note that this discourse draws attention to the progress made thus far; the survivor is in the café, already feeling confident about repeating the same task. Such awareness of being able to tolerate and control anxiety is often a turning point in the session on which the survivor can build up further progress. In addition, linking success to some sort of a reward, such as celebrating success with close ones, might reinforce motivation for further progress during the session. In the rare case where the whole session cannot be completed due to intense anxiety, there is no cause for concern; whatever progress achieved thus far is likely to have some impact on the survivor. The survivors can be asked simply to repeat the exercise in the same café (or similar public places) and continue tackling the more difficult aspects of the situation until they achieve complete success.

Live exposure to a feared situation may bring back trauma memories in some cases with severe trauma exposure, particularly those who witnessed close ones suffering acts of atrocities or some form of violent and painful death during the trauma events. Flooding of such painful memories into the mind may at times be quite overwhelming, both for the survivor and the therapist. The survivor may burst into tears and start to relate the trauma story to the therapist. In such situations allowing the survivor some time to relate the story is useful. While providing emotional support, the therapist can facilitate recall of distressing memories by asking brief prompting questions about the story. In relating their story, survivors often find a unique opportunity to express a wide range of emotions experienced during and after the traumatic events, such as fear, horror, helplessness, regrets, shame, guilt, and anger. Thoughts or beliefs associated with these emotions do not need special attention, as they are likely to change during treatment without additional cognitive interventions. The survivor can be asked to focus mentally on the most distressing details and retain the trauma images in their mind for as long as they can. At some point the survivor will notice that these trauma images no longer evoke the same distress. They often describe this experience with a feeling of great relief, using expressions like "*huge weight lifted off my chest.*" This is often a turning point in treatment, because learning to confront and tolerate distressing memories is likely to have a lasting effect in the long term. We observed that such change leads to a substantial reduction not only in re-experiencing symptoms but also avoidance of trauma-related situations. Depending on the material to be covered the session might go well beyond the allocated time. So, it is best to be prepared for this contingency.

Treatment of cases without fear as the prominent problem

So far we have focused more on cases where fear is the prominent problem. This is because most trauma events involve a threat to life and fear is likely to be the most prominent problem in people with such a trauma experience. Nevertheless, some people may develop traumatic stress after exposure to events that are not associated with perceived threat to life. For example, witnessing other peoples' trauma experiences, sights of devastation, grotesque scenes (e.g. mutilated bodies, mass graves) during a war or exposure to disturbing scenes during rescue efforts after a devastating disaster may have a traumatic impact, even though such exposure does not involve a direct threat to life. As many ordinary civilians participate in rescue efforts after a mass trauma event, care providers are likely to see people with traumatic stress resulting from such trauma exposure. The principles of treatment are the same in such cases. Treatment focuses on distress evoked by trauma memories and associated avoidance. The following case of an earthquake survivor who participated in rescue efforts after the 1999 earthquake in Turkey demonstrates that trauma-induced distress responds to exposure in the same way as conditioned fear. It also highlights how treatment effects generalize and facilitate a self-help process that eventually leads to full recovery.

Case vignette #3

Ali was a 27-year-old male who sought treatment from our community center in the disaster region with post-traumatic stress complaints. He had experienced the earthquake in the epicenter region and he and his family survived the earthquake without any harm. He participated in rescue efforts along with other members of the community and had exposure to a wide range of intensely distressing scenes, such as people dead or dying under rubble, cries for help, severely injured people, mutilated bodies, etc. His most distressing experience concerned an occasion when he stepped on something soft under the rubble, which turned out to be the body of a dead person. He developed PTSD and avoidance of the locations where he participated in rescue efforts. As he had to walk to work passing by these locations every day, he was unable to go to work. He decided to seek help.

Ali had no problem in understanding the treatment rationale, as he was acutely aware of the fact that he was not able to work because of his problem. He readily agreed to treatment. Among the various locations where he had participated in rescue work, we chose to go to the site where he had stepped on the dead body, because he thought if he were able to overcome the impact of this event he would be able to deal with other distressing events on his own. He was asked to spend some time on the plot of land where the building used to be (the rubble had been cleared away), focusing his thoughts on the events that occurred on that occasion. He initially experienced a flooding of trauma memories into his mind, which made him very distressed. He was encouraged to stay there, not avoiding distress and challenging his problem by mentally focusing on the most distressing aspects of his experience. In 30 minutes, he was no longer able to retrieve any distressing memories. After the session, he felt confident enough to tackle similar situations on his own. He was asked to conduct similar sessions at the other sites where he participated in rescue efforts. At 1 month follow-up, having complied with treatment instructions, he had completely recovered and resumed work.

In some survivors emotions such as anger, blame, or guilt may be the prominent features of the clinical picture. Such emotions are closely associated with cognitive effects of trauma (e.g. attributions of responsibility for trauma to self or other people, disillusionment with people, etc.), as evidence (Başoğlu et al., 2005; Şalcıoğlu, 2004) suggests. In such cases exposure to trauma reminders also means exposure to cues that trigger these emotions. Indeed, this is why survivors often verbalize such emotions during an exposure session, as noted earlier. Such cognitive effects of trauma and associated emotions do not impede recovery with behavioral treatment (Foa et al., 2005; Marks et al., 1998; Paunovic & Öst, 2001), as our studies of CFBT have also demonstrated (reviewed in Chapter 6; see also Chapter 9 for more discussion of this issue). Thus, it is best to treat such survivors with exposure first and then re-assess their psychological status to see whether additional cognitive interventions are needed to deal with any residual problems associated with such emotions. In our experience, this was hardly ever necessary.

Treatment termination

Treatment can be terminated when clinically significant improvement occurs in the survivor's condition. Such improvement often corresponds to 60% or more reduction in traumatic stress and depression scores and *much or very much improved* ratings on the self- and assessor-rated Global Improvement Scale. This is usually achieved within the first 4 weeks of treatment. We should note, however, that treatment of more complicated cases (e.g. those with severe depression, grief reactions, severe flashbacks, comorbid anxiety disorders, and substance abuse) may require 8 to 12 sessions with more therapist involvement in treatment. In addition, treatment sessions may need to be delivered twice weekly in some of these cases for closer monitoring of treatment compliance and progress.

In circumstances where therapist time needs to be used sparingly treatment can be terminated earlier when about 40% reduction occurs in traumatic stress symptoms, which usually corresponds to *moderately improved* rating on the Global Improvement Scale. Such early improvement is a fairly reliable indicator of longer term outcome. Early treatment responders could be asked to continue their exercises on a self-help basis and make further contact only in case of problems. A 3-month follow-up would be useful in ascertaining treatment success in such cases.

Issues in treatment

In this section we briefly review various strategies in dealing with cases that present with severe depression, suicidal ideas, severe flashbacks, comorbid anxiety disorders, substance abuse, psychotic reactions, and various medical conditions. As treatment of prolonged grief requires a fairly detailed description, it is presented in Chapter 5.

Comorbid depression

Pre-treatment depression does not constitute a problem for therapy, provided that it does not interfere with treatment. As depression is most often secondary to traumatic stress, it improves with reduction in traumatic stress (evidence reviewed in Chapter 6). Thus, in most cases additional interventions targeting depression are unlikely to be necessary. However, in a small minority of cases, depression might be sufficiently severe to undermine treatment motivation or interfere with treatment procedures. As such cases are likely to be less compliant with self-exposure instructions, they might benefit from a more intensive treatment involving two- or three-weekly therapist-administered exposure sessions until sufficient recovery in PTSD and depression symptoms allows the survivor to continue treatment with self-exposure.

Choice of antidepressants versus CFBT as first-line treatment in cases with severe depression depends on the circumstances of the setting. In our own practice we hardly ever have to use antidepressants as a first-line intervention. It might perhaps be considered in other circumstances, where intensive CFBT is not feasible. However, considering the limitations of antidepressants in treating PTSD and depression (reviewed in Chapter 8), particularly the problem of relapse after discontinuation of medication, it would be advisable to consider CFBT at some stage.

In cases where antidepressants are considered before CFBT, three points are important to bear in mind. First, the purpose of drug treatment needs to be explained clearly to the survivor. It is important to avoid presenting antidepressants as a cure for traumatic stress problems in view of their limited effects (Albucher & Liberzon, 2002; Friedman et al., 2000; Van Etten & Taylor, 1998; see also review of antidepressants in Chapter 8). It is important to tell the survivor that the drug is simply meant to provide some relief for them so that they can participate in psychological treatment. They also need to know that they will be using the medication for a limited period of time and that they will stop taking it after psychological treatment begins. Such an explanation is likely to help them attribute improvement to their own efforts during psychological treatment, rather than to the tablets. External attributions may undermine the efficacy of psychological treatment and facilitate relapse after treatment (see Chapter 6 for more discussion of this issue). Second, there is no need to wait until drug treatment is completed; CFBT can be initiated as soon as the survivor feels ready for it. This is often possible after a few weeks of drug treatment. This not only avoids unnecessary loss of time but also makes it easier for the survivor to discontinue medication when the time comes. Finally, gradual drug taper can be started as the survivor makes progress in treatment and regains sense of control (usually in about 4 weeks). We recommend that the medication is completely discontinued before the end of psychological treatment, so that the survivor can attribute improvement to psychological treatment rather than to the drug.

Suicidal ideas

Suicide risk in mass trauma survivors is an important issue to bear in mind, considering reports (Chou et al., 2003; Yang et al., 2005) of elevated suicide rates among earthquake survivors. Although we have not come across any serious suicide attempts throughout our work, we found suicidal ideas (as assessed by the

TSSC-E) in 19% of 4332 survivors screened during five field surveys (analysis based on pooled data from Başoğlu et al., 2002; Başoğlu et al., 2004b; Livanou et al., 2002; Şalcıoğlu et al., 2003; Şalcıoğlu et al., 2007b). Suicidal ideas in earthquake survivors may appear fairly soon after a major earthquake, particularly when the aftershocks are most frequent. Suicidal ideas (as assessed by the DRS) were also common among war survivors, reported by 20% of our study participants (Başoğlu et al., 2005). Also worth noting is that suicidal ideas might occur even in the absence of severe depression, possibly as a result of the overwhelming fear and helplessness effects of trauma. Indeed, while suicidal ideas were more common in earthquake and war survivors with probable depression (44% and 64%, respectively), they were also reported by 8% of the earthquake and 15% of the war survivors without probable depression. In most cases suicidal ideas are likely to disappear with treatment. However, in cases with serious suicidal risk (e.g. specific plans for suicide and/or previous suicide attempts) treatment is best conducted in a controlled environment (e.g. in a psychiatric facility).

Comorbid anxiety disorders

When other anxiety disorders accompany traumatic stress reactions, they may complicate the clinical picture by aggravating helplessness responses and interfering with treatment compliance. These conditions may need additional interventions, particularly in cases where the onset of an anxiety disorder antedates the trauma. In such cases trauma may have exacerbated the condition. When the onset of an anxiety disorder postdates the trauma, traumatic stress is often the precipitating factor and thus treating this problem might lead to an improvement in the comorbid condition. We have seen a 13-year-old female earthquake survivor with hand-washing and checking rituals, for example, who improved after treatment without requiring an additional intervention for this problem.

Comorbid anxiety disorders can be treated together with traumatic stress by prescribing additional self-exposure exercises for avoided situations. Panic disorder with agoraphobia, specific phobias, social phobia, and obsessive-compulsive disorder are most often associated with behavioral avoidance of particular situations and quite responsive to exposure-based interventions. Specific phobias are most common in earthquake survivors, often relating to earthquakes, buildings, public transport, enclosed spaces, tunnels, bridges, elevators, heights, swimming, or crowded places from which escape is difficult. In such cases additional exposure tasks relating to avoided situations can be prescribed. Increased sense of control resulting from self-exposure to trauma cues may help overcome other phobias in some cases. For example, an earthquake survivor who recovered from traumatic stress with treatment went on to treat her snake phobia without any specific therapist instructions in this regard. Panics without behavioral avoidance can be treated by exposure to internal and external cues that trigger panics and conducting exposure to such cues. As in treatment of traumatic stress, CFBT of other anxiety disorders does not involve any cognitive restructuring or other anxiety management techniques.

Psychosis

Severe traumatic events may induce transient psychotic states or even precipitate a psychotic process in some predisposed people with or without a previous history of psychotic illness. In such cases the first-line intervention is naturally to bring the psychotic state under control using drugs. Once this is achieved, however, CFBT is likely to be useful in reducing traumatic stress and enhancing the survivor's resilience, thereby making further psychotic breakdowns less likely in possible future exposures to traumatic stressors. CFBT may need to be administered in such cases using a more graduated exposure to avoid destabilizing the person in a post-psychotic state. The following example from a case study (Başoğlu, 1998) illustrates how behavioral treatment can be administered in post-psychotic cases.

Case vignette #4

A 25-year-old tortured African refugee in the United Kingdom was admitted to a psychiatric hospital for psychotic illness, presenting as persecutory delusions, auditory hallucinations, and aggressive and violent behavior. Diagnosed as unspecified paranoid psychosis, he was treated with haloperidol for 2 months. After his psychotic symptoms abated he was referred as an inpatient to the first author for behavioral treatment of his PTSD. He had PTSD symptoms that antedated the onset of psychosis, including nightmares, distress on being reminded of the trauma, avoidance of trauma reminders, difficulty talking about the trauma, and social withdrawal. Treatment was initiated while he was still on haloperidol. Treatment first involved getting him to talk about this trauma in a limited and graduated fashion. Emotional arousal was not intense enough to cause concern. Nevertheless, the trauma material was covered in three sessions, after which he was able to talk to people about his torture experience freely. As homework, he was asked to read all newspapers in the ward and cut clippings of news about human rights abuses and file them. He would then read the news in the next session and discuss them with the therapist. As homework he also read every day a 40-page document on the political events in his country, which he found particularly distressing. Although distress associated with trauma cues did not disappear completely, he no longer had difficulty talking about his trauma, reading newspapers, watching TV, or engaging in any other activity that reminded him of his trauma. His PTSD symptoms, including nightmares, disappeared completely. The change in his psychological state was also noted by the ward staff. After seven sessions in 3 months, medication was discontinued and he was discharged from the hospital. At 3-month follow-up, he was free of any psychotic or PTSD symptoms.

Substance abuse

Substance or alcohol abuse is another comorbid condition that might interfere with treatment by blocking experience of anxiety or distress during self-exposure. When it is secondary to trauma, treating traumatic stress might also improve this condition. In such cases, however, CFBT needs to be combined with a substance withdrawal program. As the survivor begins to withdraw from the substance, anxiety and other traumatic stress symptoms subdued by the substance are likely to emerge, so it is important that CFBT is initiated during this period. Regular monitoring of progress is often helpful in ensuring that the timing and pace of both procedures are correctly administered. In some severe substance abuse cases an inpatient detoxification program might be necessary, followed by psychological treatment.

Flashbacks

Although flashbacks are not uncommon in mass trauma survivors, severe flashbacks with complete dissociation and lack of awareness of surroundings that are likely to pose a safety risk are quite rare. To put this issue in perspective, we found flashbacks in 15% of the earthquake survivors in a study (Başoğlu et al., 2001) conducted during the first 6 months of the disaster. None of these cases had 'extremely severe' flashbacks according to the Clinician-Administered PTSD Scale (CAPS; Blake et al., 1990). In another study (Şalcıoğlu, 2004) of 387 earthquake survivors conducted mean 20 months post-earthquake, 14% had flashbacks, which were extremely severe in only one case (0.3%). Among 1358 war survivors (Başoğlu et al., 2005), on the other hand, 8% had flashbacks but they were extremely severe in only four cases (0.3%).

Flashbacks do not necessarily pose a problem for therapy and generally should not be considered as a counter-indication for exposure treatment. Indeed, flashbacks can be triggered by a wide range of cues in survivors' natural environment with or without treatment. Furthermore, flashbacks never posed a problem for treatment in our work with earthquake survivors, other than occasionally making self-exposure a bit more difficult to conduct for the survivor. Their frequency substantially declined with improvement in other symptoms. Nevertheless, some potentially problematic cases may need additional therapist attention. Once this problem is overcome, treatment can proceed as usual. When flashbacks are reported, the following questions would be useful in identifying potentially problematic cases:

- *Have you ever tried to harm yourself or others during the (flashback) event or afterwards? Have you ever felt an inclination to do so?*
- *Have you ever got yourself into harmful situations during the (flashback) event because you were not aware of what was going on around you (for example, having an accident or provoking fights with other people)?*
- *Did you ever go missing from home for days and were then found somewhere and had no recollection of where you were or what you did during that time?*

In cases with mild to moderate brief-lasting flashbacks, a simple self-management strategy might suffice. As the first step in dealing with this problem, the survivor needs to be informed that flashbacks are disturbing but essentially harmless phenomena. This may come as a relief for those survivors who may interpret them as a sign of 'losing their mind.' Helping the survivor understand that the symptom is controllable is also useful. The following instructions might help bring the symptom under control:

⇒ *Try to monitor your flashbacks and work out what triggers the symptom. It could be a sight, sound, smell, word, thought, image, emotion, or anything that reminds you of your trauma experience. Make a list of the situations that trigger them. When you encounter these situations, be aware that the symptom may appear.*

⇒ *When you realise that the symptom is about to appear, sit down to one side. Breathe deeply and regularly. Focus on what is happening around you. Try to watch carefully what people are doing, what they are saying. Or try to focus your attention on something. For example, look carefully at an object near you and study its shape, colour and texture. Pick it up and feel what kind of emotion it produces. Focus all your attention on this object.*

⇒ *You could carry a small bottle of cologne with you. If you do, pat some cologne on your face and hands and focus on feeling refreshed. You could also carry a string of worry beads with you. As the symptom begins, hold the beads and start counting them in two's or three's. Focus on the prayer beads and be careful not to make a mistake when counting.*

⇒ *You may find other effective ways of focusing your attention elsewhere. These could be things like walking, telling yourself where you are, the date and time, or humming a tune.*

⇒ *Talk to your family about your situation and tell them about this symptom. If the symptom appears while you are with them, they can help 'bring you back to reality.' They could do this by touching you or telling you where you are.*

Identifying the cues that trigger flashbacks and interrupting the dissociation process by focusing attention on the '*here and now*' when the cues are encountered may help the person regain sense of control over the symptom. Once this is achieved the symptom is not likely to pose any problem in self-exposure exercises. As treatment progresses and other traumatic stress symptoms begin to improve, flashbacks often reduce in frequency and intensity.

In severe cases that pose a safety risk, the problem may need to be handled by the therapist in a controlled setting. Some survivors experience flashbacks when they relate their trauma story in some detail. In such cases getting the survivor to relate the trauma story in a guided fashion might be helpful in identifying particular trauma memories that trigger flashbacks. When the first signs of a flashback begin to emerge, the survivor is asked to stop and fight back dissociation by using the 'grounding' techniques described above (e.g. focusing attention on the therapist or objects in the room, patting cologne on the face, counting beads, etc.). Once dissociation recedes, the survivor is asked to focus on the particular memory (or imagery) that triggered the flashback, retain it in mind for as long as possible while also making an effort not to lose touch with reality, and interrupt the process short of a full-blown flashback. This process is repeated until the survivor is able to control the symptom or the trauma memory no longer triggers it. At some point a full-blown flashback might occur. Once it is over, treatment is resumed, focusing again on the particular memory that triggered the flashback. The point of this exercise is to increase the survivor's tolerance of distress evoked by trauma memories so that it no longer triggers flashbacks. Note that this exercise can also be conducted during live exposure to trauma reminders that trigger flashbacks, if the latter can be identified. Such reminders might include, for example, the location where the trauma was experienced, sights of devastation in the environment, TV pictures of violence or disaster, etc. Therapist-guided graduated exposure to such situations in the way described above can be helpful.

Comorbid medical conditions

CFBT is different from traditional exposure treatment in not involving prolonged periods of exposure to highly anxiety-evoking situations. When delivered on a self-administered basis, survivors often deal with their avoidance problems at their own pace and in a rather graduated fashion. Thus, it involves relatively less risk with respect to various medical conditions that might be affected by heightened levels of anxiety, such as cardiovascular disorders, hypertension, and pregnancy. Nevertheless, when such cases are encountered, it is advisable to seek advice from a specialist regarding the risks involved. In cases that pose a risk, exposure can be conducted at a slower pace under the guidance of the therapist.

Treatment of children

Evidence from two pilot studies (Şalcıoğlu & Başoğlu, 2008; see also Chapter 6) suggests that CFBT is also useful in children. We used CFBT more extensively with child earthquake survivors, so we describe the treatment in reference to earthquake trauma. As we found group settings particularly useful in delivering treatment to children aged 8 to 14, we describe the application of CFBT in groups. Individual treatment of children is much the same as group treatment, so it is not described separately here. It is best to work with groups of about 10 children, although circumstances might require work with larger groups (e.g. in schools) in the early aftermath of a disaster.

Treatment procedures are essentially the same as those described for adults. Before the session an assessment using the child version of the SITSES and the FAQ is useful in having an idea about the severity of fear and related traumatic stress problems in the group. The first step involves getting the children to talk about their fear problems for a while until they all understand that everyone has similar problems. Discussing their questionnaire ratings can be useful in focusing their attention to fear-related problems. Then the treatment rationale is presented, while also tapping their response to the idea of confronting feared situations (e.g. sleeping alone or in the dark) instead of avoiding them. Some children may readily agree with the treatment idea and display expressions of courage in challenging their fear. It is best to encourage such children to express themselves fully, so that they serve as a model for others. Some of the children may have a story to tell about having overcome their fears (or phobias) in the past by confronting them. Giving such children a chance to tell their story and praising their courage often encourages children to overcome their fear. The final step involves getting the children write down their exposure tasks in the form of homework (e.g. "*I will sleep alone at night; I will stay alone at home when my parents are away,*" etc.). In group settings children are quite competitive in seeking approval and reward from an authority figure – a tendency that can be utilized in enhancing their treatment motivation throughout treatment. Thus, the session could be ended with a comment such as "*let us see who will beat their fear first.*"

In the next session problems are re-assessed using the SITSES-C and the FAQ to examine progress. In cases where there is no improvement, the most likely reason for failure is non-compliance with treatment. As in adults, high levels of anxiety might have been the problem, in which case more graduated exposure or easier tasks can be considered. Involving the family in treatment so that they can provide support and encouragement with homework exercises can also be helpful. In cases where the parents or other family members have similar fear-related traumatic stress problems, the whole family might need to be treated together with the child. This is important, given that children are quite susceptible to displays of fear in the family. Six to 10 sessions are likely to be sufficient for improvement in most children. Available evidence shows that six sessions in 3 weeks results in over 50% improvement in traumatic stress problems. It is worth noting that faster improvement can be achieved in children by a single session of Earthquake Simulation Treatment, a variant of CFBT described below.

Single-session applications of treatment in earthquake survivors

These interventions include single-session CFBT administered individually or in groups and single-session Earthquake Simulation Treatment. As noted in the Introduction, single-session applications of CFBT were developed for post-earthquake circumstances where regular treatment attendance is difficult for survivors. Furthermore, treatment may need to be delivered in groups due to demands for help from large numbers of survivors.

Single-session CFBT

As single-session CFBT is delivered in much the same way as the first session of full-course treatment, it will not be detailed further here. Single-session CFBT differs from full-course treatment only in not involving weekly monitoring sessions. After an agreement on the treatment rationale is achieved, the survivor is given general anti-avoidance instructions and some focused exposure exercises relating to some of the avoidance behaviors endorsed in the FAQ. They are asked to use the endorsed FAQ items as guidance in setting self-exposure tasks. It is best to give them a copy of the self-help manual (Appendix C), as this provides them with structure in treatment, an opportunity for self-assessment of progress, and useful information about dealing with possible problems in treatment. As detailed in Chapter 6, 80% of the survivors are likely to benefit from single-session treatment, while 20% may fail to improve because of their difficulty in initiating self-exposure on their own.

Single-session group CFBT

In survivor shelters or 'tent cities' we often delivered CFBT to groups of 20–30 survivors in large tents or prefabricated community centers or to families in their tents. While on occasion we had to deliver it to even larger groups, it is best to try to limit groups to 20–30, as they are more manageable. The treatment session could be delivered within one hour but it is best delivered in one to two hours. The treatment steps are the same as in individual treatment. First, survivors' SITSES and FAQ ratings are obtained before the session and the ones with highest scores are identified.

Opening the session

In the first few minutes make a brief introduction regarding the purpose of the meeting as follows:

> Now that you have finished filling in the questionnaires we can begin the session. We are all here to discuss the problems we have been experiencing since the earthquake and how to go about dealing with them. First, let me give you some idea about the problems people in this group have been experiencing. Let us see what kind of problems have been marked in the questionnaire. I have here, for example, the ratings of Ms. X [a survivor with high scores on the TSSC-E and the FAQ]. She is having problems with sleeping, memory and concentration … and she is unable to do many things in her daily life because of fear of earthquakes. Perhaps she could tell us more about her problems.

Such an introduction will immediately focus the group's attention on a problem that survivors are often most keen to talk about, i.e. fear. Give Ms. X a chance to talk about her problems. She will most likely start relating her trauma story, e.g. where she was during the earthquake, what she did to protect herself what she witnessed, etc. Allow some time for her story but do not let it go on for too long. There will be others waiting to tell their story. Always bear in mind that the purpose of the session is not to facilitate sharing of trauma stories. Try to avoid long trauma stories and make an effort to keep the group's attention on the problems marked on the questionnaires. Allow more time for group members who provide demonstrative examples of the debilitating effects of fear. For example, if someone has had to quit work because of fear, give them a chance to talk about their problem. When someone mentions such a problem, conduct a small poll in the group to find out how many of them are experiencing similar problems. Do not spend more than 15 minutes on this stage. The purpose of this introduction is to define the problem for the group and draw their attention to distress or fear as the cause. With this introduction everyone will also know that they are not alone in experiencing fear-related problems. End this phase of the session with a brief explanation of how trauma induces distress and fear and how such emotions lead to the problems marked on the questionnaires.

Explaining the treatment rationale

A useful strategy in explaining treatment rationale is to help survivors draw their own conclusions about the best way of dealing with fear, rather than didactically telling them what to do. There are likely to be several people who have had past experience of dealing with various fears. There will be some who had a phobia, for example, who overcame the problem by confronting their fear. Others may have had a past trauma (e.g. a road traffic accident, physical assault, etc.), from which they recovered by using the same strategy. Ask the group who had such fears at some point in their lives and recovered using this method. When someone volunteers this information, allow the person to talk about their experience. If necessary, get another person to relate their story. In groups people usually relate such stories with a sense of victory and pride. They not only provide very useful real-life examples of recovery from fear but also instill hope and courage in others. Once this process is completed, there may not even be a need to go into much detail about the treatment rationale. The answers to their questions they have been waiting to hear from the therapist are already obvious. You may compound this with a rhetorical question, e.g. "*Now that you have heard these stories, who wants to tell the group the best way of dealing with fear?*" At least a few of them will raise their hand and volunteer the answer the group needs to hear. The treatment rationale is now clear. If anyone disagrees with it, you can deal with their arguments as

described earlier for individual treatment. Once this is done, the path is clear for the next phase.

Defining treatment goals and encouraging self-exposure

As in individual treatment, the FAQ data are used to exemplify treatment goals. If possible, provide everyone with a copy of the questionnaire they filled in. Ask them to mark the avoidances that cause most problems in their life and prioritize them in order of their importance. These will be their homework tasks. The rest of the session is much the same as in individual treatment. There will not be time to tailor the treatment according to needs of each group member but this can be done with one or two survivors to demonstrate how the treatment should be conducted. When this is completed, ask the group if they have understood the treatment and if they have any questions.

Closing the session

In closing the session, distribute copies of the self-help manual, explain its purpose, and advise the group to read it and follow the instructions. You can end the session with the following statements:

> Now that you know what to do about your problem, the choice is yours: you either do something to beat your fear or it will beat you. You need to understand clearly that success or failure in treatment depends entirely on you. If you make sufficient efforts to overcome your problems, your chances of recovery are high. Almost all people who fail in treatment do so because they do not carry out their homework exercises. You may experience some setbacks along the way but you need not worry about them as long as you keep making an effort. I suggest you help each other with your exercises. Also, try helping your family, friends, and neighbors with what you have learned here.

In groups there are likely to be some particularly smart and articulate persons who understand the treatment very well, show strong motivation, and display remarkable enthusiasm and talent for helping others. They can be recruited as co-therapists to help others with their treatment exercises.

Single-session Earthquake Simulation Treatment

Earthquake Simulation Treatment was developed to maximize the impact of single-session CFBT. Various

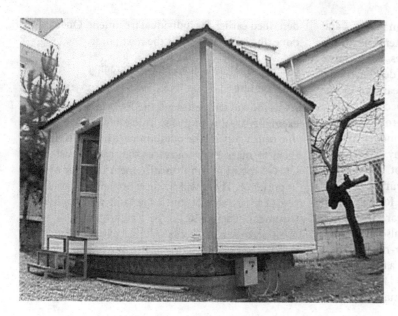

Figure 4.3 Earthquake simulator: outside view.

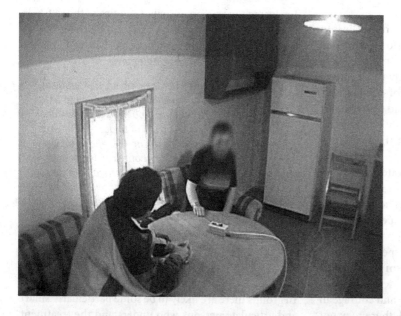

Figure 4.4 Earthquake simulator: inside view.

considerations that led to its development are detailed in Chapter 6. In brief, it was expected to be a more potent form of CFBT in involving exposure to simulated earthquake tremors (i.e. unconditioned stimuli) rather than trauma reminders (i.e. conditioned stimuli). An earthquake simulator was designed and constructed for this purpose (shown in Figure 4.3 and Figure 4.4).

The earthquake simulator sits on a shake table that can simulate earthquake tremors on nine intensity levels. The movements are controlled by computer software in accordance with various earthquake scenarios. The treatment session is designed to enhance the survivor's sense of control over both the tremors and the anxiety or distress evoked by them. For example, the survivors are allowed to start and stop the tremors at any time and change their intensity by using a mobile control switch (see Figure 4.4). The session lasts one hour, starting with the lowest intensity level and going one level up as the survivor gains sense of control over the tremors. The session often evokes fear in response to the tremors, as well as bringing back distressing memories of traumatic events experienced during the earthquake. Treatment is terminated when the survivor feels no longer intensely distressed by the tremors and memories of the trauma.

As this intervention provides the most striking examples of how a single exposure session facilitates subsequent treatment, it is worth presenting two case vignettes. These cases are among the 31 participants of our controlled study of Earthquake Simulation Treatment (Başoğlu et al., 2007), all treated by the second author. Case vignette #5 was selected as an example of a 'moderately severe' case of PTSD (e.g. CAPS score of 57), whereas Case vignette #6 was selected as an example of an 'extremely severe' case of PTSD (CAPS score of 92), severity defined according to CAPS score ranges proposed by Weathers et al. (2001). The latter was the most severe case of PTSD in the study sample.

Case vignette #5

Hasan was a 38-year-old male, married with three children. He worked as a construction worker before the earthquake. Although his house had not sustained severe damage he reported intense fear during the earthquake. He participated in rescue work after the earthquake and thus was also exposed to intensely disturbing scenes of people trapped under rubble. He had severe re-experiencing symptoms relating to these events. He had to quit his job because he used to work in neighboring towns and could not leave his family unattended for even short periods for fear of another earthquake. He was also unable to work on scaffoldings because even a slight shaking evoked intense fear. He had been unemployed and almost housebound for about 5 years. He supported his family with the help of relatives and friends. At assessment he had moderately severe PTSD (CAPS score 57) and depression (Beck Depression Inventory – BDI score 24).

Hasan agreed to self-exposure only with some reluctance, making the therapist feel that he would abandon treatment at the first difficulty with exposure. Nevertheless, he readily agreed to a single session of Earthquake Simulation Treatment. During the session he initially experienced intense fear. He was flooded with thoughts and images related to the events during rescue work. He stopped the

earthquake simulator three times in the first 12 minutes and actually left the simulator on the third occasion. The therapist told him that he could terminate the session if he wanted but that would mean accepting defeat. He was encouraged to give himself a chance to beat his fear once and for all and recover from his problems. He decided to resume the session and this time did not stop the earthquake simulator until the end. He was encouraged to go through the events in his mind (most of which related to the first day after the earthquake) as they occurred. At some point he started re-experiencing the events so vividly and with such intense distress that he was not even able to speak. He then burst into tears. Seeing that he was trying to relate his trauma story but could not do it in a coherent fashion, the therapist asked him simply to relive the events in his mind and not make an effort to talk. This phase lasted about 20 minutes, during which his anxiety showed substantial reduction. He stated *"I am now finished with the first day of the earthquake."* After another 10 minutes of going through the memories of the second day of the earthquake in his mind, the disturbing images completely vanished. Without being asked to do so, he got up and walked around the simulator while the tremors continued (an activity that often leads to sudden peaks in fear because of loss of postural control) in an effort to challenge his fear. When he felt in complete control and the tremors no longer disturbed him he said *"I've beaten my fear. I made the images fade away. It was like watching the same movie for the last time!"* He cried in relief, saying that his nightmare was finally over. The exposure session lasted 51 minutes. At the end of the session he stated that the experience reinforced his resolve to confront his fears (e.g. by travelling to neighboring towns, going out and leaving his family unattended at night, and entering safe buildings) that posed a serious problem in conducting his work. He had been told during recruitment in the trial that he would receive only one treatment session and that subsequent contacts would be with a different project worker for assessment purposes only. Assessments were conducted at regular intervals for 1.5 years after the session. The assessor refrained from discussing treatment issues and encouraging self-exposure to avoid confounding the impact of the initial treatment session. The improvement in CAPS and FAQ scores is shown in Figure 4.5. The scores showed a substantial decline at 2-month follow-up, reaching a low point at 3-month follow-up. At week 8 he rated himself as *much improved* on the self-rated Global Improvement Scale. He resumed work within 2 months after treatment and started a

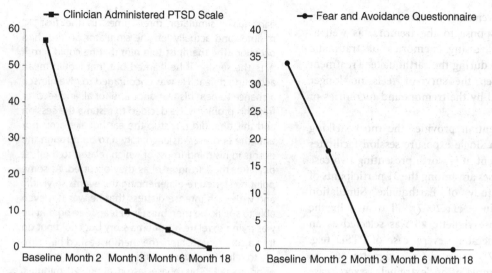

Figure 4.5 Improvement in avoidance and PTSD after a single session of Earthquake Simulation Treatment in Case #5.

new job in a neighboring city, which meant leaving his family unattended for weeks at a time. At 18 months follow-up he was *very much improved*, with a CAPS score of 0 and 92% reduction in his depression scores.

Case vignette #6

Ayşe was a 38-year-old female patient, married with two children. She was a housewife with a primary school education. Although she had not experienced physical injury or loss due to the earthquake, she reported intense fear and loss of control during the earthquake. During the week following the earthquake, she was withdrawn, stopped eating, lost weight, smoked excessively, frequently cried, barely talked, and sometimes wandered aimlessly in the streets. She was admitted to a psychiatric hospital where she received drug treatment and was discharged after a month with minimal improvement. At assessment she had severe PTSD (CAPS score 92) and was depressed (BDI score 28). Her concentration difficulty and psychomotor retardation were severe enough to interfere with assessment. Before the earthquake she was the strong figure in the family, controlling the family affairs, but she now felt totally out of control of everything in her life. She felt that she was no longer respected by her husband and children and felt very distressed about this situation. She was debilitated by anticipatory fear of a possible

future earthquake. She was constantly hypervigilant and startled by the slightest unexpected noise or movement in the environment. She avoided sexual intercourse with her husband in case she was caught unprepared by an earthquake, a problem that led to serious marital conflict. She had been in this condition for 5 years since the earthquake.

At trial entry Ayşe was assigned to waitlist control condition. During the 8-week waiting period she showed no improvement. At the end of this period she received a single session of CFBT, followed by Earthquake Simulation Treatment. The first part of the treatment session lasted longer than usual (about 90 minutes) because of her concentration difficulties. She understood the treatment rationale and agreed to try self-exposure to various feared situations (e.g. taking a bath while alone at home, sleeping with lights off, staying at home alone at night, and having sexual intercourse once a week). During the exposure session, which started at the lowest tremor magnitude level, she experienced intense fear in the beginning (rating her anxiety as 8 on a 0–8 scale) and tried to avoid distressing trauma-related thoughts and images flooding into her mind, while also distracting her attention away from the tremors. The therapist encouraged her to think about trauma experiences and to focus on the sounds and movements of the earthquake simulator. She kept the tremor intensity at the same level throughout the session to keep her distress within manageable limits. The session was terminated when a behavioral test (i.e. getting the survivor to recall the most distressing

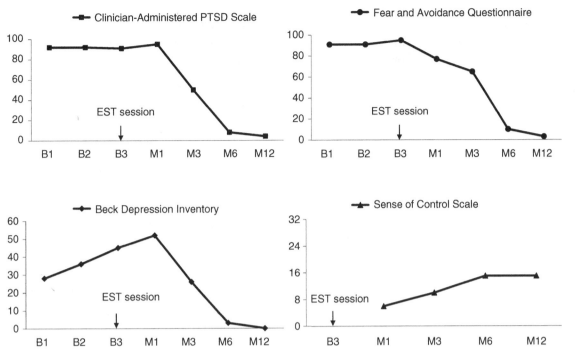

Figure 4.6 Improvement in avoidance, PTSD, depression, and sense of control after a single session of Earthquake Simulation Treatment in Case #6. B1 = First baseline assessment at trial entry at week 0; B2 = Second baseline assessment at week 4; B3 = Third baseline assessment at week 8; EST = Earthquake Simulation Treatment; M1 = 1-month follow-up; M3 = 3-month follow-up; M6 = 6-month follow-up; M12 = 12-month follow-up.

memories) demonstrated that she was able to recall the most distressing aspects of the trauma with no significant distress. After the session she reported marked increase in her sense of control and reduction in her anticipatory fear of earthquakes. Figure 4.6 shows the improvement in treatment outcome measures at follow-up.

Improvement was gradual in the first three months after the session (slight at month 1 and moderate at month 3). She was able to conduct self-exposure at a rather slow pace, because of incapacitating depressive symptoms. Nevertheless, improvement accelerated after month 3, reaching a maximum at month 6 (with 91% reduction in PTSD symptoms and 93% reduction in depressive symptoms). She was able to function normally, resumed sexual activity, and regained control over her life and family. At this point she reported having been exposed to another earthquake in the region (4.8 on the Richter scale), during which she experienced no fear or subsequent return of symptoms. At 1-year follow-up she reported almost complete recovery, with 96% reduction in PTSD and 100% reduction in depression symptoms. On a scale designed to

evaluate attributions of improvement, she attributed 60% of her recovery to the simulator experience, 40% to self-exposure exercises, and 0% to assessment or any change in life circumstances.

Case #5 demonstrates how debilitating earthquake-related fears and avoidance can be, even in the absence of severe PTSD and comorbid illness. This is also true for war and torture survivors. Case #6, on the other hand, is characteristic of very severe cases of PTSD that fail to respond to single-session CFBT, mainly because of the debilitating effects of pervasive fear and depression. When depression is secondary to persistent fear and related traumatic stress, even inpatient treatment with medication is unlikely to be useful, as her case demonstrates. The helplessness and hopelessness effects of depression can be overcome in such cases by a therapist-administered exposure session. Progress might be slow, improvement taking a few months, but they eventually recover, provided they continue with self-exposure exercises. Note that in both cases PTSD and depression started to improve with increase in their sense of control over fear (as measured by the Sense of Control Scale). Such improvement patterns were characteristic of the 31 cases that participated in our treatment study. These cases illustrate how useful a single exposure session can be in helping the survivors overcome their helplessness and initiate a self-help process.

References

Albucher, R. C. and Liberzon, I. (2002). Psychopharmacological treatment in PTSD: A critical review. *Journal of Psychiatric Research*, **36**, 355–367.

American Psychiatric Association (1994). *Diagnostic and Statistical Manual of Mental Disorders (4th Edition)*. Washington, DC: American Psychiatric Association.

Başoğlu, M. (1998). Behavioral and cognitive treatment of survivors of torture. In *Caring for Victims of Torture*, ed. J. M. Jaranson and M. K. Popkin. Washington, DC: American Psychiatric Press, 131–148.

Başoğlu, M. and Aker, T. (1996). Cognitive-behavioural treatment of torture survivors: A case study. *Torture*, **6**, 61–65.

Başoğlu, M., Ekblad, S., Bäärnhielm, S. and Livanou, M. (2004a). Cognitive-behavioral treatment of tortured asylum seekers: A case study. *Journal of Anxiety Disorders*, **18**, 357–369.

Başoğlu, M., Kılıç, C., Şalcıoğlu, E. and Livanou, M. (2004b). Prevalence of posttraumatic stress disorder and comorbid depression in earthquake survivors in Turkey: An epidemiological study. *Journal of Traumatic Stress*, **17**, 133–141.

Başoğlu, M., Livanou, M., Crnobarić, C., Frančišković, T., Suljić, E., Đurić, D. and Vranešić, M. (2005). Psychiatric and cognitive effects of war in former Yugoslavia: Association of lack of redress for trauma and posttraumatic stress reactions. *Journal of the American Medical Association*, **294**, 580–590.

Başoğlu, M., Mineka, S., Paker, M., Aker, T., Livanou, M. and Gök, S. (1997). Psychological preparedness for trauma as a protective factor in survivors of torture. *Psychological Medicine*, **27**, 1421–1433.

Başoğlu, M., Şalcıoğlu, E. and Livanou, M. (2002). Traumatic stress responses in earthquake survivors in Turkey. *Journal of Traumatic Stress*, **15**, 269–276.

Başoğlu, M., Şalcıoğlu, E. and Livanou, M. (2007). A randomized controlled study of single-session behavioural treatment of earthquake-related posttraumatic stress disorder using an earthquake simulator. *Psychological Medicine*, **37**, 203–213.

Başoğlu, M., Şalcıoğlu, E., Livanou, M., Özeren, M., Aker, T., Kılıç, C. and Mestçioğlu, Ö. (2001). A study of the validity of a Screening Instrument for Traumatic Stress in Earthquake Survivors in Turkey. *Journal of Traumatic Stress*, **14**, 491–509.

Bleuler, M. (1974). The offspring of schizophrenics. *Schizophrenia Bulletin*, **1**, 93–107.

Blake, D. D., Weathers, F. W., Nagy, L. M., Kaloupek, D. G., Charney, D. S. and Keane, T. M. (1990). Clinician-Administered PTSD Scale (CAPS) – Current and Lifetime Diagnostic Version. Boston: National Center for Posttraumatic Stress Disorder, Behavioral Science Division.

Bouton, M. E. (1988). Context and ambiguity in the extinction of emotional learning: Implications for exposure therapy. *Behaviour Research and Therapy*, **26**, 137–149.

Chou, Y.-J., Huang, N., Lee, C.-H., Tsai, S.-L., Tsay, J.-H., Chen, L.-S. and Chou, P. (2003). Suicides after the 1999 Taiwan earthquake. *International Journal of Epidemiology*, **32**, 1007–1014.

Craske, M. G., Kircanski, K., Zelikowsky, M., Mystkowski, J., Chowdhury, N. and Baker, A. (2008). Optimizing inhibitory learning during exposure therapy. *Behaviour Research and Therapy*, **46**, 5–27.

Dienstbier, R. A. (1989). Arousal and physiological toughness: Implications for mental and physical health. *Psychological Review*, **96**, 84–100.

Foa, E. B., Hembree, E. A., Cahill, S. P., Rauch, S. A. M., Riggs, D. S., Feeny, N. C. and Yadin, E. (2005). Randomized trial of prolonged exposure for posttraumatic stress disorder with and without cognitive restructuring: Outcome at academic and community clinics. *Journal of Consulting and Clinical Psychology*, **73**, 953–964.

Friedman, M. J., Davidson, J. R. T., Mellman, T. A. and Southwick, S. M. (2000). Pharmacotherapy. In *Effective Treatments for PTSD*, ed. E. B. Foa, T. M. Keane and M. J. Friedman. New York: Guilford Press, 84–105.

Hermans, D., Dirikx, T., Vansteenwegenin, D., Baeyens, F., Van Den Bergh, O. and Eelen, P. (2005). Reinstatement of fear responses in human aversive conditioning. *Behaviour Research and Therapy*, **43**, 533–551.

Livanou, M., Başoğlu, M., Şalcıoğlu, E. and Kalender, D. (2002). Traumatic stress responses in treatment-seeking earthquake survivors in Turkey. *Journal of Nervous and Mental Disease*, **190**, 816–823.

Marks, I. M., Lovell, K., Noshirvani, H. and Livanou, M. (1998). Treatment of posttraumatic stress disorder by exposure and/or cognitive restructuring: A controlled study. *Archives of General Psychiatry*, **55**, 317–325.

Mineka, S., Mystkowski, J. L., Hladek, D. and Rodriguez, B. I. (1999). The effects of changing contexts on return of fear following exposure treatment for spider fear.

Journal of Consulting and Clinical Psychology, **67**, 599–604.

Mystkowski, J. L., Craske, M. G. and Echiverri, A. M. (2002). Treatment context and return of fera in spider phobia. *Behavior Therapy*, **33**, 399–416.

Paunovic, N. and Öst, L.-G. (2001). Cognitive-behavior therapy vs exposure therapy in the treatment of PTSD in refugees. *Behaviour Research and Therapy*, **39**, 1183–1197.

Rodriguez, B. I., Craske, M. G., Mineka, S. and Hladek, D. (1999). Context-specificity of relapse: Effects of therapist and environmental context on return of fear. *Behaviour Research and Therapy*, **37**, 845–862.

Rowe, M. K. and Craske, M. G. (1998). Effects of an expanding-spaced vs massed exposure schedule on fear reduction and return of fear. *Behaviour Research and Therapy*, **36**, 701–717.

Rutter, M. (1985). Resilience in the face of adversity: Protective factors and resistance to psychiatric disorder. *The British Journal of Psychiatry*, **147**, 598–611.

Şalcıoğlu, E. (2004). *The effect of beliefs, attribution of responsibility, redress and compensation on posttraumatic stress disorder in earthquake survivors in Turkey*. PhD dissertation. Institute of Psychiatry, King's College London, London.

Şalcıoğlu, E. and Başoğlu, M. (2008). Psychological effects of earthquakes in children: Prospects for brief behavioral treatment. *World Journal of Pediatrics*, **4**, 165–172.

Şalcıoğlu, E., Başoğlu, M. and Livanou, M. (2003). Long-term psychological outcome for non-treatment-seeking earthquake survivors in Turkey. *Journal of Nervous and Mental Disease*, **191**, 154–160.

Şalcıoğlu, E., Başoğlu, M. and Livanou, M. (2007a). Effects of live exposure on symptoms of posttraumatic stress disorder: The role of reduced behavioral avoidance in improvement. *Behaviour Research and Therapy*, **45**, 2268–2279.

Şalcıoğlu, E., Başoğlu, M. and Livanou, M. (2007b). Post-traumatic stress disorder and comorbid depression among survivors of the 1999 earthquake in Turkey. *Disasters*, **31**, 115–129.

Van Etten, M. L. and Taylor, S. (1998). Comparative efficacy of treatments for post-traumatic stress disorder: A meta-analysis. *Clinical Psychology & Psychotherapy*, **5**, 126–144.

Vansteenwegen, D., Hermans, D., Vervliet, B., Francken, G., Beckers, T., Baeyens, F. and Eelen, P. (2005). Return of fear in a human differential conditioning paradigm caused by a return to the original acquistion context. *Behaviour Research and Therapy*, **43**, 323–336.

Vansteenwegen, D., Vervliet, B., Iberico, C., Baeyens, F., Van Den Bergh, O. and Hermans, D. (2007). The repeated confrontation with videotapes of spiders in multiple contexts attenuates renewal of fear in spider-anxious students. *Behaviour Research and Therapy*, **45**, 1169–1179.

Weathers, F. W., Keane, T. M. and Davidson, J. R. T. (2001). Clinician-administered PTSD scale: A review of the first ten years of research. *Depression and Anxiety*, **13**, 132–156.

Yang, C. H., Xirasagar, S., Chung, H. C., Huang, Y. T. and Lin, H. C. (2005). Suicide trends following the Taiwan earthquake of 1999: Empirical evidence and policy implications. *Acta Psychiatrica Scandinavica*, **112**, 442–448.

Assessment and treatment of prolonged grief

5

Mass trauma events, such as wars and natural disasters, not only expose people to severe trauma but also lead to bereavement and grief in many survivors. Among the earthquake survivors we came into contact with during our fieldwork in Turkey, 12.5% had lost at least one first-degree relative (based on 3905 survivors from five field surveys in the epicenter region; Başoğlu et al., 2004; Başoğlu et al., 2002; Livanou et al., 2002; Şalcıoğlu et al., 2003; Şalcıoğlu et al., 2007). Grief is a natural reaction that usually resolves to a large extent within about 6 months under normal circumstances. Therefore, natural grief reactions do not require treatment. In some people, however, it may last much longer, even many years. In a study (reviewed below) of 120 earthquake survivors who lost a first-degree relative, 31% had prolonged grief about 4 years after the loss. Such cases of prolonged grief may require treatment. Prolonged grief is often comorbid with PTSD, because most bereaved survivors have also experienced traumatic events, including witnessing the painful death of their close ones. Indeed, in the above study, 68% of the cases with prolonged grief also had PTSD. In this chapter we present a brief assessment and treatment strategy for survivors with prolonged grief.

Assessment of prolonged grief

Grief Assessment Scale and Behavior Checklist for Grief

We developed two instruments for assessment of prolonged grief reactions. The first one is a self-rated *Grief Assessment Scale* (GAS; Appendix A), which includes 20 items based on the diagnostic criteria for complicated grief proposed by Prigerson et al. (1999) and 10 items relating to prolonged grief reactions we commonly observed during our fieldwork. This scale mostly includes items relating to various cognitive and emotional effects of bereavement, such as anger, disbelief, bitterness, reluctance to accept loss, detachment from others, loss of trust in people, guilt, feeling empty, loneliness, yearning for the deceased, crying, insecurity, etc. Each item is rated on a scale of 0–2 (0 = never, 0 = sometimes, 1 = often, 2 = always).

The second instrument, *Behavior Checklist for Grief* (BCG; Appendix A), focuses on two types of grief-related behaviors that we frequently encountered during our fieldwork. The first type is characterized by behavioral avoidance of reminders of the deceased, whereas the second one involves persistent and repetitive behaviors of a ritualistic character (e.g. similar to the rituals in obsessive-compulsive disorder), such as frequent visits to the cemetery, keeping the deceased's belongings or pictures out in the open, frequent talking about the deceased, etc. The BCG has 15 items measuring the severity of avoidance and ritualistic behaviors in the last week on a 0–3 scale (0 = not at all, 1 = slightly, 2 = fairly, 3 = very much).

The psychometric properties of the GAS and the BCG were examined in a sample of 120 earthquake survivors who lost their first-degree relatives. Each instrument was administered as both a self- and clinician-rated scale to examine the validity of each item. The clinician rated the items on both scales without seeing the respective self-ratings. In the absence of established diagnostic criteria for prolonged grief, the clinician made a clinical judgment to determine '*caseness*' (i.e. whether the grief problem was sufficiently severe and functionally disabling to justify treatment) based on all information available from the clinical interview.

In comparing the self- versus clinician-rated versions of the GAS items, the criterion for symptom presence was set to an item score of 1 or higher (i.e. often / always), thus taking a rating of 'sometimes' as indicating symptom absence. A conservative approach in defining symptom presence was deemed desirable, considering that some grief reactions last for long periods on a low intensity level without causing significant functional impairment. This criterion also served to increase the sensitivity of the scale while preserving reasonable specificity in predicting need for treatment. High-scale sensitivity was also deemed important because many survivors with grief reactions did not regard their condition as requiring treatment, unless the problems were sufficiently severe to cause significant disruption in their daily functioning. Table 5.1 shows the sensitivity, specificity, correct classification rates, and kappa values of the GAS items with respect to clinician ratings.

Twenty-six items of the self-rated GAS had satisfactory sensitivity, specificity, and correct classification rate. Agreement between self- and assessor-ratings was moderate (i.e. kappa values between 0.40 and 0.59) for 10 items and strong (i.e. kappa values between 0.60 and 0.79) for 12 items. Several factors were responsible for low (or lack of) agreement on eight items. Relative to the respective clinician ratings, the survivors overestimated five symptoms (items #7, #16, #23, #24, #25) and underestimated two (items #22 and #29). The endorsement rate for one item (#26) was extremely low in both self- and assessor-ratings.

The GAS had good internal consistency (Cronbach's alpha = 0.94). The scale total scores correlated significantly with clinician-rated scale scores ($r = 0.87$, $p < 0.001$). The scale also showed high correlations with the Clinician-Administered PTSD Scale (CAPS; Blake et al., 1990; $r = 0.70$, $p < 0.001$), Traumatic Stress Symptom Checklist (TSSC; Başoğlu et al., 2001; $r = 0.84$, $p < 0.001$), and Beck Depression Inventory (BDI; Beck et al., 1979; $r = 077$, $p < 0.001$). The survivors who were judged by the clinician as in need of treatment had higher mean total scores than those who were not (mean = 23, SD = 13 vs. mean = 6, SD = 8, respectively, $p < 0.001$). A score of 25 on the self-rated GAS had a sensitivity of 0.86 and specificity of 0.81 with respect to the clinician's judgment of caseness, correctly classifying 82% of the cases ($\kappa = 0.51$, $p < 0.001$). In addition, this cut-off score yielded sensitivity of 0.79 and specificity of 0.98 with respect to a diagnosis of complicated grief based on the criteria proposed by Prigerson et al. (1999)(correct classification rate = 95%, $\kappa = 0.80$, $p < 0.001$). These findings supported the criterion based validity and concurrent validity of the GAS.

Similar analyses were conducted to examine the psychometric properties of the BCG. Symptom presence on the clinician-rated version of the scale was defined as a score of 2 and above, thus regarding a rating of 'slightly' as indicating symptom absence. This conservative approach in defining symptom presence was deemed necessary, because the BCG is used in identifying grief behaviors that are targeted in treatment. We then examined the optimum cut-off point for each self-rated item that yielded the best concordance rate with the respective clinician's rating. Table 5.2 shows the sensitivity, specificity, correct classification rates, and kappa values of the BCG items with respect to the clinician ratings.

Note that 12 items show optimal concordance with the respective clinician ratings when symptom presence is based on the cut-off point of 2. For three items relating to avoidance a cut-off of 1 yielded better sensitivity and specificity values (although κ values improved when cut-off points were set to 2). Overall, the BCG items had satisfactory concordance with the clinician ratings. Consistent with this finding, the total scores of the self- and clinician-rated versions of the scale were highly inter-correlated ($r = 0.84$, $p < 0.001$). The scale also has good internal consistency with Cronbach's alpha of 0.81.

The BCG correlated highly with both the self- and clinician-rated versions of the GAS ($r = 0.72$ and $r = 70$, respectively, all p's < 0.001), CAPS ($r = 0.63$, $p < 0.001$), TSSC ($r = 0.71$, $p < 0.001$), and BDI ($r = 0.62$, $p < 0.001$). Furthermore, the survivors judged by the clinician as having significant grief problems requiring treatment had higher BCG scores than those rated as not having significant grief problems (mean = 18, SD = 6 vs. mean = 8, SD = 6, respectively, $p < 0.001$). These findings supported the criterion and concurrent validity of the scale. A total score of 17 had sensitivity of 0.78 and specificity of 0.84 with respect to the clinician's judgment of caseness (82% correct classification, $\kappa = 0.55$, $p < 0.001$).

As the BCG was designed to measure two types of grief behaviors, we conducted a principal components analysis to examine whether avoidance and ritualistic behaviors formed distinct clusters. The analysis did indeed reveal two components that showed a clear separation between these two types of grief behaviors. This analysis does not, however, imply that survivors always display either one type of grief reactions or the other. Of the 37 survivors who met the caseness criterion, six clearly had both types of grief reactions. We do not yet know what this distinction implies for the psychological mechanisms of grief or why some

Table 5.1 Concordance between self- and clinician-rated Grief Assessment Scale items

	SE	SP	CC	κ[1]
1. I feel bitter for having lost him/her.	100	90	91	0.62
2. I go to places that he/she used to go in the hope that I might find him/her there.	100	96	96	0.53
3. I feel detached/estranged from others after his/her death.	91	91	90	0.73
4. I feel that a future without him/her will always be empty and pointless.	80	87	86	0.61
5. His/her death makes me feel like a part of me has died.	86	79	82	0.65
6. I cry when I think about him/her.	93	76	80	0.55
7. I cannot accept the fact that he/she is dead.	88	69	70	0.19
8. I have lost trust in people because of his/her death.	59	87	81	0.46
9. I feel lonely without him/her.	87	78	82	0.62
10. I do things that remind me of him/her in day to day life (for example, keeping his/her pictures or belongings out in the open, thinking or talking about him/her, visiting his/her grave, etc.).	73	83	80	0.56
11. I feel that life is empty or meaningless without him/her.	87	90	89	0.73
12. I feel guilty when I enjoy myself.	100	85	87	0.58
13. I acquired some of his/her harmful habits or behaviors (e.g. smoking or drinking).	100	98	98	0.66
14. I yearn for him/her.	91	71	80	0.61
15. I have physical complaints (e.g. headaches, pains, etc.) that started after his/her death.	71	82	80	0.49
16. I see him/her stand before me.	100	92	92	0.15
17. I feel as if my feelings have died after his/her death.	79	81	81	0.50
18. I feel I have no control over my life.	82	93	92	0.69
19. I cannot stop thinking about him/her.	79	84	82	0.61
20. I feel helpless without him/her.	83	87	86	0.57
21. I have physical complaints that he/she used to have when he/she was alive.	67	97	96	0.43
22. I cannot do things that remind me of him/her in day to day life (for example, looking at his/her pictures, visiting his/her grave, talking about him/her, etc.).	39	90	75	0.33
23. I hear his/her voice.	–	94	–	–
24. I cannot believe that he/she is dead.	100	75	76	0.26
25. I blame myself for not having tried hard enough to save him/her.	83	83	83	0.27
26. I feel angry with him/her because he/she left me.	0	97	97	0.00
27. I have dreams of him/her.	90	84	85	0.43
28. I feel envious of people who have not lost their loved ones.	91	79	82	0.62
29. I feel angry for having lost him/her.	46	91	86	0.33
30. I feel insecure because of his/her death.	80	93	92	0.66

SE = Sensitivity, SP = Specificity, CC = Correct Classification, κ = Measure of agreement.
[1] For all κ's $p < 0.001$ except for items 16 ($p < 0.01$), 23 (ns), and 26 (ns).

people display one or the other type of grief reactions or whether this finding can be replicated in other cultural settings. We do know, however, that such distinction is useful in treatment, because the two types of grief reactions require somewhat different behavioral interventions. It is thus worth bearing this distinction in mind in assessment of bereaved survivors.

The BCG is comparable to the GAS in all its psychometric properties, suggesting that a behavioral focus in assessment is just as informative in determining treatment need as a broader assessment involving

Table 5.2 Concordance between self- and clinician-rated Behavior Checklist for Grief items

	OC	SE	SP	CC	κ[1]
1. I feel like seeing his/her belongings out in the open.	2	71	88	85	0.50
2. I have difficulty looking at his/her pictures.	2	71	89	86	0.56
3. I avoid going to the place where he/she died.	2	78	93	89	0.72
4. I feel like seeing his/her pictures out in the open.	2	71	86	82	0.54
5. I feel like going to the places where we used to go together.	2	100	85	87	0.53
6. I have difficulty mentioning his/her name.	2	93	97	97	0.86
7. I avoid meeting his/her friends.	2	67	93	88	0.59
8. I have difficulty cooking/eating the meals that he/she used to like.	2	60	89	87	0.38
9. I avoid visiting his/her grave.	1	100	81	83	0.38
10. I have difficulty listening to the music he/she liked.	2	77	94	92	0.65
11. I feel like talking about him/her.	2	85	85	85	0.58
12. I have difficulty going to the places where we used to go together.	1	88	74	76	0.40
13. I avoid talking about him/her.	1	75	69	70	0.30
14. I have difficulty looking at his/her belongings.	2	74	95	91	0.68
15. I feel like visiting his/her grave.	2	78	81	80	0.56

OC = Optimum cut-off for self-rated scale items, SE = Sensitivity, SP = Specificity, CC = Correct Classification, κ = Measure of agreement.
[1] For all κ's p < 0.001.

cognitive and emotional manifestations of grief. Furthermore, compared with the GAS (or any other similar measure), its validation in other cultures might be easier, considering that cognitive and emotional manifestations of grief are likely to show greater variability across cultures. The GAS might be useful, however, in clinical practice and intervention outcome research, particularly when there is a need for more detailed assessment of treatment effects on a wider range of grief symptoms.

It is worth emphasizing the fact that both the GAS and BCG are not meant as diagnostic instruments for prolonged grief. Rather they are designed as measures to help the clinician in assessing survivors' treatment needs. We believe the latter issue is more important in post-disaster work, given that diagnostic measures pertaining to mental health outcomes of natural disasters are not always reliable indicators of survivors' need for treatment, as discussed in Chapter 3. Finally, we should note that both instruments can be used in different trauma groups, as their items are not worded with reference to a specific trauma event. However, because these scales have so far been tested only with earthquake survivors, their psychometric properties may need to be verified in war and torture survivors.

Treatment of prolonged grief

As noted earlier, some survivors of mass trauma events may have both PTSD and prolonged grief. In such cases, these conditions can be treated concurrently in the same program by giving self-exposure instructions relating to both conditions. In some survivors particular distress cues may relate to both fear and grief reactions. For example, the location where the person experienced both the trauma and loss of close ones involves both types of distress cues. If, however, the survivor finds it too difficult to work on both problems at the same time, they can tackle them in turn, starting with the one they find relatively easier to deal with and then turning to the other one. In some cases grief may need priority attention, as it may complicate treatment of PTSD by undermining motivation for treatment.

Step 1: identifying problem behaviors

The first task in treatment is to identify grief-related avoidance and ritualistic behaviors that need to be targeted during treatment. The BCG is often very useful for this purpose, as it includes the most common grief behaviors associated with prolonged grief. When this instrument is used to elicit this information, it is important to bear in mind that the survivor may have other idiosyncratic forms of grief behaviors not covered by the questionnaire. This information could be captured by questions such as "*Are there any other situations or activities that you avoid because they bring back distressing memories of your loved one?*" or "*Are there other things that you keep doing because they remind you of your loved one or because they keep his/her memory alive?*"

Step 2: explaining treatment and its rationale

Avoidance behaviors are treated with exposure to avoided cues in much the same way as in treatment of traumatic stress, whereas ritualistic behaviors require response prevention. The latter is a behavioral intervention used in treating obsessive rituals. Obsessive rituals (e.g. hand washing) are often triggered by cues (e.g. perceived dirt in hands) and serve to reduce the anxiety evoked by the cue. Preventing such rituals is thus a form of exposure to anxiety evoked by the cue. Response prevention has also been shown to be effective in treating prolonged grief (Boelen et al., 2007). The treatment and its rationale could be explained as follows:

> I can see from your initial assessment results that you still have substantial grief-related problems. Most people recover from grief after 6–12 months to the extent that they can resume reasonably normal functioning. If you look carefully, you will see that this is the case with most people who lost their loved ones during the earthquake. People usually respond to sudden loss with initial shock and disbelief but then they accept the loss and go through a period of grief. They eventually recover from grief and return to a reasonably normal life. Some people, however, find it difficult to accept the reality of their loss and develop behaviors that may block natural grief process. Such behaviors are usually of two types. Some people avoid particular situations or activities that bring back distressing memories of the loss. For example, they may avoid visits to the cemetery, talking about the lost one, looking at his/her pictures, or going to the location where s/he died. Others may repeatedly engage in certain activities to keep the memory of the lost one alive at all times. For example, they may feel like talking about the lost one all the time, make frequent visits to his/her grave, keep his/her pictures all around the house, avoid giving away his/her clothes or other belongings, and keep his/her room exactly as it was before the event. Such behaviors are ritualistic in quality; one feels an urge to engage in them, which is often difficult to resist because this causes distress. Some people may display both types of grieving behaviors.
>
> This treatment will help you change these behaviors so that you can complete your grief. You can do this by not avoiding situations that bring back memories of your loss and by not engaging in ritualistic behaviors. You may experience distress in the process but you will learn to tolerate and control it. This will help you get over your grief once and for all. Just think how this problem has taken control over your life. You will need to decide whether you want to live with this problem or do something about it. If you choose the latter option, you will need to conduct exercises to overcome your distress caused by the activities listed in this questionnaire [Behavior Checklist for Grief]. I will help you with this process. You are free to carry out your exercises at your own pace, tackling them gradually or one step at a time, if you like. Most people recover within 10 weeks, so you will need to complete your exercises within this time. We will then choose one final homework task to mark the end of your mourning and also of your treatment.

Some points concerning the treatment rationale deserve attention here. Prolonged grief is presented as a condition that occurs when the natural grief process is blocked by cognitive, behavioral and emotional avoidance of the painful reality of loss. The treatment is presented as a means of helping the person to come to terms with the reality of the loss so that s/he can complete the natural grief process. This is achieved by exposure to cues that evoke distress, grief, or other loss-related emotions. Thus, as in treatment of traumatic stress, the intervention has a sharp behavioral focus and involves only live exposure. In Part 1 we discussed our observations pointing to the important role of risk taking and confronting feared situations in natural recovery from traumatic stress. Our observations suggest that similar behavioral processes also play an important role in natural recovery from grief. It is worth briefly summarizing these observations and how they inspired certain aspects of our treatment of grief.

In many cultures the mourning process is associated with a wide range of elaborate ceremonies and rituals (Rosenblatt, 2008) that appear to facilitate grief. For example, funeral ceremonies might serve to facilitate acceptance of the loss by providing exposure to the sight of the loved one's dead body, other people's emotional reactions to the loss, and the burial process as further evidence of separation from the loved one. The sight of a dead body ingrained as the last visual memory of the loved one might be particularly important in this respect, which might perhaps explain why the relatives of the deceased are often actively encouraged to see the body before burial (or why the body of the deceased is displayed in an open coffin during the funeral ceremony in some Christian cultures). Perhaps the most fascinating example we have come across in this respect concerns a tradition in some rural regions of Turkey, which involves the recruitment of a group of professional 'mourners' (termed *ağıtçılar* in Turkish). These are usually women with no relation to the deceased and their sole task is to display overt (and often exaggerated) grieving behaviors (e.g. crying loudly in a chorus, talking about how good the deceased was, how he or she will be missed, etc.) during the funeral ceremony and the days that follow. Such tradition appears to be designed to facilitate the grieving process in the bereaved. Following burial, visits by friends and neighbors paying their condolences provide ample opportunities for talking about the deceased and crying. Furthermore, neighbors often take over domestic duties, such as cooking and cleaning, for some days to relieve the bereaved of everyday work, which seems to ensure that grieving proceeds in a focused fashion uninterrupted by distractions. Social codes concerning the mourning process also appear to be geared towards facilitating grieving in the bereaved. Certain mourning behaviors (e.g. dressing in black) are deemed appropriate and expected, while others (e.g. appearing joyful, laughing, listening to music, singing, or engaging in other entertainment activities) are met with disapproval and discouraged. Finally, grieving is a time-limited process. Social codes encourage mourning for a particular period of time, after which the bereaved is expected to resume normal life. In Turkey, for example, there are certain religious rituals that mark the end of the mourning period, which is often designated as the 40th day of the loss. There is even a descriptive term that refers to completion of the mourning process (i.e. *kırkı çıkmak*) meaning *completion of the 40th day*.

These are merely a few examples which suggest that human response to loss has evolved throughout

history in ways to help them overcome the impact of loss. Many of the grief rituals and social processes that serve to facilitate resolution of grief are essentially behavioral in nature, as noted earlier. Accordingly, we have incorporated some of these processes into our treatment approach. This explains in part why the treatment is presented as a means of facilitating the grieving process and helping the person complete the natural grief cycle by confronting the distress associated with the loss. Furthermore, in an effort to recreate the time-limited nature of the natural grief process, a time frame is set in agreement with the client for the whole treatment process. A time frame implies that there is a beginning and an end to the grieving process and that the person is expected to discontinue mourning and resume normal life, once this process is completed. Defining a closure event for the grief process is often helpful in marking the end of the grief process. Such closure is best defined by an exposure task that is most difficult to achieve and / or one that is with most symbolic significance for the person. This could be, for example, removing the deceased person's belongings from sight or giving them away. Similarly, a final cemetery visit could be arranged, together with other close ones and in a ceremonial fashion, to mark the end of the grieving process.

A potential problem in engaging the client in the idea of treatment deserves mention here. Some people regard their grief process as natural, no matter how prolonged and disabling their grief might be. We have seen survivors with such intense grief (usually associated with child loss) that they simply did not care about their own disaster-related problems, psychological or other, or the adverse impact of grief on their life functioning. Such survivors were reluctant to accept treatment for their grief problems. We often tried to negotiate a deal with such cases, asking them to give the treatment a try (e.g. conducting one or two exposure tasks) and then decide whether or not they want to continue with treatment. This strategy worked in most cases, as they found the early impact of treatment sufficiently rewarding to continue with treatment.

Step 3: defining exposure tasks and giving self-exposure instructions

Once an agreement is reached on the need for treatment, the next step is to define the exposure tasks and provide self-exposure instructions. The BCG would be useful in defining the treatment tasks. As a general rule, behaviors endorsed as 'fairly' or 'very much' need attention in treatment (though the item cut-off points indicated in Table 5.2 could also be taken into account). It is best to make a list of the endorsed behaviors and the exposure tasks targeting them. The BCG items define the following tasks:

Tasks relating to avoidance behaviors

- Looking at loved one's pictures
- Looking at loved one's belongings
- Cooking/eating the meals that loved one used to like
- Going to the place where loved one died
- Meeting with loved one's friends
- Talking about loved one
- Visiting loved one's grave
- Listening to the music that loved one liked
- Going to the places where the survivor used to go together with loved one

---

Tasks relating to ritualistic behaviors

- Removing loved one's pictures from sight or stop looking at them
- Removing loved one's belongings from sight or stop looking at them
- Not going to the places where the survivor used to go together with loved one
- Not talking about loved one
- Not visiting loved one's grave

The list is likely to include both avoidance and ritualistic behaviors, although some people may display more behaviors of one type than the other. Note once again that the BCG is not an exhaustive list of grief behaviors. It is thus important to make sure that any problem behaviors not included in the scale are listed under the 'Others' item and included in the list of exposure tasks. Once the list of problem behaviors is drawn up, the survivor is told that the aim in treatment is to change these behaviors by (a) not avoiding the activities that cause distress and (b) not engaging in ritualistic behaviors that maintain grief reactions. The following explanation about the treatment process is often useful:

You can start working on your tasks in any order you like. If you like, you can start with the easier ones and,

when you feel you can tolerate distress better, move on to more difficult ones. Look at your task list and decide which ones are the easiest and which ones are more difficult to achieve. You can also break a difficult task into easier steps. For example, if you are keeping your lost one's pictures or belongings out in the open so that you can see them all the time, you can begin your task by removing these items one by one, instead of all of them at once. Or you can remove them in a particular order, starting with the 'easier-to-remove' items first. Similarly, you can give away his/her belongings one by one, starting with the easiest items first. If you feel you cannot stop cemetery visits at once, you can reduce their frequency gradually. You may experience a certain amount of distress in achieving each task but this is natural and not undesirable. Remember always that this will help you to learn to tolerate the distress caused by your loss so that you can complete your grief in a natural fashion. The distress you experience in executing these tasks may include feelings of anger, blame, or guilt. Executing these tasks may also make you feel guilty because they may come across to you as giving up on your lost one or as betraying his/her memory. This is natural and most grieving people have such thoughts and feelings. You will recover from such emotions as your treatment progresses and you will most likely feel different about the issues that bring about these emotions.

Note also that the aim of treatment is not to deprive you of all memory of your lost one forever. It is normal to keep some pictures of the lost one in the living room or make cemetery visits from time to time, as most people do. These tasks are simply designed to help you come to terms with your loss. When the treatment is over and you are no longer distressed by the thought of removing them from your sight, you can put back some of the pictures in your living room.

Bear in mind that there is a time frame for this treatment. It is designed for a maximum of 10 weeks, as most people are able to complete their tasks within this period. Plan your treatment accordingly. Consider the number of tasks you have. If you have 10, for example, this means you can complete all tasks in 10 weeks by working on one task each week. You can, however, work on as many tasks as you want each week and complete the treatment even earlier. This is entirely up to you.

Subsequent sessions

Subsequent treatment sessions are conducted in much the same way as in treatment of traumatic stress. The sessions involve an initial assessment using the BCG, a review of progress in the last week, verbal praise for any progress achieved, troubleshooting for problems encountered, and defining new exposure tasks. As the exposure tasks can increase the person's distress levels in the early phase of treatment, strong encouragement and emotional support might be needed during this time to avoid premature termination of treatment.

In some cases a therapist-assisted exposure session might be necessary to help the survivor with some difficult tasks. Visiting the site where the loved one died, for example, is a difficult task for most people, particularly when the person has witnessed the death of the lost one. The survivor may break into tears and start talking about the trauma experience during the session. This is often an emotionally taxing experience for both the survivor and the therapist. During the session the therapist needs to maintain a certain emotional distance from the event and help the survivor, if necessary, to relive the experience by getting them to talk about the deceased and the events that led to his/her death. Getting the person to relate the story several times often helps. Such sessions are often conducive to a sense of great relief on the part of the survivor (often expressed as "great burden lifted off my chest"), significantly facilitating the treatment process thereafter. Note that such a live exposure session also involves strong elements of imaginal exposure (e.g. to memories of the trauma and loss). In our experience such imaginal exposure taking place in the context of live exposure is more potent than imaginal exposure sessions conducted in a clinical setting. Indeed, this is one of the reasons why we do not see the need for routine use of imaginal exposure in treatment.

It is often helpful to get other surviving family members or close friends involved in treatment so that they understand the treatment rationale and help the survivor through the process. In some cases they may sympathize with the survivor's grief and find it difficult to understand the treatment rationale. When not informed sufficiently about the principles of treatment, other family members may prevent the execution of certain tasks, such as removing the belongings of the deceased from sight or giving them away, for example. Because of the highly emotional nature of such tasks, they may have an entirely different meaning for those not involved in or aware of the treatment process.

As the survivor begins to make progress with their tasks, they often notice an increased sense of well being within the first few weeks of treatment. They are more able to tolerate the distress associated with the reminders of their loss, less preoccupied with memories of the deceased, more acceptant of the reality of their loss, and experience sufficient improvement in grief symptoms to function better in daily life. These changes are often noticed by their family and friends. At this point it is important to encourage the survivor to make an effort to resume normal life activities. For example, they can begin to take better care of themselves and their appearance, attend social gatherings, meet with friends, or do other things that they previously enjoyed doing. Such activities could also be prescribed as behavioral tasks. Such tasks could help the survivor regain interest in these activities. If these activities are avoided because of associated guilt, the survivor should still make an active effort to engage in them, as guilt often reduces in the process.

Defining closure for grief

The event that represents closure of the grieving process is often defined towards the end of the treatment. The following question might be helpful in identifying this event: "*What is it that you can do as one last thing that will mean finally accepting the loss of your loved one and separating from him or her?*" This could be a small family gathering or a religious or other ceremony at the cemetery, a final visit to the location where the loved one died, giving away his/her belongings (or a particular item among them), or any other activity that carries a special meaning for the person. The important point here is that this final task is perceived as the most appropriate one to mark the end of the mourning process. The timing of this event is also important. When the survivor has come to terms with the reality of their loved one's loss, gained sufficient control over avoidance and ritualistic mourning behaviors, and began to resume normal life activities, it is time for closure. To avoid any misunderstanding regarding the meaning of closure (and pre-empt any resistance to the idea), it is worth reminding the survivor at this point that closure does not mean forgetting about their loved one or separating from his/her memory forever. It simply means that their grief is now completed in the way that it should have naturally resolved in the first place.

Case vignettes

Two case vignettes are presented below to highlight treatment of prolonged grief comorbid with PTSD. Because these vignettes relate to a married couple whose treatments were conducted concurrently (by the second author), they are presented together. These survivors were the first two cases recruited for a randomized controlled treatment study of prolonged grief and PTSD, which was launched 3.5 years after the earthquake (but terminated after the recruitment of the 8th case due to staff shortage).

Case vignettes

Fatma and Mustafa were a 45-year-old married couple with two children. They experienced the earthquake in the epicenter region and their house collapsed during the tremors. They were left under the rubble with their two sons. Mustafa managed to get out of the rubble within half an hour and rescue his wife and older son after 7 hours of work. However, he failed to rescue his 14-year-old son, whose body was recovered after two days. They both sustained moderately severe physical injuries. The loss of their only house and all belongings meant a severe financial blow for the family. After the earthquake they went to their home town outside the Marmara region and buried their son there. Fatma did not see her son's body before burial.

At the time of the assessment the couple were living in a flat in a government-built housing site for homeless survivors. Assessment and treatment sessions were conducted at their home. They had difficulty acknowledging their son's death, felt lonely, and had strong yearnings for him. They felt like a part of them had died with their son and life without him looked empty and pointless. They had intrusive thoughts about their son, which made them cry frequently. Sometimes they felt like they saw their son in the house or heard his voice. Mustafa also had strong feelings of alienation, bitterness and anger, blaming the building contractors and the local government for the collapse of their house. He felt guilty for not being able to rescue his son and reported feelings of loss of control over life. These problems adversely affected their marital relationship, as they had grown emotionally distant and withdrawn from each other. Fatma had sought treatment soon after the earthquake and received antidepressant treatment for 6 months without much improvement. Mustafa, on the other, had never sought treatment, though he took diazepam for a few weeks upon the advice of some neighbors.

Although Fatma and Mustafa displayed some similar behavioral manifestations of grief, they also differed in some ways. For example, they both wanted to keep their son's belongings in the living room, avoided cooking or eating the food their son used to like, and felt like going to the places they used to go with their son. On the other hand, while Fatma frequently talked about her son, Mustafa had difficulty doing so. Fatma avoided going to the site where her son died, whereas Mustafa made frequent visits to that location. Mustafa had moderately severe depression (BDI score 29), whereas Fatma had no depression (BDI score 7). In addition, Fatma developed psoriasis on both arms after the earthquake, which was diagnosed as a stress-related problem by a dermatologist.

Fatma's treatment (case #1)

Fatma's first treatment session took 110 minutes. She readily agreed to treatment after explanation of the treatment rationale. Exposure instructions were given separately for grief and traumatic stress symptoms. Exposure tasks for grief included (1) cooking and eating her son's favorite dishes, (2) going to places they used to go together, (3) removing his only two belongings salvaged from the rubble (e.g. a blanket and a key-ring) from the living room, and (4) visiting the site where he died. Exposure tasks for traumatic stress were (1) staying alone at home at night, (2) entering concrete buildings, (3) using elevators, and (4) going to a market place named '17th of August' (the date of the 1999 earthquake). Compliance with exposure tasks was assessed by the therapist at weekly sessions.

At the second session Fatma expressed doubts about her need for treatment, stating that the way she lived with her son's death did not cause any problems. Although she found the first session helpful, she did not carry out her homework assignments because she did not have the time. Her reluctance with treatment seemed to be related to her failure in initiating self-exposure exercises. The therapist explained the treatment rationale again, particularly emphasizing the negative impact of her problems on her relationship with her husband. She agreed to give treatment a chance. This session took 90 minutes.

After the second session she initiated self-exposure exercises, albeit gradually in the beginning,

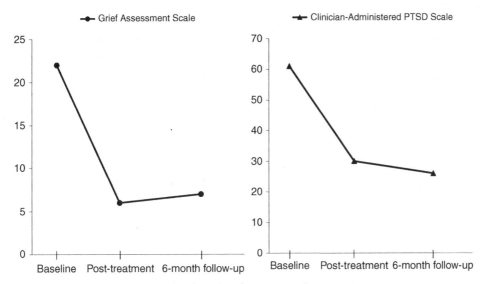

Figure 5.1 Improvement in PTSD and prolonged grief symptoms in Case #1.

and showed steady improvement thereafter. At subsequent assessments she reported feeling much better and stated that she was looking forward to treatment sessions with her therapist. After the sixth session therapy sessions were terminated and she was asked to continue with her self-exposure exercises. Treatment response on the GAS and CAPS (Blake et al., 1990) is shown in Figure 5.1.

At 6-month follow-up, grief-related avoidance and ritualistic behaviors reduced by 48%, grief symptoms by 68%, fear and avoidance behaviors (as assessed by *Fear and Avoidance Questionnaire*) by 76%, and PTSD symptoms by 57%. When symptom presence was defined as an item rating of 1 (often) or 2 (always), 9 of the 13 grief symptoms present at pre-treatment were absent at follow-up. She accepted her son's loss, did not perceive life as empty and meaningless, stopped doing things to bring back her son's memories, no longer had hallucination-like experiences of seeing him or hearing his voice, and felt less lonely, emotionally numbed, and envious of people who have not lost their loved ones. Although she still thought about her son frequently and cried from time to time when she did, her thoughts had lost their intrusive and distressing quality. However, she continued to yearn for her son and still felt like part of herself had died with her son. Nevertheless, she rated herself as 'much improved' on the *Global Improvement Scale* and also reported marked increase in sense of control over her symptoms, as well as in her self-confidence, beliefs in coping, and ability to overcome these problems (as measured by the *Sense*

of Control Scale). There was also improvement in her social and family functioning. The 1-month follow-up assessment was conducted around the time of her son's birthday, which also coincided with an earthquake in 2003 that caused some devastation and casualties in the eastern part of Turkey. Although these two events had an emotional impact on her, she did not relapse, suggesting that the treatment effects were stable despite further encounters with stressor events. Interestingly, psoriasis on her arms also started to improve after the third session and disappeared almost completely by the end of treatment. She attributed this recovery to improvement in grief-related problems.

Mustafa's treatment (case #2)

During the first session Mustafa said he regarded his grief as normal and did not see the need for treatment, despite the fact that he rated it as causing severe distress and marked disability in his social, occupational, and family life. When the therapist explained how the treatment could be useful in dealing with grief-related avoidances and ritualistic behaviors, he said he would not have any difficulty in changing these behaviors. The therapist persuaded him to try some exposure exercises and see how he would feel about treatment afterwards. He agreed and the following exposure tasks were defined: (1) to talk about his son, (2) to go to his son's school,

(3) to stop looking at his picture, and (4) to stop visiting the site where he died. His exposure tasks in relation to traumatic stress were (1) to enter avoided (safe) buildings, (2) to go to locations where many buildings collapsed, (3) to participate in discussions about earthquakes, and (4) to talk about his earthquake experiences. He came to the second session having conducted all exposure tasks. He was surprised to see how much difficulty he had in executing these tasks. The therapist explained the treatment rationale once again and, having understood it better this time, Mustafa showed more motivation for treatment. He was compliant with most exposure tasks set in the subsequent sessions, but he could not remove his son's only remaining photograph from the living room or stop looking at it occasionally during the day. Improvement was gradual but steady and by 6-month follow-up he had no difficulty with any of his exposure tasks, except for stopping looking at his son's photograph. Treatment outcome on main measures are shown in Figure 5.2.

At 6-month follow-up his grief-related avoidance and ritualistic behaviors reduced by 41%, grief symptoms by 69%, depression by 93%, earthquake-related fears and avoidances by 80%, and PTSD by 56%. Using the same criterion for symptom presence as in Fatma's case, 19 of the 28 symptoms present at pre-treatment had improved at follow-up. He accepted his son's loss, thought less about him, did not engage in activities that brought back his memories, no longer blamed himself for not having been able to

rescue him, and felt less guilty when he did something he enjoyed doing. There was also marked improvement in emotional numbing, bitterness, alienation from others, loss of trust in people, physical complaints (e.g. headaches, pains, etc.), and feelings of helplessness. He no longer had hallucination-like experiences of seeing him or hearing his voice and had only occasional dreams about him. On the other hand, he continued to yearn for his son and feel like part of himself had died, lonely, insecure, angry for having lost his son, and envious of people who had not lost close ones. Although he had some worsening in his condition after the 2003 earthquake in eastern Turkey, which coincided with his son's birthday, his symptoms returned to post-treatment levels by 6-month follow-up. He rated himself as 'much improved' on the *Global Improvement Scale* and reported marked increase in his sense of control over the problem.

As we could not complete the treatment study with prolonged grief cases, it is difficult to pinpoint an optimal time frame and number of sessions required for significant clinical improvement in such cases. Although we obtained reasonably good results in an average of four sessions in our work with bereaved survivors (detailed in the next section below), relatively difficult cases, such as Mustafa, may require a few more sessions. In such cases, PTSD and grief

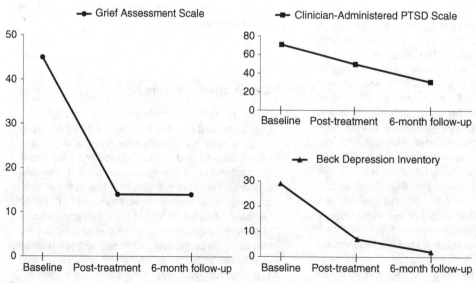

Figure 5.2 Improvement in PTSD, depression, and prolonged grief symptoms in Case #2.

problems require equal attention, which would mean defining different exposure tasks for both conditions and monitoring them. It may also be difficult to treat one condition without treating the other, because of possible interactions between traumatic stress and grief reactions. Witnessing the death of a loved one while trapped together under a collapsed building, for example, is likely to have more psychological impact than losing a loved one without being exposed to the same events. The former experience is likely to lead to at least three types of responses in the person: fear associated with exposure to the life-threatening event, distress induced by witnessing the death of the loved one, and grief associated with the loss. Treatment in such cases needs to involve exposure to particular situations that evoke all three types of responses. In our experience, best results are obtained with exposure sessions at the site of the incident. It is worth noting here that frequent ritualistic visits to the incident site, as in the case of Mustafa, do not constitute exposure, because the latter needs to be conducted as a purpose-driven exercise with the specific intention of confronting and overcoming the problem. In addition, knowledge about how an exposure session should be conducted (e.g. by challenging distress, avoiding distraction strategies, staying in the situation until sense of control develops, etc.) is an important factor that distinguishes therapeutic exposure from other encounters with distress cues, whether coincidental or serving another purpose. This implies that, in survivors like Mustafa, ritualistic visits to the incident site could be turned into therapeutic exposure by altering the purpose and meaning of the visits for the person.

The case vignettes demonstrate the difficulty in engaging some survivors in the idea of treatment. As noted earlier, a useful strategy to overcome resistance to treatment is to convince the person to conduct one exposure session and find out how it makes them feel. The impact of the first session is often sufficient to enhance motivation for treatment. This is often a more effective method than any other motivational enhancement strategy. These two cases also demonstrate the fact that a rather proactive or even assertive therapist approach in engaging initially reluctant survivors in treatment is well justified. Indeed, once the treatment process started, both Fatma and Mustafa were more than happy to have accepted treatment, from which they benefited a great deal.

Preliminary evidence of treatment effectiveness

In addition to eight case studies, there is some preliminary evidence from an uncontrolled study (Başoğlu et al., 2003) pointing to the efficacy of Control-Focused Behavioral Treatment (CFBT) in prolonged grief. This study involved 231 earthquake survivors who sought treatment for traumatic stress from our community center in the disaster region. Of these, 36 also had grief reactions at a mean of 13 months post-earthquake. Based on clinical judgment, grief problems were deemed sufficiently severe in 17 cases to require attention in treatment. Grief was due to loss of a child in six cases (35%), a parent or sibling in six (35%), and a second-degree relative or friend in five (30%). In 10 survivors (four with probable PTSD according to the TSSC-E) grief problems were predominant and thus all self-exposure tasks related to grief symptoms. In seven cases (five with PTSD) self-exposure tasks related to both PTSD and grief symptoms. The survivors received mean four treatment sessions (range 2–8). Table 5.3 shows treatment outcome on main study measures at the last available assessment in 17 cases. As treatment response did not significantly differ between cases treated for grief symptoms and those treated for both PTSD and grief, they were pooled for analysis.

Because this study was conducted before the development of grief scales, grief symptoms were not measured. However, the difficulty or avoidance associated with main exposure tasks relating to grief behaviors was measured by a self-rated 0–8 scale (0 = no difficulty / avoidance, 8 = extreme difficulty / avoidance). Other measures included BDI (Beck et al., 1979), Work and Social Adjustment (Mundt et al., 2002), and Patient's Global Impression – Improvement (PGI) and Clinician's Global Impression – Improvement (CGI; Guy, 1976). Improvement in these measures provides an idea about the effect of treatment targeting grief reactions. Treatment effect sizes were large, percentage of improvement in measures ranging from 43% to 75%. The substantial reduction in the ratings of difficulty / avoidance associated with self-exposure tasks (averaged across four main tasks) shows that the survivors complied with treatment instructions (also ascertained by weekly assessments of compliance). The overall improvement rate (much / very much improved) was 59% (n = 10) according to PGI and 82% (n = 14) according to CGI. [The difference in PGI and CGI ratings reflected a general (possibly culturally

Table 5.3 Treatment outcome in survivors with prolonged grief (n = 17)

Measures	Mean (SD)	% change	Effect size[1]
Traumatic Stress Symptom Checklist (0–51)			
Baseline	34.7 (11.4)		
Last available assessment	18.5 (8.8)***	47	1.55
Fear and Avoidance Questionnaire (0–105)			
Baseline	37.3 (19.3)		
Last available assessment	14.8 (14.4)***	60	1.29
Beck Depression Inventory			
Baseline	18.3 (7.6)		
Last available assessment	10.4 (5.5)***	43	1.16
Exposure task ratings (0–8)[2]			
Baseline	6.6 (0.7)		
Last available assessment	1.7 (1.4)***	75	4.32
Work and Social Adjustment (0–32)			
Baseline	14.9 (8.2)		
Last available assessment	6.7 (6.6)***	56	1.08

[1] Cohen's d with Hedges correction for small sample size.
[2] Averaged rating of difficulty / avoidance associated with four main self-exposure tasks.
*** p < 0.001.

determined) tendency of the survivors to underestimate their treatment gains (Başoğlu et al., 2003).] These 17 cases did not significantly differ from the 197 survivors in any of their pre-treatment clinical ratings and in their response to treatment. Comparing those who lost a child with those who lost a parent / sibling or a second-degree relative, no differences were found in outcome. Four of the six survivors who had lost a child reported much or very much improvement. These findings, though not conclusive, provide some support for the effectiveness of CFBT in prolonged grief, consistent with findings from studies of other exposure-based treatments of prolonged grief (Boelen et al., 2007; Mawson et al., 1981).

Comparison of CFBT with other grief treatments

It is worth comparing CFBT with some other cognitive and exposure-based treatments used with prolonged grief cases to illustrate the differences in their focus. For example, a recent randomized controlled study (Shear et al., 2005) compared interpersonal psychotherapy with complicated grief treatment (CGT) in non-trauma-exposed people with prolonged grief. The latter treatment involved cognitive interventions, imaginal

exposure, and live exposure. The treatment was administered in mean 16 sessions (range 7–19) in mean 19.4 weeks. In this study CGT was more effective than interpersonal psychotherapy. The overall response rate according to the CGI was 51%. A response rate of 82% based on the same measure in our study (Başoğlu et al., 2003) reviewed in the previous section suggests that a treatment focus on grief behaviors is sufficient for improvement. This is also consistent with other studies (Mawson et al., 1981) showing that exposure alone is sufficient in achieving improvement in grief.

Further support for this point comes from another study (Boelen et al., 2007), which not only used a more focused approach in treatment but also compared cognitive restructuring with exposure treatment. In this study 54 bereaved persons with complicated grief were assigned to one of three treatment conditions: six sessions of cognitive restructuring and six sessions of exposure treatment (CR + ET), these two conditions administered in reverse order (ET + CR), and six sessions of supportive counseling. Both active treatments were superior to supportive counseling, while the ET + CR condition was better than CR + ET. Comparing ET versus CR alone, six sessions of ET led to more improvement than six sessions of CR and adding ET to CR contributed more to improvement than adding

CR to ET. Moreover, dropout rates were higher in the CR condition. The percentage of reduction in the total scores of the 19-item version of the Inventory of Complicated Grief (Prigerson et al., 1995) at follow-up in the CR + ET group was 27% in intent-to-treat analyses and 44% in completer analyses. The respective figures for the ET + CR group were 39% and 48%, respectively. The effects sizes yielded by ET + CR at post-treatment in completer and intent-to-treat analyses (1.80 and 1.29, respectively) were comparable to the respective figures of 1.64 and 1.35 reported by Shear et al. (2005). This study also suggests that exposure treatment is more effective than cognitive restructuring in treating grief symptoms, though this finding needs replication in other studies. It is also worth recalling at this point studies of PTSD (Foa and Rauch, 2004; Paunovic and Öst, 2001), which showed that exposure treatment leads to cognitive change, even when cognitions are not targeted by specific cognitive restructuring techniques. Finally, it is also worth noting that CFBT differs from both treatments described by Shear et al. (2005) and Boelen et al. (2007) in not involving imaginal exposure. Yet, an improvement rate of 82% in our study (Başoğlu et al., 2003) suggests that equally good results can be obtained using live exposure alone. Imaginal exposure could be used exceptionally in cases with difficulty in initiating self-exposure.

Concluding remarks

In this chapter we presented a brief assessment strategy for grief designed to assist care providers to identify survivors in need of treatment after mass trauma events. The grief scales provided here are by no means in their finalized form and more work is needed to examine their usefulness in other survivor populations. Available psychometric data suggest that some GAS items are redundant and the scale could be shortened by omitting them. Nevertheless, we provided the entire set of items as an item pool for readers who might want to explore their cross-cultural validity. It is also worth noting that many of the cognitive items of the scale are not directly relevant to behavioral treatment. As noted earlier, The BCG is more useful in this respect and easier to validate across cultures.

The preliminary evidence pointing to the efficacy of CFBT in prolonged grief is consistent with findings from other studies showing that exposure-based interventions are useful in treating prolonged grief (Boelen et al., 2007; Mawson et al., 1981). Consistent with similar findings from our treatment studies of traumatic stress, this evidence also suggests that a treatment focusing solely on grief-related behaviors is also likely to improve cognitive symptoms of grief. Moreover, live exposure alone appears to be sufficient for improvement, and imaginal exposure, which is a fairly elaborate technique that relies heavily on therapist skills, may not be needed as a first-line intervention in grief treatment. An intervention that relies primarily on self-exposure not only requires less therapist involvement in therapy but is also suitable for dissemination on a self-help basis. This is indeed why we included a grief treatment module in the second version of our self-help manual (Appendix C).

References

Başoğlu, M., Kılıç, C., Şalcıoğlu, E. and Livanou, M. (2004). Prevalence of posttraumatic stress disorder and comorbid depression in earthquake survivors in Turkey: An epidemiological study. *Journal of Traumatic Stress*, **17**, 133–141.

Başoğlu, M., Livanou, M., Şalcıoğlu, E. and Kalender, D. (2003). A brief behavioural treatment of chronic post-traumatic stress disorder in earthquake survivors: Results from an open clinical trial. *Psychological Medicine*, **33**, 647–654.

Başoğlu, M., Şalcıoğlu, E. and Livanou, M. (2002). Traumatic stress responses in earthquake survivors in Turkey. *Journal of Traumatic Stress*, **15**, 269–276.

Başoğlu, M., Şalcıoğlu, E., Livanou, M., Özeren, M., Aker, T., Kılıç, C. and Mestçioğlu, Ö. (2001). A study of the validity of a Screening Instrument for Traumatic Stress in Earthquake Survivors in Turkey. *Journal of Traumatic Stress*, **14**, 491–509.

Beck, A. T., Rush, A. J., Shaw, B. F. and Emery, G. (1979). *Cognitive Therapy of Depression*. New York: Guilford Press.

Blake, D. D., Weathers, F. W., Nagy, L. M., Kaloupek, D. G., Charney, D. S. and Keane, T. M. (1990). *Clinician-Administered PTSD Scale (CAPS): Current and Lifetime Diagnostic Version*. Boston, MA: National Center for Posttraumatic Stress Disorder, Behavioral Science Division.

Boelen, P. A., De Keijser, J., Van Den Hout, M. A. and Van Den Bout, J. (2007). Treatment of complicated grief: A comparison between cognitive-behavioral therapy and supportive counseling. *Journal of Consulting and Clinical Psychology*, **75**, 277–284.

Foa, E. B. and Rauch, S. A. M. (2004). Cognitive changes during prolonged exposure versus prolonged exposure plus cognitive restructuring in female assault survivors with posttraumatic stress disorder. *Journal of Consulting and Clinical Psychology*, **72**, 879–884.

Guy, W. (1976). *ECDEU Assessment Manual for Psychopharmacology: Publication ADM 76–338* (DHEW Publ No ADM 76–338). National Institute of Mental Health, US Department of Health, Education, and Welfare, 218–222.

Livanou, M., Başoğlu, M., Şalcıoğlu, E. and Kalender, D. (2002). Traumatic stress responses in treatment-seeking earthquake survivors in Turkey. *Journal of Nervous and Mental Disease*, **190**, 816–823.

Mawson, D., Marks, I. M., Ramm, L. and Stern, R. S. (1981). Guided mourning for morbid grief: A controlled study. *The British Journal of Psychiatry*, **138**, 185–193.

Mundt, J. C., Marks, I. M., Shear, M. K. and Greist, J. H. (2002). The Work and Social Adjustment Scale: A simple measure of impairment in functioning. *British Journal of Psychiatry*, **180**, 461–464.

Paunovic, N. and Öst, L.-G. (2001). Cognitive-behavior therapy vs exposure therapy in the treatment of PTSD in refugees. *Behaviour Research and Therapy*, **39**, 1183–1197.

Prigerson, H. G., Maciejewski, P. K., Reynolds, C. F., Bierhals, A. J., Newsom, J. T., Fasiczka, A., Frank, E., Doman, J. and Miller, M. (1995). Inventory of complicated grief: A scale to measure maladaptive symptoms of loss. *Psychiatry Research*, **59**, 65–79.

Prigerson, H. G., Shear, M. K., Jacobs, S. C., Reynolds, C. F., 3rd, Maciejewski, P. K., Davidson, J. R., Rosenheck, R., Pilkonis, P. A., Wortman, C. B., Williams, J. B., Widiger, T. A., Frank, E., Kupfer, D. J. and Zisook, S. (1999). Consensus criteria for traumatic grief: A preliminary empirical test. *The British Journal of Psychiatry*, **174**, 67–73.

Rosenblatt, P. C. (2008). Grief across cultures: A review and research agenda. In *Handbook of Bereavement Research and Practice: Advances in Theory and Intervention*, ed. M. S. Stroebe, R. O. Hansson, H. Schut and W. Stroebe. Washington, DC: American Psychological Association, 207–222.

Şalcıoğlu, E., Başoğlu, M. and Livanou, M. (2003). Long-term psychological outcome for non-treatment-seeking earthquake survivors in Turkey. *Journal of Nervous and Mental Disease*, **191**, 154–160.

Şalcıoğlu, E., Başoğlu, M. and Livanou, M. (2007). Post-traumatic stress disorder and comorbid depression among survivors of the 1999 earthquake in Turkey. *Disasters*, **31**, 115–129.

Shear, K., Frank, E., Houck, P. R. and Reynolds, C. F., 3rd (2005). Treatment of complicated grief: A randomized controlled trial. *Journal of the American Medical Association*, **293**, 2601–2608.

An overview of treatment efficacy and mechanisms of recovery

In this chapter we review the evidence from a series of five treatment studies that tested the effectiveness of several variants of Control-Focused Behavioral Treatment (CFBT) and discuss the possible role of sense of control in recovery from traumatic stress. These studies altogether involved 339 earthquake survivors. Also worth noting is the fact that we used CFBT in our routine outreach care delivery to more than 6000 survivors in Turkey, about 1500 of whom were people who sought treatment from our community center in the disaster region. Thus, the study findings reviewed in the chapter were replicated in a much larger survivor population than the samples of these studies. These studies are presented in chronological sequence with a brief review of the various considerations that led to each study. Also reviewed in this chapter are the differences of CFBT from other exposure treatments.

An open trial of control-focused behavioral treatment

The first study that tested CFBT was an open clinical trial (Başoğlu et al., 2003b), which was launched 8 months after the earthquake at a time when occasional aftershocks were still occurring. It involved 231 survivors with traumatic stress symptoms, 167 (72%) of whom had PTSD. In an effort to develop an intervention that could be delivered with as little therapist time as possible, this study was designed to examine the minimum number of sessions required for significant clinical improvement. Accordingly, treatment duration was flexible and the sessions were discontinued when significant clinical improvement occurred. The survivors were given a mean of 4.3 (SD = 2.6) treatment sessions. Exposure tasks were defined in relation to most socially disabling avoidance behaviors (e.g. staying alone at home, entering concrete buildings, etc.). The initial treatment sessions lasted about 90 minutes, while the subsequent sessions were delivered in 45 minutes. Figure 6.1 shows the probability of improvement after each session based on a survival analysis.

Among survivors with PTSD, the probability of improvement was 76% after one session and 88% after two sessions, reaching 100% after four sessions. Significant clinical improvement in this study corresponded to a reduction of mean 57% in PTSD symptoms, 69% in avoidance behaviors, 50% in depression symptoms, and 71% in assessor-rated work and social disability. The mean number of sessions required for improvement was 1.7. All PTSD and depression symptoms improved, suggesting a 'patholytic' treatment effect. The percentages of improvement ranged from 74% to 77% for the re-experiencing symptoms (symptom rated as absent), 79% to 86% for the avoidance / numbing symptoms, 64% to 83% for the hyperarousal symptoms, and 71% to 85% for the depression symptoms. No baseline variable (including severity of trauma, PTSD, and depression) predicted treatment outcome due to little variability in the outcome measures. Improvement was maintained in 74 of 75 survivors who had 3- to 9-month follow-up, despite ongoing threat to safety caused by aftershocks and expectations of another major earthquake, suggesting increased resilience against earthquake-related traumatic stress.

Exposure treatment is thought to be less effective in reducing the 'negative' symptoms of PTSD, such as amnesia, emotional numbing, and detachment (Keane et al., 1989). Our findings did not support this view. Of particular interest was the treatment effect on psychogenic amnesia. To confirm this finding, we conducted in-depth interviews with about 10 participants of this study and found that reduction in fear and traumatic stress was indeed accompanied by significant recovery of lost memories relating to various aspects of the trauma.

In this study 80 (35%) survivors received psychotropic drugs in addition to CFBT, including sertraline (n = 43), fluoxetine (n = 11), and others (n = 26).

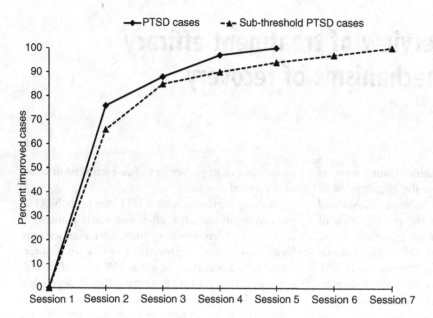

Figure 6.1 Cumulative proportion of improved cases in cases with PTSD and sub-threshold PTSD.

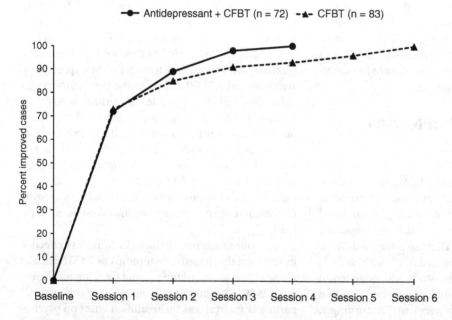

Figure 6.2 Cumulative probability of improvement with CFBT alone and CFBT combined with antidepressant treatment.

Antidepressants were used only for depression with serious suicidal intent. In cases where severe depression undermined motivation for psychological treatment, CFBT was started after a few weeks of drug treatment. Care was taken to maintain a therapeutic dose for 6 months, whenever possible. Figure 6.2 shows the cumulative probability of improvement

(based on a survival analysis) in survivors who received antidepressants in addition to CFBT, compared with those who received only CFBT. The analysis included only survivors that met the diagnosis of PTSD (eight excluded due to missing data).

Figure 6.2 shows no substantial differences between the drug and non-drug groups in the cumulative proportion of improved cases. Additional antidepressant treatment did not speed up recovery, despite the fact that 47% of the survivors met the diagnosis of comorbid depression. This was because improvement in both PTSD and depression occurred in the CFBT only group within 3–4 weeks before the drug effect reached its maximum. Although this finding does not imply drug ineffectiveness, it suggests that antidepressant treatment is not a useful addition to CFBT, even in cases with comorbid depression, because of relatively rapid recovery achieved by CFBT.

Although this study showed that CFBT could be confidently delivered in one or two sessions, it was unclear as to whether the survivors would have improved as much after a single treatment session, if they knew that they were not going to see the therapist again for monitoring and review of progress. This was an important question, given that many survivors were not able to attend treatment more than once due to increased demographic mobility after the disaster, daily survival problems, and economic difficulties. This issue was addressed in a randomized controlled clinical trial (Başoğlu et al., 2005) of a single session of CFBT.

A randomized controlled trial of single-session CFBT

This study involved 59 participants with chronic PTSD and was launched 30 months after the earthquake. The participants were recruited from among the residents of two housing sites built for homeless survivors and self-referrals to our community care center in the epicenter region. All survivors had high levels of earthquake exposure. The treatment was delivered in a single session lasting about 60 minutes. In an effort to limit the participants' expectations from treatment to a single session, they were informed that they would receive only one treatment session and subsequent contacts would be for assessment only. Subsequent follow-up sessions were limited to assessment only (by a staff member other than the therapist) and no further self-exposure instructions were given.

Although treatment compliance was not systematically measured in this study, follow-up assessments of progress made it clear that 90% of the participants complied with self-exposure instructions. Significant treatment effects were found on all measures at post-treatment, with self-rated global improvement rates of 49% at week 6, 80% by week 12, 85% by week 24, and 83% by 1–2-year follow-up. Much of the improvement

occurred during the first 12 weeks and stabilized thereafter. At the final follow-up assessment (1–2 years in most cases, last observation carried forward) fear and avoidance reduced by 69%, paralleled by 59% reduction in PTSD symptoms. All PTSD and depression symptoms showed significant improvement. As in the previous study, the relapse rate was very low, with only one survivor losing treatment gains during follow-up. This study showed that CFBT could be effectively delivered in a single session, without the usual monitoring component of traditional behavior therapy (e.g. reinforcement, verbal praise, troubleshooting, diary-keeping, setting of new homework exposure tasks, etc.).

In our review of the learning theory model of traumatic stress in Part 1 we had hypothesized that 'risk-taking' behaviors, such as not avoiding feared situations, reduce helplessness responses, thereby leading to recovery from traumatic stress. This formulation implied a certain sequence of events during the improvement process. If the intervention (e.g. treatment rationale and encouragement for risk-taking behaviors) enhances sense of control over fear, then the first change event one would expect early in treatment is *reduced behavioral avoidance* of feared situations. Second, if there is an association between reduced behavioral avoidance (which implies increased sense of control), then one would expect a generalized effect of reduced avoidance on all other traumatic stress responses, including PTSD and depression. We tested these hypotheses by examining which symptoms improved first early in treatment (e.g. at week 6) (Şalcıoğlu et al., 2007). Among all PTSD symptoms, behavioral avoidance was the only symptom that showed a significant between-group treatment effect at week 6. Significant improvement in the other PTSD symptoms appeared at subsequent follow-up assessments, reaching a maximum at week 24. Recovery rates (symptom absent) at week 24 ranged from 60% to 89% for the majority of the PTSD symptoms, indicating generalized improvement. Compared to those who recovered from behavioral avoidance, those who still had the symptom at week 24 were more likely to have intrusive memories, nightmares, distress upon reminders, physiological reactivity, avoidance of trauma-related thoughts, loss of interest, hypervigilance, startle, insomnia, memory and concentration difficulty, emotional numbing, and detachment. Thus, improvement in 12 PTSD symptoms was associated with improvement in avoidance. Compared to avoidant survivors, those who recovered from avoidance showed twice as much reduction in total Clinician-Administered PTSD Scale (CAPS; Blake et al., 1990) scores (excluding behavioral and cognitive avoidance symptoms). These findings clearly supported the critical role of reduced behavioral avoidance in recovery from helplessness and associated traumatic stress responses. Although helplessness responses (or sense of control over fear) were not directly measured in this study, the strong associations among fear, avoidance, helplessness, and hopelessness responses documented in Chapter 1 suggest that reduced avoidance most probably indicated enhanced sense of control over fear in this study. This is also supported by the fact that depressive symptoms as measured by the Beck Depression Inventory (Beck et al., 1979) reduced by 51% at week 24. The possible role of increased sense of control in improvement with CFBT will be discussed further later in this chapter.

An experiment with Earthquake Simulation Treatment

Although the first two studies found high rates of global improvement with one or two sessions of CFBT, the extent of reduction in PTSD symptoms was about 60% in both studies, suggesting that the survivors still had some residual symptoms. Furthermore, in the second study, participants with more severe fear, PTSD, depression, and social disability improved less, mainly because of their difficulty in conducting self-exposure. Thus, it appeared that the intervention fell short of providing sufficient encouragement for self-exposure in survivors with initially higher levels of illness severity. In a further effort to maximize the effectiveness of the behavioral treatment program, an experiment was conducted with 10 survivors who had PTSD according to CAPS to examine whether exposure to simulated earthquake tremors (*Earthquake Simulation Treatment*) would enhance sense of control over fear and thereby facilitate subsequent self-exposure to fear cues (Başoğlu et al., 2003a). This experiment was inspired by our observations of panic responses in survivors to earthquake-like shaking or ground vibrations, such as those created by passing trucks in locations close to highways. In addition, as noted in Chapter 1, people with previous experience of such shaking movements (e.g. sailors) showed less fear responses to aftershocks and more rapid reduction in fear with repeated exposures to aftershocks. These findings suggested that simulated unconditioned stimuli (i.e. earthquake tremors) could

be used as fear cues in exposure treatment to enhance sense of control over real earthquake tremors.

Earthquake Simulation Treatment was described in detail in Chapter 4. The sessions lasted one hour, starting with the lowest intensity level and going one level up as the survivor gained sense of control over the tremors. About 80% of the treatment session time was spent at the lowest intensity levels (corresponding to approximately 3- to 4-magnitude tremors on the Richter scale). Treatment was terminated when the survivor felt in control of his/her anxiety or distress. After the session, no specific self-exposure instructions were given so that the effect of the treatment session alone on sense of control could be examined in the long term. It was hypothesized that the intervention alone (without therapist encouragement and instructions for self-exposure to feared situations) would achieve sufficient decrease in helplessness responses, thereby reducing behavioral avoidance of earthquake reminders and other traumatic stress reactions.

Assessment conducted immediately after session termination revealed substantial reduction in anticipatory fear of earthquakes and distress associated with trauma memories. Assessments at weeks 2, 4, 8, and 12 showed a steady decrease in avoidance of feared situations, resulting in 66% reduction in total Fear and Avoidance Questionnaire (FAQ) scores at the last follow-up. This was paralleled by 71% reduction in PTSD and 66% reduction in depression symptoms. Eight survivors were markedly and two slightly improved at week 12 according to a self-rated global improvement scale.

These findings were important in suggesting that exposure to simulated earthquake tremors was highly effective in reducing behavioral avoidance. The fact that avoidance was reduced without any therapist instructions for self-exposure reflected increased sense of control over fear. A greater reduction in PTSD symptoms than in the previous two studies also attested to the potency of the intervention. This implied that adding a component of live exposure to single-session CFBT was likely to enhance the effectiveness of the latter, particularly in survivors with difficulty in initiating self-exposure.

A randomized controlled trial of Earthquake Simulation Treatment

The effectiveness of a combined approach using a single session of exposure to simulated earthquake tremors and self-exposure instructions was examined in a randomized controlled study (Başoğlu et al., 2007) involving 31 survivors with chronic PTSD. The study sample was drawn from the same population of earthquake survivors with high trauma exposure as in the previous studies. The study was launched about 4 years after the earthquake. Between-group treatment effects were examined at week 8, after which the control group was crossed over to receive the same treatment.

Treatment was delivered in two steps. At the first step the treatment and its rationale were explained, exposure tasks were defined, and self-exposure instructions were given. The second step involved Earthquake Simulation Treatment. The participants were informed that this intervention was designed to enhance their sense of control over earthquake tremors and also to demonstrate to them how they can overcome their fears. The session was conducted in the same way described earlier (mean session duration 33 minutes, SD = 18, range 9–70 minutes).

Assessment at post-session indicated that 30 of the 31 participants rated the session as fairly to very similar to their experience of the August 17 earthquake. This finding is of interest because 29 of the participants experienced simulated tremors at levels lower than 4, which corresponded to a magnitude of about 6 on the Richter scale. Nevertheless, most survivors found the tremors very similar to the August 17 earthquake, which had a magnitude of 7.4. We had originally thought that the magnitude of the simulated earthquake was likely to be a critical factor in perceived similarity to the original earthquake experience (and thus in improvement) but we were wrong. Higher tremor magnitudes were required in only two survivors, who did not experience significant distress at levels lower than 4.

Thirty participants found the experience fairly to very useful and felt satisfied with the treatment. Eighteen (72%) participants reported marked to very much reduction in their anticipatory fear of future earthquakes. The treatment effects at week 8 were significant on all measures of fear, PTSD, depression, and self- and assessor-rated global improvement. Clinically significant improvement rates (Jacobson and Truax, 1991) were 52% at week 4, 72% at week 12, 92% at week 24, and 92% at 1–2-year follow-up. Among the improved cases at week 12, only one showed relapse during further follow-up.

In this study treatment effect on sense of control was measured by a Sense of Control Scale (SCS;

Appendix A) with five items tapping change in fears, sense of control over feared situations, and courage, self-confidence, and belief about ability to cope in feared situations, each rated on a 0–3 scale (0 = no change or worsening, 3 = much increased/decreased). The mean SCS scores (range 0–15) ranged from 8.3 (SD = 3.6) at week 4 to 11 (SD = 4.1) at 1–2-year follow-up, indicating marked to much increase in sense of control over fears. The SCS correlated significantly with reduction in CAPS scores at all follow-up assessments, thus evidencing an association between increased sense of control and improvement in PTSD. Increased sense of control also meant enhanced resilience, as suggested by the fact that 11 of the 13 survivors who experienced an earthquake some time after the treatment reported much less fear than usual during the tremors.

A meta-analytic comparison of studies of CFBT

Table 6.1 shows a comparison of findings across the four studies in terms of percentage of improvement in clinical ratings, effect sizes, and the rates of global improvement. In all studies treatment had a patholytic effect on all problem areas (including impairment in work, social, and family functioning) reducing not only fear and PTSD but also depression. The effect sizes on the PTSD measures were larger in the studies involving Earthquake Simulation Treatment than in studies of self-exposure alone. Compared with self-exposure instructions alone, combined treatment achieved greater reduction in PTSD (59% vs. 79%, respectively) and better end-state functioning, with greater improvement in symptoms of irritability, loss of interest, nightmares, distress related to trauma reminders, emotional numbing, sense of foreshortened future, sleeping difficulty, and memory / concentration difficulty (Başoğlu et al., 2007). Unlike in Study 2, pre-treatment illness severity did not predict treatment outcome, suggesting enhanced treatment effects in cases with high pre-treatment anxiety.

Comparison of CFBT with other treatments for PTSD

Figure 6.3 shows a comparison of mean effect size in the four studies of CFBT with those reported in a

Table 6.1 Effect sizes in clinical trials of Control-Focused Behavioral Treatment[a]

	Study 1[b] (n = 143)	Study 2[c] (n = 51)	Study 3[d] (n = 10)	Study 4[e] (n = 25)
Clinician Administered PTSD Scale	–	1.80	2.58	3.51
Traumatic Stress Symptom Checklist	1.92	1.95	2.59	–
Fear and Avoidance Questionnaire	1.97	1.90	2.07	2.29
Beck Depression Inventory	1.22	1.13	1.56	2.47
Work and Social Adjustment – Assessor	1.84	–	–	2.91
Work and Social Adjustment – Self	1.35	1.19	–	–

[a] Cohen's d at last assessment available.
[b] Self-exposure instructions (mean 4.3 sessions). Analyses based only on cases with PTSD to allow comparison with the other studies.
[c] Single-session CFBT involving self-exposure instructions.
[d] Single-session of Earthquake Simulation Treatment.
[e] Single-session CFBT combined with Earthquake Simulation Treatment.

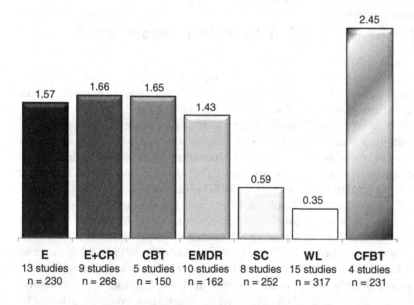

Figure 6.3 Comparison of control-focused behavioral treatment with other treatments in mean treatment effect sizes. E = Exposure treatment; E + CR = Exposure and cognitive restructuring; CBT = Cognitive-behavior therapy; EMDR = Eye movement desensitization and reprocessing; SC = Supportive Counselling; WL = Waiting list; CFBT = Control-focused behavioral treatment.

meta-analysis (Bradley et al., 2005) of trauma-focused intervention studies in PTSD. For this comparison we selected treatment protocols that were more commonly used in intervention trials. The mean effect size on PTSD in studies of CFBT was substantially larger than the mean effect sizes reported for other treatments. It is also worth noting that the effect sizes for other interventions reflect outcome in participants who completed a given treatment. The effect size for CFBT, on the other hand, is based on the more conservative last-observation-carried-forward approach which includes all cases whether or not they completed treatment. In other studies the average length of treatment was 15.64 hours (SD = 10.52), ranging from 3 to 52 hours, compared to 60 minutes for CFBT and 120 minutes for CFBT combined with Earthquake Simulation Treatment (excluding assessment).

It is worth noting that these comparisons are unlikely to reflect differences in severity of PTSD across samples, given that a mean CAPS score of 66 in Study 2 and 63 in Study 4 was similar to those in some studies (e.g. 58 in Ehlers et al., 2003 and 63 in the exposure group of Marks et al., 1998). Although these scores were lower than those reported in some other studies (e.g. 69 in Bryant et al., 2003; 71 in Tarrier et al., 1999; 80 in Schnurr et al., 2003; 98 in Paunovic and Öst, 2001), CFBT was effective in cases with CAPS scores up to 92 in Study 4. It is worth noting that CAPS scores between 60 and 79 reflect severe PTSD, while scores above 80 means extremely severe PTSD, according to the CAPS score ranges proposed by Weathers et al. (2001) for interpreting severity of PTSD.

The findings reviewed so far highlight the potency of an intervention that focuses solely on fear and avoidance. It is important to clarify an important issue at this point to avoid a common misunderstanding about CFBT. As is evident from the studies reviewed so far, therapist-delivered CFBT has three variants: (1) full-course CFBT delivered on average in four sessions, (2) single-session CFBT, and (3) single-session CFBT combined with therapist-assisted exposure. The term 'single-session CFBT' sometimes leads to the incorrect impression that the improvement achieved by the intervention occurs *within* the session. When the session does not include therapist-delivered exposure, CFBT is a self-administered intervention and the therapist's role is limited to explaining the treatment rationale and conveying sufficient sense of control to enhance motivation for treatment. What actually accounts for improvement in traumatic stress in the long term is active efforts on the part of the client after the session (or between sessions, if the treatment involves multiple sessions) to confront feared situations and, consequently, reduced behavioral avoidance. Thus, the initial session merely initiates a self-help process the therapeutic effects of which take about 3 months to reach a maximum. The following section provides more evidence concerning the self-help element in treatment.

CFBT delivered through a self-help manual

The role of self-instigated exposure in natural recovery from trauma was discussed in Part 1 of this book. The treatment studies demonstrated that the impediment in natural recovery process caused by helplessness responses could be overcome by simple encouragement for self-exposure in a brief session. These findings implied that the intervention could be as effectively delivered through media other than a therapist (e.g. self-

help manuals), provided that the essential elements of therapy are adequately conveyed to survivors. Despite these encouraging results, however, there were some challenges in developing a self-help tool. As is common knowledge to experienced behavior therapists, the most difficult task in exposure treatment is to engage the patient in the idea of exposure to feared situations and ensure compliance with treatment. Indeed, about 30% of patients with anxiety disorders either refuse or drop out from exposure treatment, even when the intervention is delivered by a therapist (Marks, 2002). In some cases substantial discussion with the client might be necessary to identify and overcome helplessness cognitions, convey self-confidence, and mobilize motivation for change. The interactive nature of the therapist–patient relationship can be of critical importance in such cases. Furthermore, effective explanation of the treatment rationale requires some persuasive discourse and this is best achieved through personal contact with the person. Unquestioning obedience to the authority of care providers (e.g. "*doctor knows what's best for me*") in some cultures may also facilitate this process. Thus, developing a stand-alone self-help tool that is capable of achieving the same cognitive and motivational impact of one hour of therapist contact poses a major challenge. This might indeed explain in part why stand-alone self-help tools for anxiety disorders are extremely rare (Newman et al., 2003). It might also explain two failed attempts (Ehlers et al., 2003; Scholes et al., 2007) to demonstrate the usefulness of self-help in PTSD.

We have explored this issue by developing a highly structured self-help manual (Appendix C) that closely paralleled the treatment program used in Study 1. It consisted of six sections providing information on (1) PTSD and depression symptoms, (2) self-assessment using the Traumatic Stress Symptom Checklist, (3) principles of treatment and suitability for treatment, (4) self-assessment of fear and avoidance behaviors using the FAQ and instructions on how to define exposure tasks, (5) administering self-exposure sessions, blocking cognitive or behavioral avoidance or distraction strategies, coping with anxiety, panic or flashbacks, monitoring fear cues, and dealing with problems encountered during the first week of treatment, and (6) evaluating progress in treatment, defining new

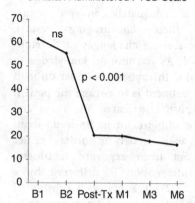

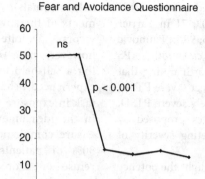

Figure 6.4 Treatment response to a self-help manual. B1 = Baseline 1; B2 = Baseline 2; Post-Tx = Post-treatment; M1 = 1-month follow-up; M3 = 3-month follow-up; M6 = 6-month follow-up.

exposure tasks, and dealing with problems encountered during the subsequent weeks of treatment.[1] The highly structured nature of the manual allowed its use as a 'stand-alone' treatment tool with minimal or no therapist contact.

Although we did not have an opportunity to test the manual in a randomized controlled study, we conducted a series of eight single-case experimental studies to examine whether the manual effectively delivered the treatment rationale, instigated self-exposure, and provided sufficient guidance throughout the treatment among survivors who read it. The study design included two baseline assessments separated by 1 month of waiting period, followed by the delivery of the manual. Post-treatment assessment was at week 10 and subsequent follow-ups were at 1, 3, and 6 months post-treatment. The mean CAPS and FAQ scores before and after treatment are shown in Figure 6.4.

The CAPS scores showed only mean 10% improvement during the baseline period, which was not significant. This is similar to the improvement rates we observed during the 6 and 8 weeks of waiting periods in our controlled studies reviewed earlier. It is also worth noting that this study was conducted 4.5 years after the earthquake with survivors who had chronic PTSD. A substantial reduction was noted in all ratings from the second baseline to post-treatment, ranging from

63% to 73%. Treatment effects were significant on all measures, with effect sizes at the last assessment on the CAPS (Cohen's d = 2.12), FAQ (Cohen's d = 2.62), and Work and Social Adjustment Scale (Cohen's d = 2.65) comparable to those achieved by therapist-delivered treatment (see Table 6.1). About 70% reduction was noted in behavioral avoidance and PTSD symptoms, with 91% improvement in work, social, and family adjustment. Using the criterion (Jacobson and Truax, 1991) of 2 SD or more improvement since baseline, 7 (88%) cases showed improvement in PTSD. At the same assessment 7 (88%) cases achieved good end-state functioning, which was defined as a CAPS total score of 19 or less indicating absence of PTSD (Weathers et al., 2001). This study suggested that the manual could be a useful means of delivering treatment after an initial assessment. Preliminary evidence from a pilot study (reviewed in Chapter 7) suggested that it might also be useful in some cases as a stand-alone self-help tool when distributed in the community without therapist contact.

Treatment studies with children

The effectiveness of CFBT in children was tested in a pilot study (Şalcıoğlu and Başoğlu, 2008) involving 23 school age children with PTSD at 20 months post-disaster. Treatment was delivered twice-weekly in groups across six sessions after a variable waiting period ranging from 1 to 18 weeks. While no significant improvement was found during the waiting period, the children showed 50% reduction in PTSD and 55% reduction in earthquake-related fears at post-treatment. These findings suggested that CFBT has promise in treatment of child earthquake

---

[1] This description pertains to the first version of the manual that we tested in the field. The manual provided in Appendix C is a revised, shortened, and streamlined version of the original. It also includes a module on treatment of prolonged grief, which was not included in the first version.

survivors. This is not surprising, given that earthquake-induced PTSD in children is mediated by the same process as in adults, i.e. loss of control over fear. Thus, encouraging children to overcome their fear through self-exposure facilitates their recovery from post-traumatic stress. Children relate very well to the rationale of the treatment (e.g. 'beat fear') and generally display greater compliance with self-exposure instructions than do adults.

The therapeutic effects of exposure to feared situations in children were indeed observed in another pilot study (Şalcıoğlu and Başoğlu, 2008) involving Earthquake Simulation Treatment. This study involved a series of eight multiple-baseline experimental case studies with four boys and four girls (aged 8 to 13) treated in the same session. While no significant improvement was noted during an initial 2 to 5 weeks of waiting period, both fear and PTSD symptoms showed 52% reduction at 1–2-month post-treatment follow-up. On a self-rated global improvement measure, 5 children (63%) reported much / very much improvement, 2 slight improvement and 1 no change. Parental assessment indicated similar improvement in school and family functioning.

Mechanisms of recovery: anxiety reduction or increased sense of control?

The findings reviewed so far might not come as a surprise to behavior therapists who have long known the important role of avoidance in anxiety disorders. We have long known from previous research that avoidance is often associated with overall illness severity in anxiety disorders (Başoğlu et al., 1988; Başoğlu et al., 1994b) and reduction in avoidance through exposure treatment leads to improvement in most patients with anxiety disorders (Marks and Dar, 2000), including PTSD. What needs explaining, however, is the high potency of an intervention that focuses solely on fear and behavioral avoidance. This becomes a compelling question in the light of its efficacy comparable to that of other relatively more intensive and lengthy exposure-based treatments, even when delivered in a single session. Could this be explained by the treatment focus on sense of control rather than on habituation? Phrased differently, does a treatment focus on sense of control achieve better results than a focus on habituation? The ideal way of

addressing this question would be a direct comparison between CFBT and traditional exposure treatment. Such a study has not yet been conducted. However, several alternative approaches might also be informative in this regard. For example, one might address the question whether increase in sense of control over fear can occur without reduction in fear during exposure. If increase in sense of control and habituation are not two sides of the same coin, then demonstrating the relative independence of the two phenomena would also be informative. Furthermore, one could also examine the relative contributions of increased sense of control and habituation in anxiety to general improvement (or a subjective sense of well-being) as reported by patients.

Habituation is the waning of a defensive response on repeated stimulation (Marks, 1987). It is a universal phenomenon that exists not only in humans but also in sub-human species in the phylogenetic scale, including the invertebrates (Marks, 1987). For example, a snail retreats into its shell when touched on the head but habituates to this stimulus with repeated touching and ceases to respond. Based on the extinction model of anxiety reduction, Marks (1987) argued that exposure should continue until substantial anxiety reduction occurs. Newer emotional processing models of fear reduction (Foa and Kozak, 1986; Foa and McNally, 1996) posit that the initial fear response and the extent of fear reduction within and across exposure sessions are indicators of successful emotional processing that determine the outcome of exposure therapy. A recent review of the processes of change in exposure treatment (Craske et al., 2008) found no conclusive evidence to suggest an association between treatment outcome and the intensity of initial fear and the extent of fear reduction during and between sessions. The authors concluded that within-session habituation appears to be mediated by mechanisms that are different from those responsible for long-term outcomes.

Habituation may not necessarily result in an increase in sense of control, unless exposure is conducted as a motivation-driven effort aimed at achieving control over fear and the outcome is attributed to personal efforts (e.g. "I did it all by myself without any help") and generalized to future encounters with similar stressors (e.g. "I will be able to deal with similar situations in the future"). Evidence from a study (Marks et al., 1993) of exposure and alprazolam treatment of panic disorder and agoraphobia indeed supports this point. In this study patients received either alprazolam or placebo combined with either exposure treatment or relaxation as a psychological placebo. Psychological treatments were terminated at week 8 and drug taper took place between week 8 and week 16. Blindness as to the drug condition was maintained until the end of the taper period. Patients who had improved at week 8 were given a Tablet Attributions Questionnaire that measured their treatment attributions, sense of control over their problem, and expectations of coping without treatment. The effect of sense of control on long-term outcome was thus examined using a prospective design. At post-treatment improved patients who attributed the reduction in their anxiety to the tablets were more likely to relapse during withdrawal of medication than those who attributed their improvement to their own personal efforts during exposure treatment (Başoğlu et al., 1994a). During the taper period some patients were anxious to find out whether they were on active drug or placebo so that they could decide whether it was the drug or exposure treatment that helped them. Interestingly, having to face such uncertainty until the end of the taper period, some of them even restarted their exposure exercises (without any encouragement from their therapist), just in case their tablets turned out to be placebo at the end of the trial.

These findings are supported by a more recent study (Powers et al., 2008) of the effects of attributional processes concerning medication-taking on return of fear following exposure treatment. In this study 95 participants with claustrophobic fears were randomly allocated to 1-session exposure-based treatment, the latter combined with a placebo pill, psychological placebo, waitlist conditions. Attributions concerning tablet-taking were manipulated by further assignment of participants in exposure plus pill condition to one of three instructional sets immediately following completion of treatment and post-treatment assessment. These included presenting the pill as (1) a sedating herb that likely made exposure treatment easier, (2) a stimulating herb that likely made exposure treatment more difficult, and (3) a placebo with no effect on exposure treatment. Thirty-nine percent of the participants who received the first instructional set experienced a return of fear, compared to 0% in the other two conditions. Return of fear in the first condition was mediated by attributions of anxiety reduction to the pill. The study also found that return of fear was mediated by low self-efficacy.

These studies highlight the critical role played by sense of control in recovery from fear. They also demonstrate that fear reduction can occur without increased sense of control as a result of attributional processes. Thus, the final destination in the path to recovery from anxiety appears to be increased sense of control, rather than habituation. It is worth noting that the role of sense of control in maintaining improvement in the long term was also demonstrated in a further study involving patients with PTSD treated with exposure treatment, cognitive restructuring, and their combination (Livanou et al., 2002).

Marks and Dar (2000) noted that sense of control might be a result rather than cause of fear reduction. Several other lines of evidence suggest that this is unlikely. Most importantly, we know from considerable evidence from animal and human literature that manipulations of control (an independent variable) are causally related to fear (see reviews by Başoğlu and Mineka, 1992; Mineka and Zinbarg, 2006). In other words, fear is the outcome of loss of control and not vice versa. This is further supported by the evidence presented in Part 1 of this book pointing to the role of uncontrollability of stressors in fear and related stress responses. Second, there is no conclusive evidence pointing to an association between fear reduction and outcome of exposure treatment (Craske et al., 2008). Third, although sense of control and fear are correlated phenomena, they are also independent of each other to a certain extent. This means that a person can experience intense fear without necessarily losing control. Indeed, in our study (Şalcıoğlu, 2004) 76% of the survivors experienced high levels of fear during the earthquake but only 40% lost total control. Similarly, in our studies of war and torture survivors, although more loss of control was generally associated with more intense anxiety during trauma, the ratings of loss of control were generally lower than the ratings of anxiety intensity (e.g. see Table 2.3), suggesting that high levels of anxiety can be experienced without substantial loss of control. Resilient political activists, for example, despite not experiencing much loss of control, experienced as much anxiety as less resilient survivors in response to certain forms of torture involving physical pain. The relative independence between sense of control and fear also means that fear reduction could occur without any increase in sense of control (e.g. when fear reduction is attributed to external factors or mediated through safety signals) and, conversely, sense of control could increase without any reduction in fear. We have observed the latter in some torture survivors, who showed no fear reduction during the first exposure session but nevertheless reported a dramatic increase in their sense of control for eventually having been able to confront a debilitating fear that had plagued them for so long. The relative independence of sense of control and fear reduction is also implied by study findings (Emmelkamp and Mersch, 1982; Rachman et al., 1986) showing that phobic patients improve even when they are allowed to terminate an exposure session before complete fear reduction occurs. Conversely, additional exposure trials after complete fear reduction does not produce better outcomes than partial fear reduction in a single exposure trial (Rachman and Lopatka, 1988) and complete fear reduction does not necessarily prevent a return of fear (Rachman et al., 1987).

Perhaps one of the most informative studies with regard to the nature of the association between fear reduction and sense of control is the alprazolam / exposure treatment study of panic disorder and agoraphobia by Marks and colleagues (1993) reviewed above. In that study we demonstrated four subgroups of patients with different treatment outcomes with respect to extent of improvement in panics and behavioral avoidance: (a) no improvement in panic or avoidance, (b) improvement in avoidance but not in panics, (c) improvement in panics but not in avoidance, and (d) improvement in both panic and avoidance (Başoğlu et al., 1994b). The presence of the first and fourth sub-groups shows that fear and avoidance (an indication of lack of sense of control over fear) are highly interrelated in some cases. The second group shows that sense of control can increase without a reduction in fear. [Prospective monitoring of daily anxiety levels and panics in the same study sample showed that most panic episodes were cued by prior elevated levels of general anxiety and anticipatory fear (Başoğlu et al., 1992). Thus, the term fear in this discussion refers not only to recurring panics but also to high anxiety levels and anticipatory fear between panics.] The third group, on the other hand, demonstrated that fear reduction can occur without an increase in sense of control. Moreover, patients who improved in avoidance but not in panics were more likely to rate themselves as improved than those who improved in panics but not in avoidance. This shows that improvement in avoidance or increased sense of control has greater significance for a person than a

reduction in fear. This implies that the critical variable accounting for recovery (when defined as a subjective sense of well-being) is increased sense of control over the problem. Fear reduction appears to be neither necessary nor sufficient for recovery.

In their review of the shortcomings of the exposure principle, Marks and Dar (2000) noted that habituation does not explain the rapid improvement in some phobic patients who report no fear or avoidance from their first exposure session or why fear declines with other interventions not involving exposure, such as hypnosis, reassuring information, and placebo tablets. In reviewing the possible therapeutic ingredients common to various treatments (e.g. exposure, cognitive restructuring, coping skills training, problem-solving, stress immunization, mindfulness meditation, etc.), they posed the question *"How many roads to the Rome of fear reduction?"* Perhaps the questions they rightly raised about habituation might be more easily addressed if we search for the roads to the Rome of increased sense of control rather than habituation.

Turning to the findings from our treatment studies with earthquake survivors, it might be worth summarizing various lines of evidence in support of sense of control as the primary factor in improvement. Study 4 (self-exposure instructions + Earthquake Simulation Treatment) demonstrated significant treatment effects on sense of control, as measured by the Sense of Control Scale. Increased sense of control also strongly correlated with reduction in PTSD. Second, in Study 2 (self-exposure instructions alone) behavioral avoidance was the first symptom to improve early in treatment, reflecting increased sense of control, followed by improvement in other PTSD symptoms. Third, exposure to simulated earthquake tremors resulted in reduced behavioral avoidance without any self-exposure instructions from the therapist (Study 3). Fourth, in all four studies the treatment improved not only PTSD but also depression, consistent with the learning theory model of traumatic stress reviewed in Part 1. Finally, the treatment appeared to enhance resilience against the traumatic effects of earthquakes. Relapse rates were remarkably low in our studies (only three cases relapsed after significant improvement), despite the fact that some study participants were exposed to further earthquakes after treatment. In Study 4, 11 of the 13 survivors who experienced an earthquake some time after the treatment reported much less fear (and less loss of control) than usual during the tremors. Such immunization effects reflect learning of control over stressors (Williams and Maier, 1977).

Another factor that might have contributed to sense of control is minimal therapist involvement in treatment. As noted earlier, a single-session intervention with no further therapist involvement means that the treatment is largely administered on a self-help basis. This might enhance sense of control by facilitating attributions of improvement to personal efforts, rather than to a therapist or other external factors, such as changes in various life circumstances. This is consistent with evidence showing that internal attributions of control consolidate treatment effects and reduces the risk of relapse in trauma survivors (Livanou et al., 2002).

Lack of compliance with exposure treatment in some patients is a problem well known to behavior therapists. Indeed, Marks (2002) noted that non-compliance rates (e.g. refusal of treatment and drop-out) reached 30% among patients with anxiety disorders receiving therapist-delivered exposure treatment in outpatient settings. Non-compliance rates were less than 10% in our studies, even when the treatment was delivered in a single session without subsequent monitoring of progress and reinforcement. This might reflect the motivation-enhancing effects of the argument behind the treatment rationale (i.e. *fight your fear to take control over your life or surrender and live the rest of your life in misery and despair*). Such discourse instills courage, self-confidence, and hope in survivors and prompts them to take action against fear. The powerful nature of such discourse (frequently used by political leaders, army commanders, or leaders of political activists groups) is illustrated by the fact that it can make people engage in activities that pose a serious threat to life (e.g. combat, political activism in repressive regimes) or even involve certain death (e.g. Kamikaze pilots in World War II, suicide bombers of today). These examples highlight the fact that cognitive and behavioral control over fear is possible even in the face of real threat to safety.

The contribution of Earthquake Simulation Treatment to the effectiveness of self-exposure instructions might also be explained by its powerful impact on sense of control. This intervention involves exposure to unconditioned stimuli (e.g. earthquake tremors), albeit in simulated form, as well as distressing trauma memories. It essentially reconstructs the original uncontrollable stressors experienced during a real earthquake (e.g. a moving physical environment, sounds of moving objects, disturbing effects of tremors on vestibular system, postural control, proprioception, etc.) and thus provides opportunities for developing sense of control over a wide range of stressor cues and emotional responses evoked by them. Such exposure is likely to have a much more potent impact on sense of control than exposure to mere reminders of the trauma or conditioned fear cues that generalize to a variety of objects (e.g. clothes worn during the earthquake), situations (e.g. enclosed spaces), or activities (e.g. turning off the light when going to bed). Indeed, the impact of the intervention can be observed in survivors' responses to real earthquakes. While traumatized survivors typically show panic responses during earthquakes (e.g. some senselessly jumping out of windows during even mild earthquakes, breaking limbs or seriously injuring themselves), treated survivors often report no loss of control, despite some (reduced) fear during the event. This is indeed consistent with evidence (Mineka et al., 1999; Mystkowski et al., 2002; Rodriguez et al., 1999) showing that fear extinction is more stable when a person is treated by exposure in a context that more closely resembles the context in which fear acquisition occurred. In addition, an experience of the original uncontrollable earthquake stressors in a controllable environment where the stressors can be initiated or stopped at will might reduce perceived uncontrollability of earthquake tremors, perhaps leading to an illusion of control over them. This might explain in part the dramatic reduction in anticipatory fear of future earthquakes observed immediately after the session.

In closing this section it is also worth noting that sense of control is different from the concept of self-efficacy (Bandura, 1997) defined as belief that one's actions are likely to lead to generally positive outcomes. While there may be some overlap between the two concepts, we understand self-efficacy as a belief in one's ability to control outcomes of adverse events in general, whereas sense of control refers to belief in one's ability to control outcomes of *specific* stressor events. Thus, self-efficacy involves a generalized belief about control, while sense of control might vary from one stressor situation to another, depending on the extent of one's previous learning experiences with these (or similar) stressor situations. Accordingly, we have always measured sense of control in relation to specific stressor situations in our research work, because it is a more reliable predictor of helplessness anxiety than generalized beliefs about control in our experience. This distinction between self-efficacy and sense of control is important in understanding the basic principles of CFBT.

Control-Focused Behavioral Treatment: a new intervention or a variant of Exposure Therapy?

Given that CFBT relies heavily on exposure in reducing trauma-induced helplessness, the reader might be left wondering whether it is a new treatment or simply a variant of exposure therapy. Although some of the ways in which CFBT differs from exposure treatment are evident from its description in Chapter 4, a more systematic overview of this issue might be helpful, particularly for readers with less experience with behavioral treatment. First of all, to avoid a semantic confusion, we should note that we use the term 'exposure' throughout the book to denote a *process* or *procedure* through which certain treatment aims are achieved and not as a description of a whole treatment program.

It is reasonable to argue that a treatment for a given problem is distinct from other interventions to the extent that it is different in its (a) aims, (b) mechanisms of action, (c) techniques, and (d) procedures. Table 6.2 provides a comparison between CFBT and exposure treatment with respect to these criteria. We have chosen two common applications of exposure treatment for comparison, i.e. prolonged exposure by Foa and colleagues (2007) and exposure treatment by Marks and colleagues (1998). The details of exposure treatments have been obtained from the authors' treatment protocols. As CFBT is readily distinguishable from cognitive treatments (e.g. those used by Ehlers et al., 2005 and Resick and Schnicke, 1993) in not involving cognitive restructuring, the latter treatments are not included in Table 6.2 for comparison.

Aims in treatment

CFBT fundamentally differs from both cognitive and exposure treatments in its aim. As noted earlier, the latter treatments are aimed at anxiety reduction, whereas CFBT is designed to enhance anxiety tolerance and sense of control over traumatic stressors (i.e. resilience).[2] Resilience is a complex phenomenon that is difficult to define and operationalize. In this book

we approached this concept from a learning theory perspective, conceptualizing it as the ability to exert active control over stressor events using cognitive and / or behavioral strategies to avert the stressor event, lessen its harmful consequences, reduce associated distress, or simply tolerate anxiety when it cannot be avoided. The latter is as important as other forms of control, as people often encounter stressor events over which no other form of control is possible. This is indeed one of the reasons why treatment needs to focus on anxiety tolerance, rather than on anxiety reduction.

Resilience-building through exposure to anxiety or distress is not a novel concept, given the many examples of this process in eastern philosophical or religious thinking. For example, Buddhist training (or life style) involves elements of exposure to austere conditions and actively promotes mental control and / or tolerance of suffering. Such resilience training might well explain findings of low traumatic stress rates in Tibetan monks subjected to torture (Holtz, 1998). Examples of austerity training can also be observed in the Mevlevi Order of Islamic Sufism, where its members (i.e. dervishes) undergo, as part of their spiritual training, a 40-day period of solitary confinement in a very small enclosed space (which allows only a very uncomfortable squatting position), fasting, and praying. This process is termed 'çile doldurmak' in Turkish, which means 'to undergo a 40-day novitiate involving torment and suffering' in Mevlevi terminology. Similar resilience-building strategies are also used in the training of soldiers, commandos, special forces, or political activists. Consider, for example, the SERE (Survival, Evasion, Resistance, and Escape) program used in the training of some military personnel in the United States, which involves controlled exposure to

---

[2] CFBT can be distinguished from other treatments not just in its theoretical framework but also in its philosophical approach to the human emotion of anxiety. Anxiety reduction as an ultimate aim in therapy reflects a puritanistic view of anxiety in western cultures as an emotion that needs to be eradicated at all costs to promote human 'happiness.' Accordingly, western mental healthcare institutions have translated this puritanistic view of anxiety into a multi-billion dollar pharmaceutical industry and various schools of thought in psychotherapy, most of which strive to reduce anxiety using different methods, rather than searching for ways of enhancing people's resilience against it. It is also worth noting in this connection that the quest for anxiety reduction also ultimately serves a political purpose in preserving a certain social order by keeping the 'revolutionary' potential of anxiety under control. Try imagining social order in a society that employs no form of control over anxiety!

Table 6.2 Comparison of Control-Focused Behavioral Treatment with other exposure-based treatments

	Prolonged Exposure (Foa et al., 2007)	Exposure Therapy (Marks et al., 1998)	CFBT
Aim	Anxiety reduction	Anxiety reduction	Enhancement of resilience against anxiety
Primary method used	Prolonged exposure to anxiety cues	Prolonged exposure to anxiety cues	Exposure to anxiety cues
Presumed mechanism of improvement (treatment rationale)	Habituation and emotional processing of trauma	Habituation / Extinction of conditioned anxiety	Enhanced anxiety tolerance and sense of control
Treatment Techniques:			
Live exposure	YES	YES	YES
Imaginal exposure	YES	YES	NO
Cognitive restructuring	NO	NO	NO
Anxiety management techniques	Breathing retraining	NO	NO
Other techniques	YES[1]	NO	YES[2]
Therapist involvement in administration of treatment techniques	YES	YES	Only when needed with treatment non-compliers
Treatment Procedures:			
Number of sessions	9	10	Variable (range 1–12 sessions)
Fear hierarchy construction	YES	YES	NO
Treatment target setting	NO	YES	NO
Homework exercises (exposure or other)	YES	YES	YES in full-course CFBT NO in single-session CFBT
Diary keeping	YES	YES	NO
Monitoring of progress	YES	YES	YES in full-course CFBT NO in single-session CFBT
Prescribed frequency of live exposure	Daily	Daily	Variable, depending on client's needs
Duration of live exposure sessions	30–45 min or until anxiety is reduced by 50%	60 min	Variable / Until sense of control develops
Within-session anxiety ratings	YES	YES	NO
Conditions for ending live exposure sessions	Significant anxiety reduction	Significant anxiety reduction	Increased anxiety tolerance and control / anxiety reduction not essential

[1] Psychoeducation, brief cognitive intervention at the end of imaginal exposure session in the form of discussion and processing of traumatic memory.
[2] When necessary, CFBT may prescribe massed practice, behavioral activation for depression, and problem-solving or any other behaviors likely to increase sense of control over life.

'torture-like' procedures with a view to increase resilience against brutal interrogation techniques or torture. The underlying idea in these examples is the same: to expose a person to stressor events in a controlled fashion and environment until they learn to tolerate and control distress.

Aiming for anxiety tolerance and control is also consistent with recently emerging views of what works with exposure treatments. In view of lack of consistent evidence on the association between anxiety reduction and treatment outcome, Craske and colleagues (2008) suggested a shift from immediate fear reduction to fear toleration as a primary goal of exposure therapy. Although the role of increased sense of control in improvement achieved by cognitive and behavioral treatments has been acknowledged by some authors (e.g. Barlow, 2002), no attempts have yet been made to maximize the efficacy of these treatments by shifting their focus from anxiety reduction to enhancement of anxiety tolerance and sense of control. It is indeed such a theoretical shift that primarily distinguishes CFBT from traditional exposure-based treatments.

It might be argued that cognitive and behavioral treatments may also enhance sense of control through anxiety reduction and thus overlap with CFBT in their mechanism of action. Although this is quite possible, increased sense of control through anxiety reduction may not be the same outcome as learning to tolerate and control anxiety for reasons discussed earlier in this chapter. Helping someone realize that their expectations of danger were unrealistic (cognitive restructuring) does not necessarily make them more resilient, given that such change implies hardly anything about their capacity to tolerate and control anxiety in situations involving realistic threat to safety. In such situations, setting anxiety reduction as the ultimate goal in exposure treatment may also not have the desired impact on sense of control, unless the person is motivated to confront the feared situation without any expectations of anxiety reduction. Furthermore, because these interventions do not have a sharp focus on sense of control, whatever impact they might have on sense of control might be coincidental and thus erratic, incomplete, and unstable.

Primary treatment method and presumed mechanism of action

Both exposure treatment and CFBT rely on exposure to anxiety cues for achieving improvement. Exposure treatment, however, involves prolonged exposure until anxiety reduction or habituation occurs, whereas exposure in CFBT does not necessarily have to be prolonged and conducive to anxiety reduction. The differences in their presumed mechanisms of action also determine the way their rationale is explained to the clients. Exposure treatment focuses on habituation (e.g. *"Your anxiety will diminish if you stay in the feared situation"*), whereas CFBT emphasizes anxiety tolerance and control over its impact on important life functions (e.g. *"You will learn to tolerate anxiety by confronting it and gain control over your life"*). Accordingly, the discourse used in explaining the rationale of CFBT is specifically geared towards reducing helplessness responses, instilling hope and courage, and enhancing motivation to confront feared situations. In addition, the differences in their aims imply different definitions of successful treatment outcome. Success is defined as anxiety reduction in exposure treatment, with the implication that exposure not resulting in sufficient reduction in anxiety would be regarded as failure. CFBT, on the other hand, defines success as ability to tolerate anxiety and 'liberation' from its debilitating effects on life functioning, regardless of the extent of reduction in anxiety.

Treatment techniques

Exposure treatments involve both live and imaginal exposure, whereas CFBT involves only live exposure for reasons explained in Chapter 4 and Chapter 8. Therapist involvement in CFBT is minimal, as live exposure is self-administered in most cases. The therapist's role is limited to assessment, explanation of the treatment rationale, teaching clients how to conduct self-exposure, and prescribing self-exposure instructions. As such, it is a largely self-help intervention. Additional therapist involvement (i.e. therapist-assisted exposure and monitoring of progress) is required only in a minority of cases that do not comply with self-exposure instructions given in the first session.

Treatment procedures

Traditional exposure treatments involve 9 or 10 sessions. CFBT does not involve a pre-determined number of sessions. In earthquake survivors it involves a single session in most cases and an additional few sessions in cases that do not respond to the initial session. Treatment duration is thus variable, ranging from 1 to 4 sessions in most cases, depending on the treatment response. Our clinical experience with war and torture survivors suggests that up to 12 sessions might be needed in severe cases with depression, though evidence from case studies (see Chapter 9) also shows that a few sessions of CFBT achieve similar levels of improvement early in treatment. This issue remains to be explored further in future research.

Exposure treatments often involve fear hierarchy construction (i.e. a hierarchical ordering of exposure tasks from the least to the most anxiety-evoking), whereas in CFBT selection of exposure tasks is often left to the discretion of the survivor. Graduated exposure is used only when a person experiences difficulty in tackling a particular task. CFBT also differs from exposure treatments in involving a relatively less structured approach. For example, in the Marks and colleagues' (1998) protocol treatment focuses usually on four main treatment targets that represent the most functionally disabling problems (e.g. '*to be able to stay alone at home*'). Once these targets are defined, then exposure homework tasks are set. Exposure tasks define specific activities that are required to achieve the treatment targets (e.g. '*To stay alone at home for 2 hours during early evening*'). In addition, the clients are asked to keep a diary, regularly recording the executed tasks and rating their anxiety before and after exposure sessions. The diary is then reviewed every week and new tasks are set as treatment progresses. Treatment needs to involve multiple targets, because anxiety reduction in one situation may not necessarily generalize to another. This approach is not used in CFBT, simply because it does not aim for anxiety reduction in as many feared situations as possible. Hence, it does not involve various procedures, such as treatment target setting, monitoring of anxiety during exposure by obtaining within-session anxiety ratings, or diary keeping. Exposure tasks are utilized as a process by which anxiety tolerance and control can be achieved. Prolonged exposure to anxiety cues is not prescribed, as brief exposures until sense of control develops are deemed sufficient. Exposure sessions can be terminated when sufficient sense of control develops, regardless of the extent of anxiety reduction.

In CFBT self-exposure instructions are of a general nature, designed to normalize daily life routines (e.g. encouraging survivors not to avoid feared situations as they are encountered in daily life), and combined with instructions for more focused exposure exercises designed for maximum treatment impact on sense of control. A more structured approach involving focused exposure exercises, monitoring sessions, and therapist assistance in exposure exercises is used only in cases that do not respond to the initial intervention.

In conclusion, exposure delivered with the framework of CFBT is distinct from exposure treatment in its underlying theory, aims, presumed mechanisms of action, and treatment techniques and procedures. On the other hand, it might also be regarded as involving a modified version of exposure treatment, the efficacy of which is enhanced by a theoretical shift in its focus. Given that both arguments have some validity, decision on this issue is left to the reader's judgment.

Concluding remarks

The evidence of treatment effectiveness reviewed in this chapter needs to be evaluated within the broader framework of the literature evidence pertaining to the effectiveness of exposure-based interventions in anxiety disorders. Despite its differences from exposure treatments reviewed above, CFBT utilizes the same potent therapeutic process as traditional exposure treatments, i.e. exposure to anxiety cues. Relative to habituation-based exposure treatments, it appears to have an enhanced potency, though this remains to be confirmed by future comparative studies. Nevertheless, such comparisons aside, the potency of an intervention with a sole focus on anxiety tolerance and sense of control, even when delivered in a single session, requires an explanation. This is an important question that will need to be addressed by anxiety researchers and cognitive and behavior therapists.

The evidence reviewed here needs to be evaluated bearing in mind that CFBT was derived from the learning theory formulation of traumatic stress presented in Part 1. This formulation maintains that helplessness responses that block natural recovery in trauma survivors can be overcome by an intervention designed to enhance sense of control over anxiety. Generalized improvement in all traumatic stress reactions with such an intervention is consistent with causal associations among helplessness, PTSD, depression, and social disability hypothesized by this formulation. Thus, the evidence presented supports not only the efficacy of the intervention but also its underlying theoretical framework. The fact that the intervention prompted high rates of treatment compliance and recovery when delivered in a single session is consistent with evidence pointing to an evolutionarily determined readiness in humans to utilize risk-taking behaviors in overcoming fear. The implications of these findings for an effective mental healthcare model for mass trauma survivors will be reviewed in Part 3.

References

Bandura, A. (1997). *Self-efficacy: The Exercise of Control*. New York: Freeman.

Barlow, D. H. (2002). *Anxiety and its Disorders: The Nature and Treatment of Anxiety and Panic*. New York: Guilford Press.

Başoğlu, M., Lax, T., Kasvikis, Y. and Marks, I. M. (1988). Predictors of improvement in obsessive-compulsive disorder. *Journal of Anxiety Disorders*, **2**, 299–317.

Başoğlu, M., Livanou, M. and Şalcıoğlu, E. (2003a). A single session with an earthquake simulator for traumatic stress in earthquake survivors. *American Journal of Psychiatry*, **160**, 788–790.

Başoğlu, M., Livanou, M., Şalcıoğlu, E. and Kalender, D. (2003b). A brief behavioural treatment of chronic posttraumatic stress disorder in earthquake survivors: Results from an open clinical trial. *Psychological Medicine*, **33**, 647–654.

Başoğlu, M., Marks, I. M., Kılıç, C., Brewin, C. R. and Swinson, R. P. (1994a). Alprazolam and exposure for panic disorder with agoraphobia: Attribution of improvement to medication predicts subsequent relapse. *British Journal of Psychiatry*, **164**, 652–659.

Başoğlu, M., Marks, I. M., Kılıç, C., Swinson, R. P., Noshirvani, H., Kuch, K. and O'Sullivan, G. (1994b). Relationship of panic, anticipatory anxiety, agoraphobia and global improvement in panic disorder with agoraphobia treated with alprazolam and exposure. *British Journal of Psychiatry*, **164**, 647–652.

Başoğlu, M., Marks, I. M. and Şengün, S. (1992). A prospective study of panic and anxiety in agoraphobia with panic disorder. *British Journal of Psychiatry*, **160**, 57–64.

Başoğlu, M. and Mineka, S. (1992). The role of uncontrollable and unpredictable stress in posttraumatic stress responses in torture survivors. In *Torture and its Consequences: Current Treatment Approaches*, ed. M. Başoğlu. Cambridge: Cambridge University Press, 182–225.

Başoğlu, M., Şalcıoğlu, E. and Livanou, M. (2007). A randomized controlled study of single-session behavioural treatment of earthquake-related posttraumatic stress disorder using an earthquake simulator. *Psychological Medicine*, **37**, 203–213.

Başoğlu, M., Şalcıoğlu, E., Livanou, M., Kalender, D. and Acar, G. (2005). Single-session behavioral treatment of earthquake-related posttraumatic stress disorder: A randomized waiting list controlled trial. *Journal of Traumatic Stress*, **18**, 1–11.

Beck, A. T., Rush, A. J., Shaw, B. F. and Emery, G. (1979). *Cognitive Therapy of Depression*. New York: Guilford Press.

Blake, D. D., Weathers, F. W., Nagy, L. M., Kaloupek, D. G., Charney, D. S. and Keane, T. M. (1990). *Clinician-Administered PTSD Scale (CAPS) – Current and Lifetime Diagnostic Version*. Boston: National Center for Posttraumatic Stress Disorder, Behavioral Science Division.

Bradley, R., Greene, J., Russ, E., Dutra, L. and Westen, D. (2005). A multidimensional meta-analysis of psychotherapy for PTSD. *American Journal of Psychiatry*, **162**, 214–227.

Bryant, R. A., Moulds, M. L., Guthrie, R. M., Dang, S. T. and Nixon, R. D. (2003). Imaginal exposure alone and imaginal exposure with cognitive restructuring in treatment of posttraumatic stress disorder. *Journal of Consulting and Clinical Psychology*, **71**, 706–712.

Craske, M. G., Kircanski, K., Zelikowsky, M., Mystkowski, J., Chowdhury, N. and Baker, A. (2008). Optimizing inhibitory learning during exposure therapy. *Behaviour Research and Therapy*, **46**, 5–27.

Ehlers, A., Clark, D. M., Hackmann, A., Mcmanus, F. and Fennell, M. (2005). Cognitive therapy for posttraumatic stress disorder: Development and evaluation. *Behaviour Research and Therapy*, **43**, 413–431.

Ehlers, A., Clark, D. M., Hackmann, A., Mcmanus, F., Fennell, M., Herbert, C. and Mayou, R. (2003). A randomized controlled trial of cognitive therapy, a self-help booklet, and repeated assessments as early interventions for posttraumatic stress disorder. *Archives of General Psychiatry*, **60**, 1024–1032.

Emmelkamp, P. M. and Mersch, P. P. (1982). Cognition and exposure in vivo in the treatment of agoraphobia: Short-term and delayed effects. *Cognitive Therapy and Research*, **6**, 77–90.

Foa, E. B., Hembree, E. A. and Rothbaum, B. O. (2007). *Prolonged Exposure Therapy for PTSD: Emotional Processing of Traumatic Experiences (Therapist Guide)*. New York: Oxford University Press.

Foa, E. B., and Kozak, M. J. (1986). Emotional processing of fear: Exposure to corrective information. *Psychological Bulletin*, **99**, 20–35.

Foa, E. B., and Mcnally, R. J. (1996). Mechanisms of change in exposure therapy. In *Current Controversies in the Anxiety Disorders*, ed. R. M. Rapee. New York: Guilford Press, 329–343.

Holtz, T. (1998). Refugee trauma versus torture trauma: A retrospective controlled cohort study of Tibetan refugees. *Journal of Nervous and Mental Disease*, **186**, 24–34.

Jacobson, N. S. and Truax, P. (1991). Clinical significance: A statistical approach to defining meaningful change in psychotherapy research. *Journal of Consulting and Clinical Psychology*, **59**, 12–19.

Keane, T. M., Fairbank, J. A., Caddell, J. M. and Zimering, R. T. (1989). Implosive (flooding) therapy reduces symptoms of PTSD in Vietnam combat veterans. *Behavior Therapy*, **20**, 245–260.

Livanou, M., Başoğlu, M., Marks, I. M., De Silva, P., Noshirvani, H., Lovell, K. and Thrasher, S. (2002). Beliefs, sense of control and treatment outcome in post-traumatic stress disorder. *Psychological Medicine*, **32**, 157–165.

Marks, I. and Dar, R. (2000). Fear reduction by psychotherapies: Recent findings, future directions. *The British Journal of Psychiatry*, **176**, 507–511.

Marks, I. M. (1987). *Fears, Phobias, and Rituals*. Oxford: Oxford University Press.

Marks, I. M. (2002). The maturing of therapy: Some brief psychotherapies help anxiety/depressive disorders but mechanisms of action are unclear. *The British Journal of Psychiatry*, **180**, 200–204.

Marks, I. M., Lovell, K., Noshirvani, H. and Livanou, M. (1998). Treatment of posttraumatic stress disorder by exposure and/or cognitive restructuring: A controlled study. *Archives of General Psychiatry*, **55**, 317–325.

Marks, I. M., Swinson, R. P., Başoğlu, M., Kuch, K., Noshirvani, H., O'Sullivan, G., Lelliott, P. T., Kirby, M., Mcnamee, G. and Şengün, S. (1993). Alprazolam and exposure alone and combined in panic disorder with agoraphobia: A controlled study in London and Toronto. *British Journal of Psychiatry*, **162**, 776–787.

Mineka, S., Mystkowski, J. L., Hladek, D. and Rodriguez, B. I. (1999). The effects of changing contexts on return of fear following exposure therapy for spider fear. *Journal of Consulting and Clinical Psychology*, **67**, 599–604.

Mineka, S. and Zinbarg, R. (2006). A contemporary learning theory perspective on the etiology of anxiety disorders: It's not what you thought it was. *American Psychologist*, **61**, 10–26.

Mystkowski, J. L., Craske, M. G. and Echiverri, A. M. (2002). Treatment context and return of fear in spider phobia. *Behavior Therapy*, **33**, 399–416.

Newman, M. G., Erickson, T., Przeworski, A. and Dzus, E. (2003). Self-help and minimal contact therapies for anxiety disorders: Is human contact necessary for therapeutic efficacy? *Journal of Clinical Psychology*, **59**, 251–274.

Paunovic, N. and Öst, L.-G. (2001). Cognitive-behavior therapy vs exposure therapy in the treatment of PTSD in refugees. *Behaviour Research and Therapy*, **39**, 1183–1197.

Powers, M. B., Whitley, D., Telch, M. J., Smits, J. A. J. and Bystritsky, A. (2008). The effect of attributional processes concerning medication taking on return of fear. *Journal of Consulting and Clinical Psychology*, **76**, 478–490.

Rachman, S., Craske, M., Tallman, K. and Solyom, C. (1986). Does escape behavior strengthen agoraphobic avoidance? A replication. *Behavior Therapy*, **17**, 366–384.

Rachman, S. and Lopatka, C. (1988). Return of fear: Underlearning and overlearning. *Behaviour Research and Therapy*, **26**, 99–104.

Rachman, S., Robinson, S. and Lopatka, C. (1987). Is incomplete fear-reduction followed by a return of fear? *Behaviour Research and Therapy*, **25**, 67–69.

Resick, P. A. and Schnicke, M. K. (1993). *Cognitive Processing Therapy for Rape Victims*. Newbury Park, CA: Sage.

Rodriguez, B. I., Craske, M. G., Mineka, S. and Hladek, D. (1999). Context-specificity of relapse: Effects of therapist and environmental context on return of fear. *Behaviour Research and Therapy*, **37**, 845–862.

Şalcıoğlu, E. (2004). *The effect of beliefs, attribution of responsibility, redress and compensation on posttraumatic stress disorder in earthquake survivors in Turkey*. PhD Dissertation. Institute of Psychiatry, King's College London, London.

Şalcıoğlu, E. and Başoğlu, M. (2008). Psychological effects of earthquakes in children: Prospects for brief behavioral treatment. *World Journal of Pediatrics*, **4**, 165–172.

Şalcıoğlu, E., Başoğlu, M. and Livanou, M. (2007). Effects of live exposure on symptoms of posttraumatic stress disorder: The role of reduced behavioral avoidance in improvement. *Behaviour Research and Therapy*, **45**, 2268–2279.

Schnurr, P. P., Friedman, M. J., Foy, D. W., Shea, M. T., Hsieh, F. Y., Lavori, P. W., Glynn, S. M., Wattenberg, M. and Bernardy, N. C. (2003). Randomized Trial of Trauma-Focused Group Therapy for Posttraumatic Stress Disorder: Results From a Department of Veterans Affairs Cooperative Study. *Archives of General Psychiatry*, **60**, 481–489.

Scholes, C., Turpin, G. and Mason, S. (2007). A randomised controlled trial to assess the effectiveness of providing self-help information to people with symptoms of acute stress disorder following a traumatic injury. *Behaviour Research and Therapy*, **45**, 2527–2536.

Tarrier, N., Pilgrim, H., Sommerfield, C., Faragher, B., Reynolds, M., Graham, E. and Barrowclough, C. (1999). A randomized trial of cognitive therapy and imaginal exposure in the treatment of chronic posttraumatic stress disorder. *Journal of Consulting and Clinical Psychology*, **67**, 13–18.

Weathers, F. W., Keane, T. M. and Davidson, J. R. T. (2001). Clinician-administered PTSD scale: A review of the first ten years of research. *Depression and Anxiety*, **13**, 132–156.

Williams, J. and Maier, S. (1977). Transsituational immunisation and therapy of learned helplessness in the rat. *Journal of Experimental Psychology: Animal Behavior Processes*, **3**, 240–252.

A mental healthcare model for earthquake survivors

The various theoretical and practical features of Control-Focused Behavioral Treatment (CFBT) reviewed so far offer prospects for a cost-effective mental healthcare model for mass trauma survivors. In this chapter we review possible methods of cost-effective treatment dissemination to survivors. Because the idea of this model was developed through work with earthquake survivors, it is described in relation to earthquake trauma. This chapter consists of three sections. The first section presents an outreach treatment delivery program that incorporates several applications of CFBT, including (1) treatment delivered through a self-help manual, (2) single-session treatment involving self-exposure instructions, (2) single-session treatment involving therapist-administered exposure, and (3) full-course treatment delivered on average in four sessions. The outreach program is an important component of the mental healthcare model, because it enables delivery of care to particular targeted survivor populations, such as people who seek refuge in shelters, communities in regions most affected by the disaster, schools, factories, work places, etc. The second section reviews prospects of treatment dissemination through self-help tools, lay therapists, and mass media. The final section includes an overview of a mental healthcare model that might be useful in facilitating recovery from trauma in large survivor populations.

An outreach treatment delivery program

The aim of this program is to allow delivery of the intervention to as many survivors as possible using a largely self-help approach with minimal therapist involvement, while sparing resources for interventions that require more therapist time. To illustrate how the program works, let us consider a targeted population of 1000 survivors in the community or a shelter. Figure 7.1 shows a flowchart of the various steps in disseminating treatment to this population.

The program entails sequential administration of various assessment and intervention procedures in ways that minimize assessor and therapist time, while maximizing the number of survivors receiving care. The first step is screening of the entire survivor population for needs assessment, using a screening instrument (e.g. Screening Instrument for Traumatic Stress in Earthquake Survivors – SITSES). Our studies showed that about 50% of earthquake and war survivors in the community either request help or are identified as potentially in need of help based on screening data (see Chapter 3). At Stage 1 single-session CFBT is delivered to these survivors individually or in groups together with the self-help manual. These two treatment tools are best used together, because the therapist-delivered session might increase the chances of the manual being utilized by survivors, while the guidance provided by the manual might make treatment easier to administer.

Six weeks after the delivery of the intervention, survivors are re-assessed using the screening instrument to identify likely non-responders. Although improvement after single-session intervention reaches a maximum in about 3 months, a good treatment response within the first 4 to 6 weeks (defined as minimum 40% reduction in Traumatic Stress Symptom Checklist – Earthquake Version scores and /or at least 'moderately improved' rating on the self-rated Global Improvement Scale; Appendix A) is a fairly reliable indicator of longer term outcome. An assessment in 6 weeks is thus useful in identifying likely non-responders for further treatment without losing more time. The most common reason for treatment failure at this stage is non-compliance with treatment instructions due to high levels of anxiety.

Stage 2 involves the delivery of a therapist-administered exposure session to help non-responders overcome initial anxiety that blocks the treatment

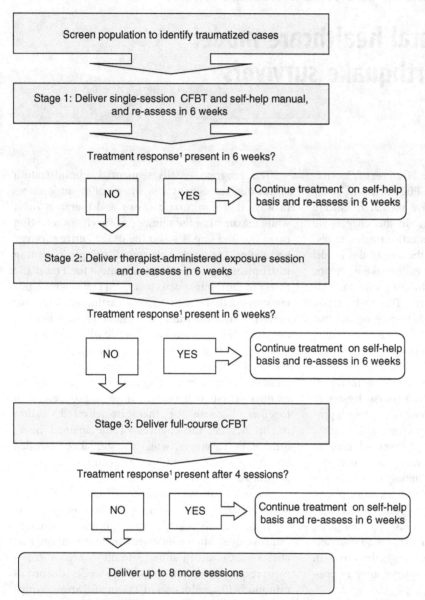

Figure 7.1 Flowchart of assessment and treatment procedures in outreach programs. CFBT = Control-Focused Behavioral Treatment. [1]Defined as at least 40% reduction in Traumatic Stress Symptom Checklist score and / or a moderately improved rating on the self-rated Global Improvement Scale.

process. In earthquake survivors we often used Earthquake Simulation Treatment for this purpose with an improvement rate of 90% (Başoğlu et al., 2007), though exposure could also involve trauma cues in the survivor's natural environment. In Chapter 4 we discussed how these trauma cues should be selected for therapist-aided exposure to maximize the latter's impact on survivors' sense of control. Once this session facilitates further self-exposure, treatment often progresses unhindered. Such cases can also be treated in groups.

Stage 3 involves full-course CFBT, which differs from single session interventions in involving a monitoring component, closer supervision of progress, and a more structured approach. The cases that improve after four sessions can be discharged from treatment and advised to continue with self-exposure exercises on their own. A follow-up assessment 3 months post-treatment, whenever possible, is useful in ascertaining good longer-term outcome. Non-responders to four-session CFBT continue to receive up to eight more sessions until recovery is achieved.

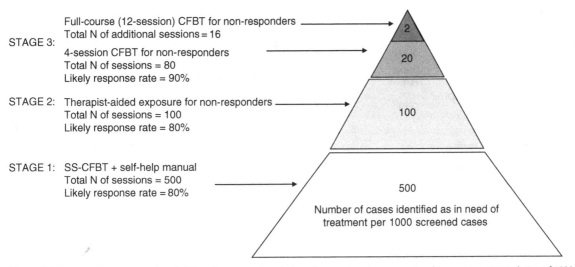

STAGE 3: Full-course (12-session) CFBT for non-responders
Total N of additional sessions = 16

4-session CFBT for non-responders
Total N of sessions = 80
Likely response rate = 90%

STAGE 2: Therapist-aided exposure for non-responders
Total N of sessions = 100
Likely response rate = 80%

STAGE 1: SS-CFBT + self-help manual
Total N of sessions = 500
Likely response rate = 80%

2

20

100

500
Number of cases identified as in need of
treatment per 1000 screened cases

Figure 7.2 Intervention stages and probability of recovery at each stage in an outreach program involving a survivor population of 1000. CFBT = Control-Focused Behavioral Treatment; SS-CFBT = Single-Session Control-Focused Behavioral Treatment.

Figure 7.2 illustrates the underlying concept of the program in a survivor population of 1000 by providing the number of therapist sessions and expected rates of recovery at each intervention stage. The numbers within the shaded parts of the pyramid indicate the likely treatment non-responders at each stage. Note that the total number of sessions and likely recovery rates at each stage are based on the assumptions that (a) treatment is delivered individually at all stages, (b) all survivors are available for treatment at each stage, and (c) all cases complete treatment at Stage 3. Evidence (Başoğlu et al., 2005b) shows that the likely response rate to single-session CFBT in 3 months is 80%. Thus, 400 cases are likely to improve at Stage 1, while 100 treatment non-responders would need Stage 2 treatment. The likely response rate to a single therapist-aided exposure session combined with self-exposure instructions at Stage 2 is also over 80% (Başoğlu et al., 2007). Thus, of the 100 treatment non-responders at Stage 1, 80 are likely to improve at this stage, while 20 would need full-course CFBT at Stage 3. When CFBT is delivered in 12 sessions evidence (Başoğlu et al., 2003) shows that 90% of the survivors improve after four sessions, while 10% need up to eight more sessions. This means that 18 of the 20 non-responders to Stage 2 intervention are likely to improve with four sessions of CFBT at Stage 3, while only two cases would require additional sessions. These figures suggest that only 4% of the survivors identified as in need of treatment through

screening during an outreach program (or 2% of all screened cases) would require full-course CFBT. The total number of therapist sessions required for 500 cases at all three stages is 696 or mean 1.4 sessions per case. These figures have important implications for cost-effective care delivery to large survivor populations.

Cost-effectiveness issues

The cost-effectiveness of CFBT is best evaluated in relation to other treatments reported to be effective. Table 7.1 compares CFBT with three other treatments commonly used with trauma survivors in terms of mean number of sessions required to deliver the treatment, cost per case, cost ratio relative to CFBT, and total cost of delivering treatment to 6000 survivors. The latter figure reflects the approximate number of earthquake survivors we treated during our outreach care delivery program in Turkey. Thus, the estimates provide a good idea about the relative costs of the four treatments when used as part of similar outreach programs. Information on mean number of sessions in CBT and EMDR is obtained from a meta-analysis of treatments for PTSD by Van Etten and Taylor (1998). As a study by Marks et al. (1998) showed that exposure treatment alone or combined with cognitive restructuring can be effectively delivered in eight sessions, this treatment (E+CR) is also included for comparison. Therapy sessions in all four

Table 7.1 Comparison of treatments for PTSD in therapist time costs

	Mean N of sessions per case	Cost per case[1] (USD)	Cost ratio relative to CFBT[2]	Cost per 6000 cases (USD)
CFBT	1.4	17.5	–	105 000
CBT	14.8	185	10.6	1 110 000
E + CR	8	100	5.7	600 000
EMDR	4.6	57.5	3.3	345 000

CFBT = Control-focused behavioral treatment; CBT = Cognitive-behavioral treatment; E + CR = Exposure + cognitive restructuring; EMDR = Eye Movement Desensitization and Reprocessing.
[1] Based on 1-hour therapist time cost in Turkey = $12.50 (average monthly psychologist salary of $2000 / 160 work hours per month).
[2] Obtained by dividing cost of each intervention by cost of CFBT.

treatments are assumed to last one hour in calculating the cost of therapist time per case. Also worth noting is that therapist time costs constitute about 70% of the total costs in such outreach programs.

As is evident from the cost ratios, the CFBT program is substantially more cost-effective than other interventions. It is 3.3 times less costly than EMDR, which is said to be the briefest intervention available for PTSD. We should note that the cost of CFBT per case is quite close to the actual therapist time cost of 32 USD per case in our outreach program in Turkey. The difference is due to the fact that the three-stage treatment model was not implemented in its present form from the outset; it evolved gradually over time as evidence pertaining to the usefulness of its various components became available.

The cost-effectiveness of the CFBT delivery model relative to other treatments could be increased further with various modifications in its components. The relatively simple nature of CFBT makes it easy to deliver in groups at all stages. In survivor shelters we usually delivered Stage 1 intervention in groups of 20 to 30 survivors. When the treatment is delivered in groups of 25 at Stage 1, the number of therapy sessions required at this stage can be reduced from 500 to 20. This means that 500 cases can be treated in a total of 216 sessions at the three stages; this yields a ratio of 0.43 sessions per case, thereby reducing the costs by 3.3-fold. Furthermore, Stage 1 intervention could also be delivered through self-help tools without any therapist involvement, if their usefulness as stand-alone tools

is established by future work. The model can also benefit from other dissemination methods discussed later in this chapter.

In this comparison we assumed equal efficacy for all four interventions. As discussed in Chapter 6 (see Figure 6.3), the mean effect size obtained by CFBT is higher than that achieved by most treatments for PTSD. Lower effect sizes mean more unimproved or partially improved cases with residual problems. Indeed, a meta-analysis of treatment studies of PTSD (Bradley et al., 2005) has shown that clinically significant PTSD symptoms persist in 47% of cases treated with exposure, 53% of cases treated with CBT, and 44% of cases treated with exposure and CBT, and 40% of cases treated with EMDR. The possible reasons for such partial treatment effects are discussed in Chapter 8. Partial improvement implies a greater likelihood of relapse, more future treatment costs, and further loss of work time and productivity. Such factors also need to be taken into account in estimating cost-effectiveness of interventions.

A further cost-effectiveness issue concerns the costs of training care providers. Current trauma treatments involve fairly elaborate procedures that rely heavily on therapist skills (e.g. cognitive restructuring, imaginal exposure, relaxation training, coping skills training, breathing training, thought stopping, guided self-dialogue, etc.) and thus require not only a certain amount of training by specialists but also additional supervision in the process of treatment delivery (Cahill et al., 2006). Aside from the problem of finding sufficient numbers of therapists for care of tens of thousands of people in the aftermath of a major disaster, such a training and supervision process is likely to incur substantial costs. Considering that CFBT is a relatively simple intervention that does not involve such elaborate procedures, dissemination of treatment knowledge to care providers is likely to be much easier and less costly.

Applications of CFBT in primary care and outpatient settings

Although the three-stage CFBT model is most likely to be used in outreach programs after disasters, it can also be implemented in primary care and outpatient settings. Although it is generally believed that trauma survivors usually do not seek help, our experience shows that this is not entirely true – at least for earthquake survivors. Of the total of about 6000 earthquake survivors who received treatment from us in 3 years, 27% actively sought help from our two community centers in the disaster region. This implies that primary and secondary care facilities may need to undertake a non-negligible portion of the task of disseminating care to disaster survivors.

The three-stage approach in treatment can be implemented in such settings in much the same way as illustrated in Figure 7.1, with one important difference. The self-help manual can be used as the first-line intervention without single-session CFBT in outpatient settings, as there is some preliminary evidence (Başoğlu et al., 2009) that about 50% of the survivors are likely to benefit from the manual when delivered after an initial contact with a therapist. Our experience has indeed shown that it is well worth giving the manual a try as the first-line intervention in outpatient settings and reserve therapist sessions for non-responders to self-help. After an initial brief assessment to establish suitability for self-help treatment, the manual can be delivered to survivors, advising them simply to read the manual and follow the instructions.

Alternative treatment dissemination methods

As any care provider with an experience of a devastating disaster would know, post-disaster circumstances necessitate treatment dissemination through every means possible. CFBT offers a variety of prospects in this respect, including dissemination through a wide range of health professionals, lay people, self-help tools, and mass media. We explored some of these dissemination methods and found them promising. Although more work is needed to establish their usefulness, a brief review of these methods here is worthwhile in pointing to directions for future research.

CFBT Delivery Manual

We prepared a CFBT Delivery Manual (see Appendix B) to facilitate treatment delivery by a wide range of health professionals, including psychiatrists, psychologists, general practitioners, nurses, social workers, and counselors with or without previous training in trauma work or behavior therapy. The manual is highly structured, providing step-by-step guidance in assessing traumatic stress problems and suitability for treatment, explaining the treatment and giving anti-avoidance instructions and homework exercises, evaluating and monitoring progress and dealing with problems in treatment, assessing and treating children, delivering treatment in groups in a single session, and assessing and treating prolonged grief.

The manual is written in as simple language as possible so that it can also be used by lay people with an adequate educational background (e.g. schoolteachers, army personnel, religious leaders, etc.). Our experience suggests that CFBT can be effectively delivered by lay people. While some survivors with severe traumatic stress problems (e.g. the tip of the pyramid in Figure 7.2) may require professional attention, what most survivors need is simple encouragement for overcoming fear. Many earthquake survivors who recover with treatment often pass on what they learned during treatment to their close ones, friends and neighbors, encouraging them not to avoid fear. To cite an example, an 8-year-old girl who was living in a survivor camp with her family and who had recovered after a single treatment session urged her father to overcome his fear of buildings so that the family could return home. She actually led him by hand several times to a building site where he practiced exposure and recovered. Similarly, many survivors who recovered using the self-help manual distributed copies of the booklet to their relatives, friends or neighbors and encouraged them to utilize it. These observations led us to recruit some recovered survivors as 'lay therapists' in survivor shelters. Some survivors who understood the treatment principles very well and who were motivated to help others were particularly suitable for this purpose. They went from tent to tent, encouraging and motivating people for self-exposure. Although treatment delivery by lay therapists remains to be explored more systematically, we believe that this dissemination method carries great potential after major mass trauma events.

Self-help manual

In Chapter 6 we reviewed the evidence regarding the usefulness of a self-help manual in delivering CFBT. When disseminated to survivors, the usefulness of a self-help manual needs to be judged according to two criteria: their *effectiveness rate* (proportion of improved users among those who read the manual and comply with treatment instructions) and their *benefit rate* (proportion of improved cases among those who receive the manual) (Başoğlu et al., 2009). Effectiveness rate is an indication of whether the intervention involves therapeutic elements and how successfully the manual delivers these elements to users, whereas benefit rate reflects not only the effectiveness of the manual but also the probability of it being read and utilized by the targeted survivor population when made available to them. Preliminary evidence suggests that when the manual is delivered after an initial assessment by the therapist, about 50% of the survivors are likely to read it and comply with instructions and, of these, over 80% are likely to recover. Although based on a small sample, this finding is important in showing that the manual delivers the treatment rationale effectively and prompts compliance with treatment instructions among survivors who read it.

We examined earthquake survivors' responses to the manual in a pilot study involving 84 survivors with PTSD who had taken part in an epidemiological study (Başoğlu et al., 2004). The manual was delivered by students to the survivors' homes with a brief information leaflet explaining its purpose (but not its content). A phone interview 3 months later found that 46 (55%) survivors read the manual, 36 (78%) found the treatment credible, and 22 (48%) complied with treatment instructions. Among the latter cases, 17 (77%) rated the manual as fairly to very satisfactory and 20 (91%) as recommendable to others and 19 (86%) rated themselves as improved on a global improvement scale, while 3 (13%) reported no change. Also worth noting is the fact that 35% of 20 survivors who found it recommendable to others actually gave copies of the manual to their friends and neighbors. Improvement did not significantly correlate with any demographic, trauma, or personal history characteristic. Among the 38 survivors who never read the manual, the reasons stated were 'did not have time' or 'neglected it' in 20 (61%), 'reminded me of the earthquake' in 2 (6%), 'interfering life events' in 3 (8%), 'lost the manual' in 3 (8%), 'concentration problems or reading difficulty' in 2 (6%), 'no problem with fear' in 1 (3%), and 'treatment with a booklet not possible' in 1 (3%) (data missing on 5 cases). Among the 24 survivors who read the manual but did not instigate self-exposure, the stated reasons were 'did not have time' in 6 (25%), 'treatment not convincing' in 5 (21%), 'prefer treatment by a therapist' in 4 (17%), 'no problem with fear' in 2 (8%), 'treatment likely to increase fear' in 2 (8%), and others (not interested, treatment not relevant to grief problem, did not read entire booklet) in 3 (1%) (data missing on 2 cases).

These findings suggest that in most cases the idea of a self-help treatment does not conflict with traditional expectations of treatment from a medical professional. Furthermore, the fact that neither reading the manual nor compliance with it related to age, gender, marital status, education, and intensity of exposure to trauma suggests these factors are not likely to influence its utilization rate.

These results suggest an effectiveness rate of 86% (19 improved cases among 22 treatment compliers) and a benefit rate of 23% (19 improved cases among 84 that received the manual). While the benefit rate may appear relatively low, its implications are better appreciated when extrapolated to tens or hundreds of thousands of survivors. It means that nearly one in four cases can be helped by simply distributing the manual in the community without any therapist contact. This proportion can be increased further by various means. For example, in outreach programs targeting survivor shelters or camps, the manual can be distributed to groups of survivors after a brief presentation and encouragement from a health professional or camp administrator. Furthermore, it can be distributed in the community with some media campaigning designed to encourage its use. It is also worth noting that the pilot study findings pertain to an earlier version of the manual, which was later shortened and streamlined for easier readability and also revised in other ways to maximize its impact. The manual provided in this book is the revised version.

Our experience suggests that self-treatment does not pose any serious risks to survivors. The manual provides emphatic instructions to contact mental healthcare providers in case of problems during treatment, such as suicidal ideas, uncontrollable rage, behavior harmful to self or others, and unmanageable panics or flashbacks. The original version of the manual instructed the survivors to contact our regional community center in case of problems. In the pilot study none of the survivors contacted us during the study period and no adverse effects were reported at the phone interview. The manual was later distributed to about 900 survivors in the disaster region and none reported any problems.

Despite the preliminary nature of evidence regarding the usefulness of the self-help manual, we believe it has much potential as a treatment dissemination tool. Evidence at least suggests that the critical ingredient of the intervention is the content of the message delivered, rather than the medium of delivery. Its effectiveness could be attributed in part to its trauma-specific and highly structured content that closely parallels therapist-delivered treatment. Indeed, a survivor noted that it makes one feel as if one is getting treatment from an invisible therapist. In our view, the usefulness of self-help approach is hardly surprising in view of our observations of natural recovery through self-instigated exposure without any contact with a therapist (see Chapter 1). This has further implications for other dissemination methods, as will be reviewed later.

The usefulness of the manual might be viewed as limited in post-disaster settings where there is a high rate of illiteracy or where people are lacking in reading habits. The latter has indeed been a problem in our work, particularly with survivors of lower socio-educational background. This does not, however, pose a serious problem for the three-stage approach as a whole, given alternative methods of treatment delivery (e.g. single-session treatments). The problem posed by illiteracy could be overcome to some extent by recruiting help from family members, relatives, or friends who can act as lay therapists by reading the manual to the survivor, encourage its utilization, and even monitor the treatment process. In addition, audio (or video) versions of the manual could be developed and used in regions where there is at least electricity (or battery-run play-back instruments).

In the aftermath of a disaster there may be occasions where a self-help manual might be the only conceivable form of psychological help for survivors, at least for a period of time. For example, there may be remote and difficult-to-access regions of the country where no form of psychological help is ever likely to reach. Printed or audio versions of the manual might be considered for such locations. Furthermore, self-help may be the only viable option in delivering psychological care to large numbers of survivors in the early aftermath of mass trauma events (e.g. first few months). Indeed, this is the stage when conditioned fear responses develop and generalize to a wide range of situations. Informing survivors about how to deal with fear at this stage might prevent chronic traumatic stress in the longer term. It is worth recalling from Chapter 6 that evidence of CFBT efficacy comes in part from studies conducted at a time when the aftershocks were continuing. Because of widespread fear caused by aftershocks, this is also the stage when demands for help from survivors are likely to be most intense. In such

circumstances, the self-help manual might be the only feasible option in meeting their demands.

Self-help tools are also needed in the post-trauma phase. Although mass trauma events initially trigger a remarkable media and public response, with aid and resources pouring in, the sad reality is that such interest rapidly fades away. As the disaster begins to disappear from media headlines, local and national governments (as well as the international community) are often more than willing to forget about the survivors. As time goes by, these factors make it increasingly difficult to find funding for outreach programs, no matter how cost-effective they might be. In such circumstances, self-help remains as the only option in delivering care to survivors.

Treatment dissemination through mass media

Perhaps the most exciting prospect afforded by CFBT is its dissemination through mass media, such as TV, radio, and newspapers. While this might come across as an ambitious idea, evidence suggests that it is well worth exploring in future research. There are three conditions that need to be met for effective mass dissemination of a behavioral intervention. First, the intervention needs to prescribe particular behaviors, which, when executed, reduce traumatic stress. Evidence reviewed in this book shows that not avoiding or self-exposure to trauma cues achieves this effect. Second, the prescribed behaviors need to be presented with a rationale that overcomes helplessness (anxiety) and hopelessness (depression) cognitions to a sufficient extent so that a person is motivated to execute the prescribed behaviors. Evidence from our treatment studies shows that CFBT rationale achieves this in 80% of the cases. Third, the treatment rationale needs to achieve the same impact, when delivered by media other than a therapist. Evidence suggests that this is possible with CFBT in about 50% of the cases, consistent with other evidence showing that the therapist is not always essential for effective delivery of fear-focused interventions in anxiety disorders (Newman et al., 2003).

Disseminating treatment through local and national TV channels might be particularly useful. Educational programs and documentaries demonstrating how treatment works are likely to help many survivors. Treatment sessions with real cases could be shown, allowing phone calls from viewers seeking advice on their problems. Popular media personalities, celebrities, charismatic opinion leaders, and community, political, or religious leaders could be invited to participate in these programs to maximize their impact. Because the treatment involves a discourse designed to instill courage and hope, such discourse from people in a position to influence public opinion is likely to be particularly effective.

A mental healthcare model for earthquake survivors

In this section we review the prospects of a mental healthcare model for earthquake survivors based on a control-focused behavioral approach to trauma. This model envisions various interventions at individual, community, and social levels and incorporates all possible means of treatment dissemination reviewed earlier. In discussing this model we assume that it is implemented by the government in an earthquake-prone country. The model reviewed here could therefore be useful for governments facing the challenging task of providing psychological care for large sectors of the population.

Successful implementation of the model requires efficient coordination and supervision of all care dissemination activities in the disaster region. This can be best achieved by appointing a committee of mental healthcare professionals with powers to coordinate and supervise all mental healthcare activities in the disaster region. This is important for not only effective implementation of the model but also for protection of survivors from various ineffective and potentially harmful interventions provided by national and international psychosocial aid groups that often rush to the disaster scene after a major disaster (see Chapter 8 for more discussion of this issue). This committee needs to have an adequate understanding of the need for evidence-based treatments in survivor care and the importance of operational research and intervention outcome evaluations in maximizing the impact of interventions at various levels. Table 7.2 shows an outline of procedures in implementing the model in pre- and post-disaster phases.

Pre-disaster phase: earthquake preparedness activities

The pre-disaster phase includes earthquake preparedness activities. The concept of earthquake preparedness is often understood as involving only reinforcement of infrastructural constructions and buildings, precautionary safety measures in buildings, and organization of rescue and relief efforts. Psychological preparedness is often neglected or, at best, limited to training people in self-protection during earthquakes. Reducing the extent of devastation and casualties caused by earthquakes might reduce their traumatic impact to a certain extent but this requires major financial resources often not available in developing countries. Such measures are of course important in protecting human life but they may not entirely prevent traumatic stress problems, given the fear conditioning effects of earthquake tremors per se. Furthermore, the psychological impact of large-scale disasters is not merely a mental health issue; it has far reaching social, economic, and political implications. Psychological preparedness efforts could be useful in reducing the impact of disasters on societies as a whole.

Disseminating treatment knowledge

The coordinating committee could oversee dissemination of treatment knowledge as widely as possible to the public, mass media organizations, and various governmental and non-governmental organizations that are likely to participate in relief efforts after a major disaster. The latter include primary and secondary healthcare facilities, disaster relief agencies, army, universities, professional associations, schools, factories, work places, and so on. The treatment manuals would not only inform these organizations and their personnel about effective dealing with traumatic stress but might also help them disseminate treatment knowledge in the aftermath of a disaster.

Securing close cooperation of media organizations in disseminating treatment knowledge through media programs is important in view of their potential role in educating the public. Helping media organizations understand how they can contribute to recovery from trauma might encourage them to play an active role in this process. Furthermore, informing them about how broadcasting of disturbing disaster scenes might augment the traumatic impact of disasters may lead them to adopt more responsible broadcasting policies.

Disseminating treatment knowledge to the public is likely to be useful in several ways. Prior knowledge of how trauma affects people and effective ways of dealing with traumatic stress can increase people's sense of control over stressors. We have seen survivors who use such knowledge even in overcoming their

Table 7.2 A mental healthcare model for earthquake survivors

Pre-disaster phase	Tools and methods	Post-disaster phase	Tools and methods
		TRAUMA PHASE	
		Organize early intervention:	
(1) Establish a committee of mental health professionals empowered to organize, coordinate, and supervise all mental healthcare services for survivors	Government action	1) Disseminate treatment knowledge through mass media	Educational programs, media campaigns
(2) Undertake earthquake preparedness efforts in at risk regions		(2) Disseminate self-help tools to public	Self-help tools
(a) Educate media and public in psychological effects of disasters and CFBT principles	Media programs + dissemination of self-help tools[1]	(3) Disseminate treatment knowledge to primary and secondary healthcare facilities, universities, schools, factories, work places, etc.	Treatment Delivery Manual + self-help tools
(b) Disseminate treatment knowledge to primary and secondary healthcare facilities, universities, schools, factories, work places, etc.	Treatment Delivery Manual + self-help tools	(4) Implement community outreach programs + coordinate activities with local healthcare facilities for care of survivors requiring medical / inpatient psychiatric treatment.	Outreach model in Figure 7.1 + other psychiatric care as needed + local healthcare facilities
(c) Screen previously earthquake exposed people to identify at-risk cases	SITSES[2]	(5) Secure early resettlement of displaced survivors	Government action
(d) Deliver interventions to enhance resilience against future earthquakes	Self-help tools + Earthquake Simulation Treatment	POST-TRAUMA PHASE	
		Organize long-term intervention programs	
		(1) Conduct periodic screening to identify cases in need of treatment and implement step 4	SITSES
		(2) Undertake earthquake preparedness programs in longer term	See pre-disaster preparation phase

[1] Self-help tools include the self-help manual and its audio and visual versions on audiocassettes, CDs, etc.
[2] Screening Instrument for Traumatic Stress in Earthquake Survivors.

various phobias without any prompting by a therapist. This knowledge can also help people in overcoming fear-induced helplessness and avoidance in the early phase of a disaster. As discussed in Part 1, people have a natural tendency to overcome fear by confronting fear cues but some need encouragement before they can take action. Treatment knowledge can also be helpful for people with previous exposure to earthquakes. In earthquake-prone countries many people are likely to have at least one past experience of an earthquake and some may still have chronic traumatic stress problems. Indeed, we have come across people with chronic problems arising from earthquakes that occurred in 1967 and 1992. Traumatic stress can persist for a long time in many earthquake survivors as fear and some related stress problems, if not PTSD

as a syndrome, even as long as 50 years (Lazaratou et al., 2008).

Enhancing resilience to earthquake tremors: Earthquake Simulation Treatment

In addition to general dissemination of treatment knowledge, more specific actions could be taken for those who are more at risk of developing traumatic stress after future earthquakes. Although it is impossible to predict the exact timing of earthquakes, the science of seismology provides some clues regarding the probable location of future earthquakes and their time frame. In Istanbul, for example, a major earthquake (magnitude of over 7 on the Richter scale) is expected anytime in the next 25 years. Such information provides an opportunity to conduct preparedness efforts in specific locations. At-risk cases could be identified using the SITSES to assess both current traumatic stress problems and those experienced in the early aftermath of the past earthquake. Given the strong association between fear and traumatic stress reactions, at-risk cases could be identified based on (a) the intensity of fear experienced during the past earthquake, (b) the severity of traumatic stress problems in the early aftermath of the earthquake, and (c) intensity of current anticipatory fear of future earthquakes. In Turkey, for example, those who had higher scores on fear and traumatic stress problems in our field surveys, assuming they are left untreated, would be at-risk cases after the next earthquake. The association between anticipatory fear and traumatic stress is so strong that it would be possible to predict possible future traumatization by simply asking the person how much anticipatory fear they experience in relation to future earthquakes. Indeed, this association appears to be very time-resistant, as suggested by a study (Lazaratou et al., 2008) conducted 50 years after the 1953 Cephalonia earthquake in Greece. In this study, 78% of the survivors still had distinct fear of earthquakes after 50 years and, compared with those who did not report any fear, they had more severe traumatic stress problems during the 6 months after the disaster (assessed retrospectively).

Several other indicators might be helpful in identifying at-risk cases among people with no previous experience of a major earthquake. Risk factors, such as female gender, proximity to an active fault line, lower education, past history of psychiatric illness, and psychological responses to previous traumatic events could be taken into account. Based on our experience, though, we think that such cases could be most reliably identified by their response to simulated tremors in an earthquake simulator. We have observed that some people show an anxiety response to this experience similar to that of earthquake-exposed individuals, albeit at a lower level of intensity. We have also seen people who felt reluctant to undergo such experience in anticipation of distress. Such people may be at greater risk of developing traumatic stress after earthquakes.

Once such people are identified, Earthquake Simulation Treatment is likely to be the most effective way of enhancing their resilience. This intervention naturally requires the availability of earthquake simulators that are specifically designed for this purpose. Despite its cost implications, this intervention is highly cost-effective in the long term, considering the overall economic cost of traumatic stress problems in society and their treatment. Mobile earthquake simulators (mounted on a truck, for example) could be used to deliver the intervention in at-risk regions. As the intervention can be administered in groups, about 100 people could be treated in a day using a medium size earthquake simulator. Using such mobile teams, the intervention could be delivered to various institutions (e.g. schools, factories, work places, etc.). The business sector could be encouraged to share the economic costs of this intervention, making them aware of the fact that a future disaster will also traumatize their employees and cause significant loss of productivity. Indeed, after the earthquake in Turkey, businesses, such as banks, companies, and factories were among the first to seek help for their traumatized employees.

It is worth noting here that Earthquake Simulation Treatment is fundamentally different in its effects from currently existing earthquake preparedness programs (e.g. in the United States or Japan) that are designed to train people in self-protective behaviors using an earthquake simulator. Such programs might be helpful in teaching people what to do during an earthquake but they may not necessarily enhance resilience against the fear-inducing effects of earthquakes. Mere exposure to earthquake tremors may not have the desired resilience-building effect, unless it is a motivation-driven exercise with the specific aim of challenging and overcoming distress or fear. Thus, when not used in accordance with a treatment protocol, exposure to earthquake tremors might not only fail to enhance resilience but also sensitize some vulnerable people to earthquake tremors. Moreover, such possible undesirable effects aside, training in self-protective behaviors might not be of much use during a real earthquake, if the person cannot control intense fear or panic responses. Such responses can be so intense, even during mild aftershocks, that some people jump out of windows, risking their lives and often seriously injuring themselves.

Post-disaster phase

The implementation of the model during the post-disaster period involves the same treatment dissemination methods and tools as in the pre-disaster phase. This is because the same treatment knowledge can be useful in both prevention and treatment of traumatic stress. In the post-disaster phase, however, treatment dissemination efforts need to be more intensive and directed at larger target populations, due to the large numbers of people awaiting psychological care. The activities in the post-disaster period broadly fall under two headings: trauma phase and post-trauma phase. The trauma phase is defined as the period starting with the initial major shock and ending with the complete cessation of aftershocks. This phase may last as long as 1 year, depending on the duration of seismic activity in the region. The CFBT model does not make a distinction between acute and chronic trauma phase as defined by DSM-IV (American Psychiatric Association, 1994) in terms of timing of interventions, because the mechanisms of traumatic stress are the same in both phases. Thus, it envisions early interventions at all levels in post-disaster circumstances. Conceptually, the trauma period provides the best opportunities for learning of control over most traumatic stressors, i.e. ongoing aftershocks. This is consistent with our findings reviewed in Chapter 6 showing that controlled exposure to unconditioned stimuli (e.g. simulated earthquake tremors) achieves stronger resilience effects than exposure to conditioned stimuli (i.e. trauma reminders). Thus, helping people resume their normal life by not avoiding feared situations during a period of ongoing aftershocks is likely to have greater impact on their sense of control. We should stress the fact that normalizing life does not mean resettlement in homes in the very early phase of the disaster, when it may not be safe to do so. Rather, it implies exercising control over irrational conditioned fears that seriously interfere with important life activities. Fear conditioning occurs quite rapidly in the aftermath of earthquakes, so early intervention is important before helplessness and hopelessness responses set in.

Dissemination of treatment knowledge through mass media

We briefly described earlier how treatment knowledge can be disseminated through educational programs in mass media. The early aftermath of devastating earthquakes is often characterized by chaos and a state of shock accompanied by widespread fear, grief, helplessness, and hopelessness in people. With its discourse designed to convey courage, dispel feelings of helplessness, instill hope, and enhance motivation to fight fear and distress, CFBT is particularly well suited for this phase of disasters. Dissemination of such

discourse through mass media is conceived as a first-line intervention in such circumstances, because this is the quickest means of delivering help to survivors at a time when they need it most. Sometimes political leaders use a similar discourse after major disasters in an effort to convey similar messages, as illustrated by the following Associated Press news wire (Ang, 2008) about 2 weeks after the May 2008 earthquake in China.

> In another sign that health care professionals will not reach everybody in need right away, the Ministry of Health has issued a handout of guidelines on how to help survivors, rescue workers and volunteers who have experienced the carnage. Blue flyers circulated by Sichuan health authorities offer concern and compassion from the ruling Communist Party. "When we're facing a disaster, the first thing we want to do is to continue living," it said. "That's the only way we can fight the disaster."

Notice the parallels between this discourse and the rationale of CFBT. Indeed, the first thing to do after a disaster is to *fight* the disaster and *continue living*. To achieve this, people need to know how they can overcome their fear and also need encouragement to confront their fear. Such encouragement coming from political leaders, popular media personalities, celebrities, charismatic opinion leaders, community or religious leaders could be particularly useful.

Securing early resettlement of displaced survivors

Earthquakes that cause extensive devastation often lead to displacement of people to camps, 'tent cities,' or to makeshift barracks. Many people whose homes have sustained minimal or no damage also seek refuge in such shelters because of fear. Indeed, 58% of the 15 000 people who were living in shelters 6 months after the earthquake in Turkey had a safe and inhabitable house (Committee for Tent Cities in Kocaeli: Report on the status of tent cities in Kocaeli, March 8, 2000). This figure does not include many more survivors who were living in tents or makeshift barracks next to their house. Because of generalized conditioned fear and avoidance, many displaced survivors find it difficult to resettle in concrete buildings even months after the earthquake when it is reasonably safe to do so. Indeed, in our community surveys involving 1655 earthquake survivors living in prefabricated housing compounds or residential units in the epicenter zone, the strongest predictor of relocation to shelters was behavioral avoidance, after controlling for the effects of level of damage to home and financial loss (Şalcıoğlu et al., 2008). The social environment of survivor shelters is characterized by a culture of fear and avoidance (Başoğlu et al., 2002; Şalcıoğlu et al., 2008), which reinforces avoidance and helplessness. Living conditions in these shelters are often quite difficult and entail various hazards to safety. In a study (Şalcıoğlu et al., 2007) that examined traumatic stress reactions in survivors who were resettled in permanent accommodation, we found that resettlement was associated with reduction in traumatic stress reactions. This is because living in a concrete building involves exposure to trauma cues and thus opportunities for overcoming trauma-induced fear or distress. Resettlement also means less exposure to avoidance-reinforcing social milieu of shelters. This finding, consistent with the principles of CFBT, implies that policies encouraging or enabling early resettlement in displaced survivors is likely to facilitate recovery in survivors. Such policies would also spare survivors the hardships of living under difficult conditions in camps, while at the same time substantially reducing the economic costs of looking after so many people for so long.

Government officials may not find it easy to implement such policies, particularly when they have a personal experience of earthquake trauma. Fear may color their judgment and make them feel uneasy or reluctant about the idea of early resettlement in concrete buildings, even when it is safe to do so. Furthermore, the culture of fear and avoidance that prevails in the social environment after a major earthquake may make such policies difficult to implement. Nevertheless, these problems can be overcome by helping the authorities as well as the survivors to understand the potentially beneficial effects of these policies. The authorities also need to know that reduced traumatic stress in the community also means reduced anger and resentment towards the authorities. Indeed, evidence (Başoğlu et al., 2005a; Şalcıoğlu, 2004) suggests that such emotional and cognitive effects of trauma are closely associated with traumatic stress and are likely to diminish with recovery from the latter.

Outreach programs

The implementation of outreach programs was described earlier in this chapter. These programs are conceived as a complementary measure to provide care for those survivors who do not benefit from self-help for various reasons. Although survivors in the epicenter region need priority attention in planning these programs, it is important to bear in mind that there are likely to be many people well outside this region who are traumatized by mere exposure to the tremors (evidence reviewed in Chapter 1). This implies that all people with an experience of earthquake tremors need to be screened for traumatic stress. This is obviously an enormous task but, given the availability of a screening instrument, one that is conceivable and perhaps even feasible in certain favorable circumstances. In any event all survivors in the epicenter region would need to be screened, regardless of whether or not they were directly exposed to the devastating impact of the earthquake.

Organizing long-term mental healthcare programs

A field survey (Şalcıoğlu et al., 2007) conducted 3.5 years post-disaster suggested that earthquake-induced traumatic stress may persist for at least several years after the disaster. This finding points to a need for periodic screening of survivors in the years that follow the disaster to identify cases in need of help. Traumatic stress may be maintained, reinforced, or even exacerbated by recurring earthquakes in an earthquake-prone country, even when they are of relatively low magnitude or when they occur in another region of the country. Other factors, such as media broadcasts about expected earthquakes in the region or media news about disasters occurring in other countries, might also contribute to the persistence of traumatic stress in survivors. Thus, long-term mental healthcare planning is needed in this phase, perhaps for as long as 5–10 years. Such planning is also justified by the need for earthquake preparedness efforts for future earthquakes. In countries situated in seismologically active regions, the post-disaster period following an earthquake also needs to be regarded as the pre-disaster period for the next earthquake. While major earthquakes in some regions might be decades apart from each other, this time period might also be as short as a few years or even months. In Turkey, for example, the August 1999 earthquake was followed by another major earthquake in the same region 3 months later. Treatment of chronic traumatic stress also means psychological preparedness for future earthquakes.

Concluding remarks

Some points regarding the mental healthcare model reviewed here need emphasis to avoid misconceptions.

First, it is important to understand the distinction between CFBT as a form of brief psychotherapy delivered in weekly sessions and a control-focused behavioral approach to trauma derived from learning theory. The latter entails a wide range of interventions at different levels, whereas the former is a specific application of the behavioral approach using exposure as the main procedure in reducing helplessness. Second, the model has a sharp focus on traumatic stress, because it is the causal process in a wide range of psychiatric and medical problems. Third, as detailed in Chapter 1, the model targets all health outcomes of disasters. Furthermore, it does not preclude use of other psychiatric treatments when the need arises. However, it differs fundamentally from mainstream psychiatric treatments in its learning theory-based behavioral approach to mental illnesses caused or exacerbated by traumatic stress. Because traumatic stress is the causal process in trauma-induced mental illnesses, all other traditional psychiatric treatments are conceived as *complementary* interventions. No treatment is complete without a trauma-focused intervention. In cases with trauma-induced acute psychosis, for example, drugs might control the psychosis but are not likely to reduce traumatic stress that triggered the psychosis in the first place. Case vignette #4 in Chapter 4 illustrates this point. Recurrence of illness due to continued exposure to traumatic stressors or even trauma reminders is always a possibility in such cases. Other similar examples include suicidal depression, drug and alcohol abuse problems, and various medical conditions induced by traumatic stress. Traditional psychiatric care alone is unlikely to be sufficient in such cases.

Needless to say, the model in its present form is far from complete. The treatment dissemination methods need to be explored further in future research. They also need to be tested with other forms of trauma. Nevertheless, in view of the evidence pointing to its potential in cost-effective care of disaster survivors, we presented the model in some detail so that its various components can be tested by others in different settings. Its implications for various issues in care of trauma survivors are reviewed in the last two chapters of the book.

References

American Psychiatric Association (1994). *Diagnostic and Statistical Manual of Mental Disorders (4th Edition)*. Washington, DC: American Psychiatric Association.

Ang, A. (2008, May 28). Mental trauma rampant after China earthquake. *Associated Press.* Accessed on April 28, 2010 at the Associated Press Archive at http://nl.newsbank.com/sites/apab.

Başoğlu, M., Kılıç, C., Şalcıoğlu, E. and Livanou, M. (2004). Prevalence of posttraumatic stress disorder and comorbid depression in earthquake survivors in Turkey: An epidemiological study. *Journal of Traumatic Stress*, **17**, 133–141.

Başoğlu, M., Livanou, M., Crnobarić, C., Franćišković, T., Suljić, E., Đurić, D. and Vranešić, M. (2005a). Psychiatric and cognitive effects of war in former Yugoslavia: Association of lack of redress for trauma and posttraumatic stress reactions. *Journal of the American Medical Association*, **294**, 580–590.

Başoğlu, M., Livanou, M., Şalcıoğlu, E. and Kalender, D. (2003). A brief behavioural treatment of chronic post-traumatic stress disorder in earthquake survivors: Results from an open clinical trial. *Psychological Medicine*, **33**, 647–654.

Başoğlu, M., Şalcıoğlu, E. and Livanou, M. (2002). Traumatic stress responses in earthquake survivors in Turkey. *Journal of Traumatic Stress*, **15**, 269–276.

Başoğlu, M., Şalcıoğlu, E. and Livanou, M. (2007). A randomized controlled study of single-session behavioural treatment of earthquake-related post-traumatic stress disorder using an earthquake simulator. *Psychological Medicine*, **37**, 203–213.

Başoğlu, M., Şalcıoğlu, E. and Livanou, M. (2009). Single-case experimental studies of a self-help manual for traumatic stress in earthquake survivors. *Journal of Behavior Therapy and Experimental Psychiatry* **40**, 50–58.

Başoğlu, M., Şalcıoğlu, E., Livanou, M., Kalender, D. and Acar, G. (2005b). Single-session behavioral treatment of earthquake-related posttraumatic stress disorder: A randomized waiting list controlled trial. *Journal of Traumatic Stress*, **18**, 1–11.

Bradley, R., Greene, J., Russ, E., Dutra, L. and Westen, D. (2005). A multidimensional meta-analysis of psychotherapy for PTSD. *American Journal of Psychiatry*, **162**, 214–227.

Cahill, S. P., Foa, E. B., Hembree, E. A., Marshall, R. D. and Nacash, N. (2006). Dissemination of exposure therapy in the treatment of posttraumatic stress disorder. *Journal of Traumatic Stress*, **19**, 597–610.

Lazaratou, H., Paparrigopoulos, T. J., Galanos, G., Psarros, C., Dikeos, D. and Soldatos, C. R. (2008). The psychological impact of a catastrophic earthquake: A retrospective study 50 years after the event. *Journal of Nervous and Mental Disease*, **196**, 340–344.

Marks, I. M., Lovell, K., Noshirvani, H. and Livanou, M. (1998). Treatment of posttraumatic stress disorder by exposure and/or cognitive restructuring: A controlled study. *Archives of General Psychiatry*, 55, 317–325.

Newman, M. G., Erickson, T., Przeworski, A. and Dzus, E. (2003). Self-help and minimal contact therapies for anxiety disorders: Is human contact necessary for therapeutic efficacy? *Journal of Clinical Psychology*, 59: 251–274.

Şalcıoğlu, E. (2004). *The effect of beliefs, attribution of responsibility, redress and compensation on posttraumatic stress disorder in earthquake survivors in Turkey*. PhD Dissertation. Institute of Psychiatry, King's College London, London.

Şalcıoğlu, E., Başoğlu, M. and Livanou, M. (2007). Posttraumatic stress disorder and comorbid depression among survivors of the 1999 earthquake in Turkey. *Disasters*, 31, 115–129.

Şalcıoğlu, E., Başoğlu, M. and Livanou, M. (2008). Psychosocial determinants of relocation in survivors of the 1999 earthquake in Turkey. *Journal of Nervous and Mental Disease*, 196, 55–61.

Van Etten, M. L. and Taylor, S. (1998). Comparative efficacy of treatments for post-traumatic stress disorder: A meta-analysis. *Clinical Psychology and Psychotherapy*, 5, 126–144.

Issues in care of mass trauma survivors

In the Introduction we noted that a mental healthcare model that is capable of addressing millions of mass trauma survivors around the world in a cost-effective fashion requires interventions that are (1) *theoretically sound*, (2) *proven to be effective*, (3) *brief*, (4) *easy to train therapists in their delivery*, (5) *practicable in different cultures*, and (6) *suitable for dissemination through media other than professional therapists, such as lay people, self-help tools, and mass media*. In this chapter we take a brief look at treatments commonly used in care of mass trauma survivors to assess their potential for such a model. We then review the implications of our work for care of earthquake survivors in developing and industrialized countries, prospects for mass dissemination of care after mass trauma events, current views regarding aims, levels, focus, and timing of interventions, and controversies regarding the cross-cultural validity of PTSD. In view of the rather indiscriminate use of antidepressants in treatment of mass survivors in developing countries, we also briefly review the role of these drugs in survivor care. The chapter ends with a review of implications of Control-Focused Behavioral Treatment (CFBT) for treatment of anxiety disorders in general.

State of the art in treatment of trauma survivors

Traumatic stress is by definition a fear-related process and evidence reviewed in this book shows that it is primarily mediated by loss of control over fear associated with appraisal of threat to safety. Consistent with such evidence, fear-related stress symptoms are often the most prominent features of PTSD (Başoğlu et al., 2002; Buckley et al., 1998; Livanou et al., 2002; Şalcıoğlu et al., 2003; Şalcıoğlu et al., 2007b; Taylor et al., 1998). Yet, most treatments used with mass trauma survivors, such as psychological debriefing, counseling, psychosocial

support strategies, various forms of non-directive group psychotherapy, psychodynamic interventions, insight therapy, and art or play therapy have no sharp focus on trauma-induced anxiety or fear as the primary causal process. Choice of such interventions, despite no evidence of their usefulness, reflects lack of evidence-based thinking, which is arguably the most important problem in this field (Başoğlu et al., 2009). What is sorely lacking among many care providers is an awareness of the fact that an intervention is likely to be effective to the extent that its mechanisms of action match the causal processes that underlie traumatic stress reactions. A misplaced treatment focus yields either no improvement in PTSD or at best only partial and modest effects, as demonstrated by a study (Bolton et al., 2007) of Ugandan survivors of war and displacement, who were treated for depression using group interpersonal psychotherapy and creative play, despite a wide range of anxiety- and fear-related problems.

Effective use of cognitive-behavioral treatment (CBT) and other exposure-based interventions in PTSD represents the most significant advance in trauma treatment in the last few decades. However, judged against the above criteria for post-disaster suitability, CBT has certain important shortcomings. First, as discussed further later in this chapter, there are certain theoretical issues that might limit the efficacy of CBT. Second, although CBT is considered a brief treatment, it takes an average of 15 weekly sessions (Van Etten and Taylor, 1998). As such, it is not sufficiently brief in post-disaster settings where large numbers of survivors need urgent care. Furthermore, high demographic mobility after disasters makes regular treatment attendance difficult, if not impossible, for many survivors. Third, applicability of cognitive restructuring techniques in non-western cultures is uncertain. Fourth, certain treatment procedures, such as keeping homework sheets (Foa et al., 1991; Resick et al., 2002) and heavy writing tasks (Resick et al., 2002), in exposure and cognitive therapy protocols may complicate their practicability with survivors with low levels of education that characterize populations of developing countries (Şalcıoğlu and Başoğlu, 2009). They also pose challenges of use in post-disaster or post-war settings, where survivors have to deal with day-to-day survival problems. Fifth, the relatively complex procedures involved in imaginal exposure and cognitive restructuring pose challenges in the training of therapists, particularly in developing countries. Finally and most importantly, most therapy elements are elaborate procedures that rely heavily on therapist skills and thus are difficult to deliver as self-help interventions. The fact that two studies (Ehlers et al., 2003; Scholes et al., 2007) failed to demonstrate the efficacy of a CBT-based self-help tool in acute traumatic stress reflects the difficult nature of this task.

Another widely used treatment of PTSD is Eye Movement Desensitization and Reprocessing (EMDR). This intervention is not based on sound theory and its reported efficacy might well be explained by imaginal exposure to trauma cues (American Psychiatric Association, 2004; Bradley et al., 2005; Van Etten and Taylor, 1998). Indeed, a meta-analysis (Davidson and Parker, 2001) of 13 dismantling studies in which EMDR was compared with the same procedure without eye movements has shown that eye movements are not an essential component of treatment. The potential limitations of imaginal exposure are discussed later in this chapter. Furthermore, evidence from our work strongly suggests that a three-way synergistic interaction among self-instigated exposure to trauma cues, increased sense of control over fear, and reduction in behavioral avoidance is the primary therapeutic process that accounts for generalized improvement in post-traumatic stress reactions and functional impairment. This implies that improvement in psychotherapy cannot be attributed to a particular therapist-administered intervention *during* a session before one rules out *between-session* processes as possible therapeutic factors, which might be incidental or unrelated to the intervention. Such an important treatment process variable is hardly ever examined in clinical trials involving EMDR (or any other intervention for that matter). Most importantly, EMDR is not suitable for dissemination on a self-help basis and thus has no potential for cost-effective care of large numbers

of disaster survivors, particularly in developing countries.

In recent years Narrative Exposure Therapy (NET) has been reported to be useful in treatment of war (Bichescu et al., 2007; Neuner et al., 2008; Neuner et al., 2004) and natural disaster (Catani et al., 2009) survivors. NET involves getting a detailed chronological account of the survivor's life starting from early childhood to the current day. Trauma events are discussed using the imaginal exposure procedures as detailed in other exposure protocols. The intervention is thus essentially a variant of imaginal exposure, which is a weak form of exposure with limited efficacy, as discussed later in this chapter. It is worth briefly reviewing the evidence regarding the efficacy of NET to illustrate this point. In a randomized controlled study (Neuner et al., 2004) that compared NET with supportive counseling and psychoeducation in 15 civilian war survivors, the treatment achieved 24% reduction in PTSD symptoms with a moderate effect size of 0.62 at post-treatment. NET was superior to psychoeducation but not to supportive counseling (between-groups effect size = 0.06). Furthermore, PTSD symptoms in the group that received NET returned to baseline levels at 4-month follow-up. Although significant symptom reduction was again observed at 1-year follow-up (overall 36.5%), lack of continuous assessments during the 8 months between two assessment points precludes a definitive conclusion as to whether the observed improvement is attributable to NET. In another study (Neuner et al., 2008) involving 111 war survivors, NET delivered by lay therapists (i.e. refugees trained as counselors) was compared with non-specific trauma counseling and a no-treatment control group. The treatment was delivered in six twice-weekly sessions and follow-up assessments were conducted at 3 and 9 months post-treatment. At 9-month follow-up NET achieved only moderate treatment effect compared to the no-treatment control group. The stability of this finding is uncertain, given that the control group was not assessed at the 3-month follow-up point. Furthermore, the treatment effects achieved by NET at both follow-up points were not different from the non-specific treatment offered by lay counselors. In a third and rather small study (Bichescu et al., 2007) involving 18 survivors of torture (about 40 years after the event) NET reduced a higher number of PTSD symptoms compared to a control group involving psychoeducation. However, although the treatment was delivered in 3 weeks, the only post-treatment assessment was carried out at 6-month follow-up. Lack of multiple assessments precludes a definitive conclusion about the stability of treatment effects over time. A fourth study (Catani et al., 2009) of NET involved 31 child survivors of the 2004 South-Asian Tsunami and was conducted 3 weeks after the disaster. Although NET achieved large treatment effects at both post-treatment and 6-month follow-up (1.76 and 1.98, respectively), so did the control group (meditation / relaxation). There was no difference between NET and relaxation at post-treatment (between groups effect size 0.01) and relaxation did somewhat better than NET at 6-month follow-up (between groups effect size 0.26). Although the authors argued that these recovery rates were higher than could be expected from natural recovery, the study lacked a waitlist group to control for the effects of time. This is particularly important, considering that the study was conducted in the acute phase of trauma, during which natural recovery rates are reported to be higher in the literature. In view of these findings and methodological issues, these studies cannot be regarded as providing convincing evidence regarding the efficacy of NET in war and natural disaster survivors. Furthermore, both within- and between-groups effect sizes achieved by NET in these studies are lower than those reported with other exposure protocols.

In conclusion, none of the current treatments widely used with trauma survivors satisfy all six criteria outlined above. Some of these interventions, such as CBT, EMDR, and NET, deserve credit for being trauma-focused but there are still unresolved issues pertaining to their theoretical basis, mechanisms of action, efficacy, and cross-cultural practicability. Their focus on anxiety reduction rather than on anxiety tolerance and control is a factor that might limit their efficacy. Furthermore, none of these treatments are suitable for cost-effective dissemination on a self-help basis in post-disaster settings.

Prospects for cost-effective care of mass trauma survivors

The mental healthcare model for earthquake survivors described in Chapter 7 was conceived bearing in mind the needs of developing countries. As the work was conducted in Turkey, the outcomes are highly relevant to other earthquake-prone developing countries with similar socio-cultural and post-disaster characteristics. Findings suggest that cost-effective mental healthcare of earthquake survivors is possible with brief, relatively simple, and largely self-administered interventions. Given its theoretical framework, a CFBT approach is likely to have cross-cultural applicability. Its minimal reliance on cognitive interventions confers a distinct advantage in work with survivors from a lower socio-educational background, as cognitive interventions require a reasonably well-differentiated cognitive structure on the part of the client. The structured CFBT Delivery Manual included in this book may facilitate effective treatment delivery by professional and lay therapists. Further work is underway to develop a version of this manual for war and torture survivors. Furthermore, preliminary evidence suggests that treatment can be delivered effectively through self-help tools. Although much work is still needed to validate the various components of this model, the prospects it offers are well worth exploring in future research.

Issues in survivor care in developing countries

Our experience demonstrates that it is possible to develop an effective mental healthcare approach for disaster survivors in developing countries without depending on intervention strategies imported from western countries. Uncritical acceptance and use of treatments developed in western countries is a common problem in developing countries, reflecting a cultural tendency to view everything coming from the west as 'good.' In Turkey, for example, psychological debriefing was commonly used after the 1999 earthquakes, despite lack of evidence for its effectiveness (Carlier et al., 2000; Conlon et al., 1999; Rose et al., 1999) and evidence suggesting that it may even be harmful (Bisson et al., 1997; Hobbs et al., 1996). Choice of such treatments reflects in part the influence of 'trauma experts' who rush to the disaster scene from western countries to make their 'expertise' available to the local professionals. The mental health professionals in developing countries need to bear in mind that experience in the western world with the kind of large-scale disasters that occur in developing countries is limited and that their western colleagues, however well intentioned they might be, might not always have the answers to their problems. Indeed, as noted earlier, available treatments for trauma survivors have various shortcomings that limit their usefulness in post-disaster settings in developing countries.

Mental health professionals in developing countries also need to be aware of the fact that many psychosocial aid projects established by various international groups in their country after a disaster might lack an evidence-based approach. An evidence-based approach is not yet the norm in all areas of trauma work in western countries. In Turkey we observed that most psychosocial aid projects executed, guided or advised by foreign groups (some funded by respectable international organizations) lacked a sound theoretical basis and did not involve outcome evaluation. Such projects are not only unlikely to yield useful outcomes but may also have harmful effects for survivors. Similar concerns have also been voiced about the work of international psychosocial aid groups in developing countries after the tsunami disaster in Southeast Asia (Ganesan, 2006). We have observed, for example, that psychological debriefing provided by such groups led to angry responses from many survivors, who typically said *"They opened our wounds and left without closing them. Where are they now when we need them most?"* Some even initially refused to talk to us, thinking that we knocked on their door to offer more of the same.

This issue also has important implications for governments of developing countries. After a major disaster, particularly one that attracts international media attention, foreign aid often pours into the country, along with numerous international psychosocial aid groups. While some of these groups may be genuinely motivated by a desire to provide psychological care, we have also come across in Turkey various missionary groups with a different agenda rushing into the disaster scene under the disguise of psychosocial aid. Thus, a measure well worth considering by governments is the establishment of a national advisory body that reviews and vets all proposals for psychosocial aid projects for survivors and also coordinates and monitors them. Such projects need to be assessed as to whether the proposed work is evidence-based and practicable in the particular cultural and post-disaster circumstances of the country.

Funding organizations also play a major role in use of non-evidence-based treatments by supporting psychosocial aid projects without a critical review of their potential usefulness. While such organizations may be lending support to these projects out of humanitarian concerns, they also need to be aware of the fact that their money is highly likely to be wasted on non-evidence-based, potentially useless, or even harmful projects, if they do not observe the criteria for potential usefulness of psychological treatments for disaster survivors. We have indeed observed significant amounts of financial resources being wasted on such projects during our work in Turkey and former Yugoslavia countries. At the very least, funding organizations could make their funding support conditional on two requirements to avoid wasting their resources: (a) previous evidence of treatment efficacy published in respectable professional journals and (b) evaluation of treatment outcome early in the life of the project (e.g. in a cohort of consecutively treated cases) as preliminary evidence of potential usefulness of the treatment program in a particular post-disaster setting.

Care of earthquake survivors in industrialized countries

Earthquakes are generally not considered to be a priority problem among western trauma researchers, mainly because earthquakes in industrialized countries, such as the United States or Japan, do not cause as extensive devastation and casualties as they do in developing countries. While this is generally true so far, our findings imply that earthquakes have the potential to lead to extensive conditioned fear responses and related traumatic stress problems in the community even in the absence of such devastation. Findings of some studies conducted in industrialized countries support this point. For example, in a study (McMillen et al., 2000) of 130 survivors of the 1994 Northridge California earthquake, while 13% met the criteria for PTSD, 48% had re-experiencing and arousal symptoms, despite the fact that this earthquake caused relatively few casualties. In a study (Livanou et al., 2005) of 157 survivors of the 1999 Parnitha earthquake in Greece, which caused relatively limited devastation and 143 deaths, 25% still had traumatic stress problems (most commonly hyperarousal and re-experiencing symptoms) 4 years after the disaster. Furthermore, a study (Carr et al., 1997) of the 1989 Newcastle earthquake in Australia (Richter scale magnitude 5.6), which caused 13 deaths, estimated that 18.3% of survivors exposed to high levels of threat were at risk of developing PTSD. Finally, in a study of 52 earthquake survivors conducted after the two

6.6-magnitude earthquakes that hit Iceland in 2002 4 days apart and that caused no structural damage or casualties 24% of the survivors had PTSD compared to 0% of the control group participants with no earthquake exposure (Bodvarsdottir and Elklit, 2004). Such findings might well reflect the traumatic effects of mere exposure to earthquake tremors.

It should also be born in mind that studies that focus on PTSD alone might not reflect the true extent of the mental health problems in the community. The prevalence rates of PTSD based on DSM-IV diagnostic criteria is most likely to create a misleading impression of the actual proportion of the survivor population in need of care. As indicated in Chapter 3, 35% of survivors whom we contacted through a community outreach program perceived a need for treatment, despite not meeting the criteria for PTSD. In addition, 35% of the survivors who actively sought treatment from our community center in the disaster region did not meet the criteria for PTSD. Most of these cases had sub-threshold PTSD with prominent fear-related stress problems. These figures demonstrate how misleading a diagnosis of PTSD can be in determining treatment needs in a trauma-exposed population. Furthermore, our work suggests that prevalence studies also need to explore rates of depression and anxiety disorders in earthquake survivors. Among these psychiatric conditions specific phobias or phobic fear of earthquakes need particular attention.

It is also worth questioning the general belief that earthquakes do not pose as serious a threat to life and property in industrialized countries as in developing countries. A report by the US Geological Survey (US Geological Survey, November 22, 1999) that examined the implications of the 1999 Kocaeli earthquake in Turkey for the United States is quite sobering in this regard. According to this report, much of the building stock in the United States was constructed before the importance of ductility (the ability to deform without loss of strength) was fully understood. Consequently, large numbers of reinforced concrete structures in the eastern United States, including buildings and bridges, are vulnerable to catastrophic collapse during the oscillatory motions of large earthquakes, because they have little or no ductility. The report also noted that a magnitude 7.2 earthquake on the San Francisco Peninsula would displace more than 100 000 people from their homes, while a magnitude 7.3 on the Hayward fault in California would displace 150 000

people. Recent forecasts indicate that the probability of a 6.7 magnitude earthquake in the San Francisco Bay region in the next 30 years is 70%, while the probability of an earthquake with a magnitude greater than or equal to that of the 7.4 Kocaeli earthquake is 13%. Pointing to the fact that the Kocaeli earthquake led to collapse of more than 20 000 houses (causing about 18 000 deaths according to official estimates) and displaced more than 250 000 people, the report concluded that tragedies of comparable scale are possible in the United States.

In view of the above considerations, the mental health hazard posed by earthquakes in industrialized countries might be much more serious than previously thought. Perhaps the most important implication of our work for such countries pertains to the potentially traumatic effects of earthquakes even in the absence of extensive devastation. On a more positive note, however, our work also suggests that such conditioning effects of earthquakes can be effectively countered by various earthquake preparedness efforts detailed in Chapter 7.

Social recovery from mass trauma: potential role of mass media

The learning theory model of traumatic stress posits that fear can be learned vicariously, through observing traumatic experiences of others (Mineka and Sutton, 2006). In Chapter 1 we reviewed some data to suggest that survivors' fear of earthquakes is further aggravated by TV broadcasts of horror stories and distressing pictures of people being trapped under rubble and survivors' expressions of fear, horror, or grief. This is consistent with other reports suggesting an association between greater psychological distress and TV images of mass trauma events (Ahern et al., 2002; Blanchard et al., 2004; Neria et al., 2007; Pfefferbaum et al., 2002; Schlenger et al., 2002; Silver et al., 2002). Thus, measures designed to ensure more responsible media broadcasting after disasters might prove useful in preventing high rates of traumatic stress in the community.

Perhaps the most exciting prospect with a control-focused behavioral approach is its potential in facilitating trauma recovery on a societal level and media could play an important role in this process. In Chapter 7 we discussed possible ways of mass dissemination of CFBT in the aftermath of major earthquakes. Similar considerations might well apply to other mass trauma events. For example, disasters such as the September 11 events in New York, the train bombing in Spain, and the July 2005 underground bombing in London affect not only the people directly exposed to such events but also entire societies witnessing these events on their TV screens. In the aftermath of such events many people are likely to fear and avoid various situations associated with further threat. Indeed, avoidance of underground trains was common among the survivors of the 2005 bombing of the London underground (Handley et al., 2009; Rubin et al., 2007). Similarly, 9/11 terrorist attacks led to widespread fear and avoidance behaviors in American citizens. An opinion poll (Cosgrove-Mather, 2002) of 940 randomly selected New York City residents 9 months after the 9/11 events found that 41% avoided going to some places in New York City, 33% avoided crowded public events, 36% avoided riding in subways, and 26% avoided skyscrapers. Interestingly, these figures showed no change from an earlier poll conducted 1 month after the attacks. Another nationwide poll (Associated Press, 2002; Schwarz, 2002) based on 1001 randomly selected adults from all states in the USA (except Alaska and Hawaii) found that 29% of the Americans were most concerned about flying in commercial airlines and more than 10% about attending a crowded public event and visiting New York and Washington or other big cities 11 months after the 9/11 attacks. Avoidance of air travel resulted in a 20% decline in the number of passengers in the USA in the last 4 months of 2001 (Marshall et al., 2007a).

Our work shows that a discourse that presents avoidance as a form of surrender to fear (or to those who use it as a means of achieving political ends), instills courage, hope, and self-confidence, and encourages anti-avoidance action is highly effective in reducing fear and associated traumatic stress reactions. If future research can demonstrate that such a discourse can be effectively disseminated through audio-visual media without any therapist involvement, this would imply that widespread fear and associated traumatic stress reactions in the aftermath of such events can be effectively counteracted by public and media campaigns designed to promote anti-avoidance action. The latter would simply mean leading a normal life without avoiding any situations or activities that pose an acceptable level of safety threat (e.g. using the underground as usual). It is worth recalling here that trauma-related fears often reflect the secondary conditioning effects of trauma (e.g. not using the same toothbrush that was being used during an earthquake or not wearing the same clothes) and exposure strategies usually involve situations that pose no real safety threat. Such campaigns might not only reduce fear-related traumatic stress and prevent chronic stress reactions but also psychologically prepare people against similar events in the future. Such a prospect clearly deserves further research.

Implications for intervention guidelines in survivor care

The learning theory formulation of trauma and the supporting evidence presented in this book have important implications for various issues in mental healthcare of mass trauma survivors. Some of these issues were reviewed in a 2007 article by a group of trauma specialists (Hobfoll et al., 2007). As this review is fairly representative of the current status of knowledge on treatment of mass trauma survivors, we will take the views expressed in this article as the reference point in our discussion.

Intervention aims

In their review Hobfoll and colleagues identified five empirically supported intervention principles that should be used to guide and inform intervention and prevention efforts. These include *promotion of sense of safety, calming, sense of self- and community efficacy, connectedness,* and *hope* (pp. 284), using a wide range of interventions (including but not limited to psychotherapy) on an individual, group, and community level. The authors have concluded that "*These principles will not lead to a one-treatment-fits-all approach*" (pp. 301). With its focus on helplessness and hopelessness responses, the therapeutic effects of CFBT are consistent with these guidelines. However, CFBT is fundamentally at odds with the underlying principle of these guidelines, i.e. anxiety reduction. Rather than aiming for anxiety reduction, it promotes 'risk-taking' behaviors with a view to enhancing resilience against traumatic stressors and their fear-conditioning effects. Calming is achieved as a result of increased sense of control and not mere anxiety reduction. As noted in Chapter 6, anxiety reduction as an ultimate aim in therapy reflects a puritanistic view of anxiety in western cultures as an emotion that needs to be eradicated at all costs to promote human 'happiness.' Anxiety reduction through multi-level interventions is not a realistic aim in the aftermath of mass trauma events, particularly in dispossessed populations of third world countries where people often face a wide range of problems and stressor events, including ongoing threat to their safety. Furthermore, promoting safety does not necessarily reduce traumatic stress reactions, because, as detailed in Part 1, conditioned fears are fairly resistant to extinction and persist even in situations of safety. Thus, helping survivors gain control over their generalized fear would be a more realistic aim.

A common belief is that survivors need redress and compensation of losses for recovery from traumatic stress reactions. Available evidence (reviewed in Chapter 2; see also Başoğlu et al., 2005; Şalcıoğlu, 2004) does not support this belief. Lack of an association between redress and traumatic stress reactions suggests that redress measures, even if successful in restoring sense of justice in survivors, are unlikely to have an impact on PTSD. In fact, the only controlled study (Kaminer et al., 2001) on this issue found that participation in the truth and reconciliation process in South Africa had no effect on the survivors' post-traumatic stress problems. Evidence (Foa and Rauch, 2004; Paunovic and Öst, 2001) suggests that a reduction in fear and associated post-traumatic stress responses through behavioral interventions is followed by a change in beliefs about self, others, and the world. Such evidence implies that cognitive processes leading to attribution of blame to the perceived enemy and associated feelings of anger, hostility, and vengeance might also be altered by appropriate interventions. These findings have important implications not only for mental healthcare of mass trauma survivors but also for conflict resolution, reconciliation, and social reconstruction efforts in post-war countries (Başoğlu et al., 2005). It is rather curious that such evidence is hardly ever taken into account in guidelines for mental healthcare policies for mass trauma survivors. In our view, this is an indication of how resistant such beliefs are to contrary evidence, the reasons for which are beyond the scope of our discussion here. Suffice it to say, however, that these deep-rooted beliefs, essentially a product of western thinking, achieve not much more than serving various political agendas. They have, unfortunately, also played a major role in impeding the development of effective psychological treatments for mass trauma survivors. While mass trauma survivors' need for

redress cannot be disputed on moral and / or humanitarian grounds, evidence suggests that it is not essential for recovery from traumatic stress. In any event, the fact remains that redress in the form of retributive justice or compensation of losses is not feasible or even conceivable in many countries, given their political and economic realities. This by no means implies that effective treatment of mass trauma survivors in such countries is impossible.

Levels of intervention

That mass trauma survivors need various individual, group, and community level interventions to recover from post-traumatic stress reactions is another popular view in the field. It is clear from the review by Hobfoll and colleagues (2007) that multi-level interventions are conceived as being ultimately conducive to recovery from traumatic stress reactions, the most common of which are PTSD and depression. In Chapter 6 we demonstrated that CFBT achieves substantial generalized improvement across all PTSD symptoms, hence promoting sense of safety and calmness. It also increases sense of control over traumatic stressors, as well as life in general, thereby enhancing self-confidence in dealing with post-disaster problems. Improvement in depression associated with PTSD means a reduction in hopelessness responses or increased hope. Improvement in functional impairment associated with PTSD and depression means improved family, social, and occupational functioning and hence improved 'connectedness.' Thus, CFBT, even when used as a 'single-level' intervention, achieved all five intended effects of multi-level interventions, despite various disaster-related adverse circumstances, such as extensive loss of resources, continued realistic threats to safety posed by the aftershocks, and the adverse living conditions in shelters. This is at odds with the view that "these principles will not lead to a one-treatment-fits-all approach" (Hobfoll et al., 2007, pp. 301). This apparent discrepancy can be explained by the fact that CFBT focuses on helplessness and hopelessness responses as causal processes that account for traumatic stress reactions and that it has sufficient potency to reverse these reactions and enhance resilience against traumatic stressors even when used on an individual level.

It is also important to emphasize once again that CFBT is not limited to exposure to trauma cues and can involve other interventions on different levels with a potential to reduce helplessness and hopelessness responses. The fundamental issue in treatment is to get the person to do whatever it takes to overcome feelings of helplessness and hopelessness. Exposure to trauma cues is only one technique in the arsenal of interventions available to CFBT, though arguably the most potent in enhancing sense of control in a traumatized person. While exposure alone is sufficient in reducing helplessness / hopelessness in most cases, some might need additional interventions to maximize treatment impact on their sense of control over life in general. These may include problem-solving strategies that might be required for effective dealing with real life problems, training in social skills that might be needed for reconstruction of social life and support networks, and encouragement for training in any other skills that might be helpful in reconstructing disrupted life routines or pursuing new life goals. In brief, a CFBT approach may incorporate any individual, group, or community empowerment strategy that might be useful in reducing helplessness and hopelessness and, as such, it entails a much broader scope than other forms of psychotherapy. It can also be delivered on individual, group, and community levels as part of the mental healthcare model described in Chapter 7. It is thus important to make a distinction between CFBT as a form of psychotherapy and a broader mental healthcare approach to mass trauma based on learning theory.

Focus of interventions

The foregoing discussion highlights the importance of a sound theoretical framework in understanding the mechanisms by which mass trauma events traumatize people and effective ways of treating survivors. Lack of a sound theoretical approach to mass trauma is a problem that plagues most existing mental healthcare approaches in this field. In this connection it is worth briefly reviewing the basic principles of the approach recommended by the World Health Organization (WHO). The WHO recommends a mental healthcare approach that essentially consists of making "... *basic mental health services broadly available in post-disaster countries*" (Saxena et al., 2006). Van Ommeren et al. (2005a) argued that PTSD is not the main or most important mental disorder and only "*one of a range of often comorbid common mental disorders ... that tend to make up the mild and moderate mental disorders ... after disaster.*" (pp. 1160). Stating that survivors in

non-western cultures do not often seek help for PTSD, the authors concluded that the latter is not "*the focus of many survivors of trauma*" (pp. 1160). They also expressed concern about trauma-focused approaches in treatment and advocated a "*public health perspective that considers all mental health problems, ranging from pre-existing severe mental health disorder to widespread non-pathological psychological distress induced by trauma and loss*" (pp. 1160, see also World Health Organization, 2003).

This view reflects a common belief that PTSD does not represent the full spectrum of possible outcomes of trauma exposure and therefore a trauma-focused approach in treatment is not justified or not sufficient. The fact that trauma leads to a wide range of mental and physical health outcomes is central to the learning theory model of traumatic stress reviewed in Part 1. In discussing the implications of this model for mental healthcare of earthquake survivors in Chapter 7, we acknowledged the need to provide mental healthcare for all outcomes of trauma but we also discussed the reasons why all evidence-based psychiatric treatments need to be conceived as complementary to a trauma-focused approach. To clarify what we mean by a trauma-focused approach, it is important to draw attention to the distinction between *traumatic stress as a mediating process* (involving distress, anxiety, fear, and related helplessness / hopelessness responses evoked by unpredictable and uncontrollable stressors) that leads to a wide range of mental and physical health outcomes and *PTSD as a diagnostic entity* that defines only one of the outcomes of traumatic stress. Considering the causal associations between traumatic stress and the spectrum of mental and physical illnesses, the focus in treatment needs to be on *traumatic stress* and *not on PTSD per se as a symptom constellation*. Thus, in our understanding, a trauma-focused approach entails a range of behavioral interventions – including but not limited to exposure to trauma cues – that are designed to reduce all mental and physical health outcomes of trauma by focusing on traumatic stress responses. Indeed, evidence from our studies suggests that such interventions enhance resilience against stressors, which probably accounts for the potent patholytic effect of CFBT across all problem domains. Thus, whether PTSD is the main outcome of trauma or not is an academic issue that is irrelevant to a consideration of what needs to be done to reverse the effects of trauma. Nevertheless, we should also note that there is sufficient literature evidence, including findings from our own studies, that PTSD is the most common outcome of trauma. A close association between traumatic stress and PTSD is to be naturally expected, given that the latter is simply a cluster of symptoms that directly results from traumatic stress experienced during the trauma. Thus, the view that PTSD is *one of a range of often comorbid common mental disorders*, although consistent with the learning theory model of traumatic stress, lacks perspective on the mechanisms of traumatic stress that account for the range of post-trauma mental disorders and the relative importance of PTSD among them. Concerns about a trauma-focused approach would be justified in cases where a treatment focuses on a particular outcome of trauma in total disregard for other outcomes. This is not the case with the CFBT approach, as it focuses on the causal processes involved in traumatic stress. A recommended focus on making "*basic mental health services broadly available in post-disaster countries*" (Van Ommeren et al., 2005a, pp. 1160) would essentially amount to not much more than a 'business as usual' approach after disasters, if such services are not complementary to a behavioral trauma-focused approach that effectively reverses the effects of traumatic stress.

The view that PTSD and other comorbid disorders *tend to make up the mild and moderate mental disorders* (Van Ommeren et al., 2005a, pp. 1160) after disasters is not supported by evidence from our studies as well as those of other researchers. While survivor populations show wide variability in severity of trauma-induced mental health problems, it is common knowledge to experienced care providers that a non-negligible proportion of survivors suffer from serious psychiatric conditions, including severe PTSD and depression. Evidence (reviewed in Chapter 9) shows that the mental health consequences of natural disaster trauma can be as serious as those of war and torture trauma. Regarding the severity of PTSD and associated depression, the reader is also referred to Chapter 3 on assessment where we presented data from our studies on the severity of these conditions and the extent and severity of associated functional impairment. In our field surveys involving 3912 earthquake survivors from the epicenter region, 31% rated their traumatic stress problems as fairly to extremely severe. Second, total PTSD scores were strongly correlated with the severity of overall perceived distress and functional impairment. Third, treatment-seeking behavior was closely associated with severity of traumatic stress problems. Furthermore, as

noted earlier, 35% of earthquake survivors who actively sought help from our community center in the disaster region had only sub-threshold PTSD. This could be explained in part by the fact that 'mild' traumatic stress reactions can be associated with significant social disability (e.g. loss of employment, inability to execute important daily functions, social isolation, etc.), particularly in cases with extensive behavioral avoidance of trauma reminders. These findings do not support the view that PTSD is not "*the focus of many survivors of trauma.*"

The WHO position also overlooks the fact that some survivors do not seek help does not necessarily mean they do not need help. In our epidemiological study (Başoğlu et al., 2004) 50% of the earthquake survivors who expressed a need for help for traumatic stress problems had not sought treatment before we contacted them (unpublished data). Not seeking help in such cases reflected in part the lack of sufficient treatment facilities, economic or practical problems in accessing the few available facilities, and daily survival problems in post-disaster circumstances. Our fieldwork showed that such survivors utilize psychological care services when made available to them through outreach programs. Some survivors who have highly distressing traumatic stress symptoms do not seek treatment, because they do not recognize such symptoms as problems that can be treated. Sometimes they are unable to see the connection between their trauma and stress symptoms. There are also cultural reasons for not seeking help. For example, men are often less likely to seek help than women, possibly reflecting their appraisal of help seeking as a sign of weakness. Thus, help-seeking behavior is not necessarily the primary indicator of the importance of a mental health problem. A sound mental healthcare approach needs to take into account all mental health consequences of disasters, not just those that prompt help-seeking.

Timing of interventions

Evidence shows that most people respond to mass trauma events with pervasive anxiety, fear, and related stress reactions. The view among many trauma workers, also shared by the WHO (Van Ommeren et al., 2005b), is that such responses to extreme events are 'normal' and that most people will recover from them. The fact that people display similar responses to trauma and that most of them recover does not necessarily imply that such responses are 'normal.' This is indeed similar to arguing that a virus infection is normal because most people respond to the virus when it enters their body and the symptoms that they develop are similar. Trauma often causes a marked disturbance in the psychological, physiological, and physical integrity of a person, which represents a deviation from the normal state of the organism. The psychological mechanisms responsible for 'normal' acute stress responses to trauma are essentially the same ones that account for 'abnormal' responses, such as chronic PTSD, depression, and anxiety disorders and other stress-related mental or physical illnesses that either persist or appear in the long-term. An understanding of acute traumatic stress as a 'normal reaction to abnormal events' also plays a role in the increasingly popular 'watchful waiting' approach in the early aftermath of mass trauma events. Such views imply inaction and are likely to discourage future work on prevention.

The material covered in this book suggests that much can be done in the way of psychologically preparing people for disasters and reducing acute traumatic stress in the early aftermath of trauma to prevent chronic stress problems in the long term. In Chapter 7 we discussed the rationale for early intervention in the early trauma phase, which is worth briefly summarizing here. As noted above, acute and chronic traumatic stress responses share the same mechanisms and thus are likely to respond to resilience-enhancing interventions in a similar fashion. Indeed, our naturalistic observations of natural recovery in earthquake survivors during the early trauma phase (largely facilitated by self-instigated exposure to trauma cues; see Part 1) support this point. Furthermore, some earthquake survivors in our treatment studies (e.g. Başoğlu et al., 2003a; Başoğlu et al., 2003b) were treated in the trauma phase (defined as the period starting with the initial major shock and ending with the cessation of aftershocks after about a year) and responded to treatment as much as those treated in the post-trauma phase. In addition, relapse rates in these cases were extremely low, despite exposure to further aftershocks, suggesting increased resilience against earthquake trauma. It is also worth noting that all our studies, including those that took place after the cessation of aftershocks, were also conducted in a social environment of prevalent fear resulting from expectations of yet another major earthquake expected to take place near Istanbul in the not so distant future. These

findings are also consistent with other studies (Bryant et al., 1999; Bryant et al., 2008; Foa et al., 1995) showing the effectiveness of exposure-based treatments in the early aftermath of trauma. If (a) helplessness responses account for both acute and chronic traumatic stress and (b) blocking avoidance behaviors reverses traumatic stress reactions, as our studies demonstrate, then exposure to trauma cues should be encouraged as early as possible in the aftermath of a trauma so that the development of chronic traumatic stress reactions can be prevented at an early stage.

Controversy regarding cross-cultural validity of PTSD

As the view that PTSD as a western concept lacks cross-cultural validity is one of the most controversial issues in the field of psychological trauma, it is worth saying a few words about what this view implies for the CFBT approach. Many studies (e.g. Assanangkornchai et al., 2004; Başoğlu et al., 2004; Başoğlu et al., 1994b; Cardozo et al., 2000; Cardozo et al., 2004; Chae et al., 2005; de Jong et al., 2001; Goenjian et al., 1994; Gorst-Unsworth and Goldenberg, 1998; Mollica et al., 2001; Norris et al., 2004; Pham et al., 2004; Ramsay et al., 1993; Sharan et al., 1996; Thienkrua et al., 2006; Wang et al., 2000) using PTSD measures have verified the existence of PTSD symptoms in various developing countries after different traumatic events, such as wars, torture, and natural disasters. These studies suggest that cross-cultural variation in the phenomenology of PTSD symptoms does not pose much of a problem in assessment of trauma survivors in non-western cultures. There are, however, problems with the definition of PTSD even in western countries, considering that both exploratory (Başoğlu et al., 2002; Şalcıoğlu et al., 2003; Şalcıoğlu et al., 2007b; Taylor et al., 1998) and confirmatory factor analytic studies (Anthony et al., 1999; Anthony et al., 2005; Asmundson et al., 2000; Buckley et al., 1998; King et al., 1998; Palmieri et al., 2007; Simms et al., 2002) of PTSD symptoms have so far failed to demonstrate the existence of three distinct symptom clusters as defined by DSM-IV (American Psychiatric Association, 1994). The phenomenology of particular PTSD symptoms and the particular clustering of PTSD symptoms might well show some variance across cultures and perhaps even across different types of traumatic events. Nevertheless, these issues do not alter the fact that fear and related traumatic stress responses to uncontrollable and unpredictable stressors are universal phenomena that cut across not only cultures but also species. Whether such responses should be labeled PTSD or given some other name is irrelevant to treatment. The important question is what can be done to reverse traumatic stress processes to facilitate recovery from the impact of trauma, however the latter may manifest itself in a particular culture. Given the universal nature of helplessness-induced traumatic stress, interventions designed to enhance resilience are most likely to have the same impact on people, whether in Western Europe, Tibet, or Africa.

Much of the debate on cross-cultural validity of PTSD is not based on a sound theoretical understanding of mechanisms of traumatic stress and what they imply for effective treatment. In our view, such debate, while it may provide opportunities for interesting academic discussion, unfortunately does not serve a useful purpose. It creates much confusion and frustration among care providers in developing countries who come across many cases with traumatic stress reactions in their daily practice. It also discourages trauma-focused treatment approaches and efforts to develop more effective interventions. As mental health professionals who have worked with trauma survivors in both western settings and developing countries, we are well aware of the cross-cultural differences in the perception of trauma and its effects on people. We are also acutely aware, however, of the need for interventions with a focus on the universals in human behavior and that a blanket dismissal of trauma-focused approaches in treatment is not in the interest of millions of survivors in desperate need for such interventions. Such attitudes on the part of some western trauma workers sometimes stem from an ideological position against imposition of western values on non-western cultures, which is regarded as essentially colonial in nature. While we are in total agreement with such an anti-colonial position in principle, we are also of the opinion that such a position, when imposed on non-western cultures without a thorough understanding of the underlying theoretical issues and in total disregard of scientific evidence as well as the experience of mental health professionals in developing countries, is also colonial in nature. It essentially amounts to not much more than a 'we know what is best for you' attitude displayed by western 'trauma experts' rushing into a disaster scene in developing countries.

Antidepressants in treatment of mass trauma survivors

Many psychiatrists in developing countries tend to prescribe antidepressant drugs as a first-line intervention in mass trauma survivors without due attention to alternative evidence-based psychological interventions. While this is in part due to lack of training in alternative treatments, it also reflects the influence of American psychiatry and pharmaceutical companies. It is therefore worth taking a brief look at the literature on the usefulness of antidepressants in treatment of trauma survivors.

Selective serotonin reuptake inhibitors (SSRIs) are indicated as the pharmacotherapy of choice in several clinical practice guidelines for PTSD (American Psychiatric Association, 2004; Friedman and Davidson, 2007; Friedman et al., 2000). Recently, the efficacy of newer antidepressants, including serotonin-norepinephrine reuptake inhibitors (SNRIs) and nora-drenergic and specific serotonergic agents (NaSSA) have also been examined. In addition, some atypical antipsychotic medications (risperidone and olanzapine) have been tested as adjunctive agents for refractory patients who have failed to respond to antidepressants.

The efficacy of SSRIs (sertraline, fluoxetine, paroxetine), SNRIs (venlafaxine), NaSSA (mirtazapine), and antidepressants combined with atypical antipsychotics (risperidone, olanzapine) was examined in 19 double-blind placebo-controlled randomized clinical trials of PTSD. Mean reduction in PTSD and depressive symptoms in these studies was 38% (SD = 16.5) and 32% (SD = 14.4), respectively, in cases treated with active drugs, while the corresponding rates were 28% (SD = 14.1) and 21% (SD = 13.1) in cases given pill placebo (Bartzokis et al., 2005; Brady et al., 2000; Connor et al., 1999; Davidson et al., 2001b; Davidson et al., 2003; Davidson et al., 2006a; Davidson et al., 2006b; Friedman et al., 2007; Hamner et al., 2003; Marshall et al., 2001; Marshall et al., 2007b; Martenyi et al., 2002b; Martenyi et al., 2007; Reich et al., 2004; Rothbaum et al., 2008; Tucker et al., 2001; Van der Kolk et al., 1994; Van der Kolk et al., 2007; Zohar et al., 2002). Thus, drug-placebo difference was about 10% for PTSD and depression. This pattern of improvement was also noted in effect sizes. Although the majority of the drugs achieved large pre- to post-treatment effects, so did the pill placebo. Indeed, the between-treatment effect sizes rarely exceeded the threshold (i.e. 0.50) necessary to detect a clinically significant difference between an active drug and placebo (overall mean 0.47, SD = 0.34). This is in contrast with exposure-based treatments which yield much larger effect sizes.

Also important is the fact that no studies examined relapse in drug-free follow-ups. Few double-blind placebo controlled maintenance studies involving survivors treated with SSRIs found that discontinuation of drug treatment is associated with return of PTSD symptoms (Davidson et al., 2001a; Martenyi et al., 2002a; Rapaport et al., 2002). Antidepressant treatment (paroxetine) did not improve patients who remained symptomatic after 12 weeks of exposure treatment (Simon et al., 2008). On the other hand, adding exposure treatment to SSRI treatment conferred additional benefits in patients who did not respond to previous pharmacotherapy (Otto et al., 2003; Rothbaum et al., 2006). Evidence from one of our treatment studies (Başoğlu et al., 2003b) shows that antidepressants do not contribute to improvement in PTSD when used together with CFBT (see Figure 6.2).

It is worth noting that antidepressants are also not very effective in alleviating depressive symptoms. A meta-analysis (Kirsch et al., 2008) of all clinical trials submitted to the US Food and Drug Administration for the licensing of antidepressants found that, compared with placebo, the new-generation SSRIs did not produce clinically significant improvements in patients who initially had moderate or even severe depression, but showed significant effects only in the most severely depressed patients. The findings also showed that the effect for these patients seems to be due to decreased responsiveness to placebo, rather than increased responsiveness to medication. These findings were supported by another review (Anderson et al., 2008) conducted for the purposes of revising the British Association for Psychopharmacology guidelines for treating depressive disorders with antidepressants. This review found only 20% of difference in drug versus placebo response rates with 55–65% of patients having significant residual symptoms after antidepressant treatment. Response to antidepressants increased in most severely depressed patients, which was related to decreased responsiveness to placebo. These two studies concluded that there is little reason to prescribe new-generation antidepressant medications to any but the most severely depressed patients unless alternative treatments have been ineffective.

An additional problem concerning drug trials in PTSD is that the findings have limited generalizability

because most studies involved middle-aged females sexually abused as children or Vietnam Veterans (Friedman and Davidson, 2007). There is also less evidence on the efficacy of medications in different age groups, because concerns about increased suicides among children and adolescents treated with SSRIs for depression and concerns about safety, age-related pharmacokinetic capacity, drug-drug interactions, and comorbid medical conditions in elderly people pose obstacles to pharmacotherapy research in these populations (Friedman and Davidson, 2007). Finally, when used in combination with exposure-based treatments, drugs may undermine the efficacy of the latter by facilitating attributions of improvement to the tablets rather than to personal efforts (Başoğlu et al., 1994a). In view of these findings, it is only fair to conclude that the use of antidepressants as a first-line intervention in treatment of trauma survivors can hardly be justified.

Implications for cognitive-behavioral treatment

The effects of exposure treatment on sense of control are well known to cognitive-behavioral therapists (e.g. Barlow, 2002; Marks and Dar, 2000). It is likely that some therapists observe such effects in their patients and perhaps even utilize strategies to boost their sense of control. Indeed, certain procedures used in behavior therapy (e.g. removal of safety signals during exposure) serve to increase sense of control in patients. Nevertheless, an intervention that does not have a sharp focus on the critical therapeutic processes is likely to have weaknesses. For example, the control-enhancing effects of exposure treatment are more likely to be coincidental or erratic (i.e. benefiting some but not others), and thus at times weak when the treatment focus is on fear reduction and when the attributional processes that lead to increased sense of control are not intentionally and specifically targeted and facilitated in every way possible. This might perhaps explain in part the findings from a meta-analysis of treatment studies of PTSD (Bradley et al., 2005) showing that 47% of the cases treated with exposure, 53% of cases treated with CBT, and 44% of cases treated with exposure and cognitive restructuring did not improve at the end of treatment. A sharper focus on avoidance and sense of control might enhance the efficacy of treatment, eliminate its redundant components, reduce therapist involvement (thereby enhancing self-reliance and sense of control), and thus facilitate its dissemination on a largely self-help basis.

A shift in treatment aims from anxiety reduction to enhancement of sense of control might not only enhance motivation for and compliance with treatment but also achieve greater and faster reduction in helplessness and associated stress responses. Presenting treatment merely as a means of reducing anxiety might have a limited effect on motivation. After all, as far as the patient is concerned, there are much easier ways of reducing fear than exposure treatment, such as avoiding fear-evoking situations, reliance on safety signals (e.g. carrying tablets), or taking anxiolytics. Moreover, setting anxiety reduction as the main goal in therapy against which progress is assessed and rewarded might further undermine sense of control in some patients whose anxiety fluctuates in response to various situational variables in an exposure session. This is generally true for most anxiety disorders. People with panic disorder and agoraphobia, for example, might show reduced fear in a supermarket but attribute this to the fact that the supermarket was not very crowded or that they woke up feeling generally better that day. Such characteristic 'yes but' responses (yes, I didn't panic but this was because ...) reflect insufficient sense of control, arising from the fact that anxiety cues in the same feared situation show significant variability from one occasion to another. A feared situation is never the same on two occasions in terms of its threat value. Such ever-changing nature of the fear stimuli might require repeated exposures to the same situation to ensure an adequate increase in sense of control when the patient perceives the treatment goal as reduction in fear. A control-focused approach might circumvent this problem by making treatment success contingent on lasting reversal of avoidance behavior, regardless of fear. In any event, such behavioral change and associated sense of control often lead to substantial reduction in fear. Those cases that show only partial or no reduction in fear during exposure, often regarded as treatment failures (Marks and Dar, 2000), are more likely to benefit from this approach, provided that a lasting reduction in avoidance can be achieved.

The effectiveness of a treatment involving only live exposure also raises questions about the need for certain commonly used interventions in CBT programs, such as imaginal exposure (e.g. Foa et al., 1999; Foa et al., 2005; Marks et al., 1998), cognitive restructuring (e.g. Blanchard et al., 2003; Bryant et al., 2003; Ehlers et al., 2003; Tarrier et al., 1999), and various anxiety

management techniques including relaxation training, coping skills training, breathing training, thought stopping, and guided self-dialogue (e.g. Cloitre et al., 2002; Foa et al., 1999; Glynn et al., 1999; Lee et al., 2002). Our findings are consistent with available evidence suggesting that cognitive interventions (Foa et al., 2005; Marks et al., 1998; Paunovic and Öst, 2001) or anxiety management techniques (Foa et al., 1999; Foa et al., 1991) do not confer additional benefits when used in combination with exposure.

Imaginal exposure might not be as potent as live exposure, as also noted by Devilly and Foa (2001) in their comment on the possible reasons for a relatively small effect size reported for imaginal exposure in a treatment study (Tarrier et al., 1999). Indeed, in a meta-analysis (Bradley et al., 2005) of treatment studies of PTSD, the mean effect size for interventions involving imaginal exposure combined with live exposure was twice as large as that for imaginal exposure alone (1.78 vs. 0.91; means recalculated by the present authors Şalcıoğlu et al., 2007a). The superiority of live over imaginal exposure might be explained by the fact that the former involves exposure to both past trauma memories and cues that signal future threat. For example, we have observed in our last study (Başoğlu et al., 2007) that exposure to simulated tremors in an earthquake simulator evokes not only fear of future earthquakes but also distress associated with past trauma memories, thus providing opportunities for gaining control over both types of stressors. We also noted that live exposure triggers much more vivid and wider range of trauma-related memories and imagery than would be possible in imaginal exposure. Furthermore, although imaginal exposure reduces the distress associated with trauma memories, such improvement might not generalize when it is not accompanied by increased sense of control associated with reduction in behavioral avoidance. Unfortunately, most studies have not reported treatment effects specifically on behavioral avoidance so we do not know if imaginal exposure reduces avoidance (or increases sense of control) before any actual live exposure takes place. In one of the few studies that examined this issue (Keane et al., 1989) imaginal exposure was not effective in reducing avoidance, a finding which might explain why improvement did not generalize to other symptoms, such as emotional numbing and guilt. In conclusion, our results suggest that better results could be obtained, while also saving considerable therapist time and effort, by giving priority to live exposure in therapy and using the other techniques only when the patient is having difficulty in conducting exposure. Therapist involvement in exposure could also be limited to such cases.

Finally, our findings imply that certain components of traditional behavior therapy, such as exposure homework tasks, weekly monitoring of progress, verbal reinforcement, and diary keeping are not always required for treatment success. Such time consuming practices might perhaps be reserved for more severely ill cases or those that pose problems of compliance. In setting treatment targets priority needs to be given to anxiety- or distress-evoking situations that contribute most to feelings of helplessness. Such situations are not necessarily the ones that are associated with highest levels of anxiety. Conversely, exposure does not always need to involve the most distressing cues to have significant impact on sense of control; low intensity stressors might achieve the same effect. Furthermore, repeated and lengthy exposure sessions until fear subsides might not be necessary. Exposure could be terminated when the person feels in control.

References

Ahern, J., Galea, S., Resnick, H., Kilpatrick, D., Bucuvalas, M. and Gold, J. (2002). Television images and psychological symptoms after the September 11 terrorist attacks. *Psychiatry, Interpersonal and Biological Processes*, **65**, 289–300.

American Psychiatric Association (1994). *Diagnostic and Statistical Manual of Mental Disorders (4th Edition)*. Washington, DC: American Psychiatric Association.

American Psychiatric Association (2004). *Practice Guideline for the Treatment of Patients with Acute Stress Disorder and Posttraumatic Stress Disorder*. Arlington, VA: American Psychiatric Association Practice Guidelines.

Anderson, I. M., Ferrier, I. N., Baldwin, R. C., Cowen, P. J., Howard, L., Lewis, G., Matthews, K., Mcallister-Williams, R. H., Peveler, R. C., Scott, J. and Tylee, A. (2008). Evidence-based guidelines for treating depressive disorders with antidepressants: A revision of the 2000 British Association for Psychopharmacology guidelines. *Journal of Psychopharmacology*, **22**, 343–396.

Anthony, J. L., Lonigan, C. J. and Hecht, S. A. (1999). Dimensionality of posttraumatic stress disorder symptoms in children exposed to disaster: Results from confirmatory factor analyses. *Journal of Abnormal Psychology*, **108**, 326–336.

Anthony, J. L., Lonigan, C. J., Vernberg, E. M., La Greca, A. M., Silverman, W. K. and Prinstein, M. J. (2005). Multisample cross-validation of a model of childhood posttraumatic stress disorder symptomatology. *Journal of Traumatic Stress*, **18**, 667–676.

Asmundson, G. J. G., Frombach, I., Mcquaid, J., Pedrelli, P., Lenox, R. and Stein, M. B. (2000). Dimensionality of posttraumatic stress symptoms: A confirmatory factor analysis of DSM-IV symptom clusters and other symptom models. *Behaviour Research and Therapy*, **38**, 203–214.

Assanangkornchai, S., Tangboonngam, S.-N. and Edwards, G. J. (2004). The flooding of Hat Yai: Predictors of adverse emotional responses to a natural disaster. *Stress and Health*, **20**, 81–89.

Associated Press (August 19, 2002). *Sept-11 Poll*. Accessed on March 24, 2010 at the Associated Press Archive: http://nl.newsbank.com/apab.

Barlow, D. H. (2002). *Anxiety and its Disorders: The Nature and Treatment of Anxiety and Panic*. New York: Guilford Press.

Bartzokis, G., Lu, P. H., Turner, J., Mintz, J. and Saunders, C. S. (2005). Adjunctive risperidone in the treatment of chronic combat-related posttraumatic stress disorder. *Biological Psychiatry*, **57**, 474–479.

Başoğlu, M., Kılıç, C., Şalcıoğlu, E. and Livanou, M. (2004). Prevalence of posttraumatic stress disorder and comorbid depression in earthquake survivors in Turkey: An epidemiological study. *Journal of Traumatic Stress*, **17**, 133–141.

Başoğlu, M., Livanou, M., Crnobarić, C., Franćišković, T., Suljić, E., Đurić, D. and Vranešić, M. (2005). Psychiatric and cognitive effects of war in former Yugoslavia: Association of lack of redress for trauma and posttraumatic stress reactions. *Journal of the American Medical Association*, **294**, 580–590.

Başoğlu, M., Livanou, M. and Şalcıoğlu, E. (2003a). A single session with an earthquake simulator for traumatic stress in earthquake survivors. *American Journal of Psychiatry*, **160**, 788–790.

Başoğlu, M., Livanou, M., Şalcıoğlu, E. and Kalender, D. (2003b). A brief behavioural treatment of chronic posttraumatic stress disorder in earthquake survivors: Results from an open clinical trial. *Psychological Medicine*, **33**, 647–654.

Başoğlu, M., Marks, I. M., Kılıç, C., Brewin, C. R. and Swinson, R. P. (1994a). Alprazolam and exposure for panic disorder with agoraphobia: Attribution of improvement to medication predicts subsequent relapse. *British Journal of Psychiatry*, **164**, 652–659.

Başoğlu, M., Paker, M., Paker, O., Özmen, E., Marks, I., İncesu, C., Şahin, D. and Sarımurat, N. (1994b). Psychological effects of torture: A comparison of tortured with nontortured political activists in Turkey. *American Journal of Psychiatry*, **151**, 76–81.

Başoğlu, M., Şalcıoğlu, E. and Livanou, M. (2002). Traumatic stress responses in earthquake survivors in Turkey. *Journal of Traumatic Stress*, **15**, 269–276.

Başoğlu, M., Şalcıoğlu, E. and Livanou, M. (2007). A randomized controlled study of single-session behavioural treatment of earthquake-related post-traumatic stress disorder using an earthquake simulator. *Psychological Medicine*, **37**, 203–213.

Başoğlu, M., Şalcıoğlu, E. and Livanou, M. (2009). Advances in our understanding of earthquake trauma and its treatment: A self-help model of mental health care for survivors. In *Mental Health and Disasters*, ed. Y. Neria, S. Galea and F. H. Norris. Cambridge: Cambridge University Press, 396–418.

Bichescu, D., Neuner, F., Schauer, M. and Elbert, T. (2007). Narrative exposure therapy for political imprisonment-related chronic posttraumatic stress disorder and depression. *Behaviour Research and Therapy*, **45**, 2212–2220.

Bisson, J. I., Jenkins, P. L., Alexander, J. and Bannister, C. (1997). Randomized controlled trial of psychological debriefing for victims of acute burn trauma. *British Journal of Psychiatry*, **171**, 78–81.

Blanchard, E. B., Hickling, E. J., Devineni, T., Veazey, C. H., Galovski, T. E., Mundy, E., Malta, L. S. and Buckley, T. C. (2003). A controlled evaluation of cognitive behavioral therapy for posttraumatic stress in motor vehicle accident survivors. *Behaviour Research and Therapy*, **41**, 79–96.

Blanchard, E. B., Kuhn, E., Rowell, D. L., Hickling, E. J., Wittrock, D., Rogers, R. L., Johnson, M. R. and Steckler, D. C. (2004). Studies of the vicarious traumatization of college students by the September 11th attacks: Effects of proximity, exposure and connectedness. *Behaviour Research and Therapy*, **42**, 191–205.

Bodvarsdottir, I. and Elklit, A. (2004). Psychological reactions in Icelandic earthquake survivors. *Scandinavian Journal of Psychology* **45**, 3–13.

Bolton, P., Bass, J., Betancourt, T., Speelman, L., Onyango, G., Clougherty, K. F., Neugebauer, R., Murray, L. and Verdeli, H. (2007). Interventions for depression symptoms among adolescent survivors of war and displacement in Northern Uganda: A randomized controlled trial. *Journal of the American Medical Association*, **298**, 519–527.

Bradley, R., Greene, J., Russ, E., Dutra, L. and Westen, D. (2005). A multidimensional meta-analysis of psychotherapy for PTSD. *American Journal of Psychiatry*, **162**, 214–227.

Brady, K., Pearlstein, T., Asnis, G. M., Baker, D., Rothbaum, B., Sikes, C. R. and Farfel, G. M. (2000). Efficacy and safety of sertraline treatment of posttraumatic stress disorder: A randomized controlled trial. *Journal of the American Medical Association*, **283**, 1837–1844.

Bryant, R. A., Mastrodomenico, J., Felmingham, K. L., Hopwood, S., Kenny, L., Kandris, E., Cahill, C. and Creamer, M. (2008). Treatment of acute stress disorder: A randomized controlled trial. *Archives of General Psychiatry*, **65**, 659–667.

Bryant, R. A., Moulds, M. L., Guthrie, R. M., Dang, S. T. and Nixon, R. D. (2003). Imaginal exposure alone and imaginal exposure with cognitive restructuring in treatment of posttraumatic stress disorder. *Journal of Consulting and Clinical Psychology*, **71**, 706–712.

Bryant, R. A., Sackville, T., Dang, S. T., Moulds, M. and Guthrie, R. (1999). Treating acute stress disorder: An evaluation of cognitive behavior therapy and supportive counseling techniques. *American Journal of Psychiatry*, **156**, 1780–1786.

Buckley, T. C., Blanchard, E. B. and Hickling, E. J. (1998). A confirmatory factor analysis of posttraumatic stress symptoms. *Behaviour Research and Therapy*, **36**, 1091–1099.

Cardozo, B. L., Bilukha, O. O., Crawford, C. A. G., Shaikh, I., Wolfe, M. I., Gerber, M. L. and Anderson, M. (2004). Mental health, social functioning, and disability in postwar Afghanistan. *Journal of the American Medical Association*, **292**, 575–584.

Cardozo, B. L., Vergara, A., Agani, F. and Gotway, C. A. (2000). Mental health, social functioning, and attitudes of Kosovar Albanians following the war in Kosovo. *Journal of the American Medical Association*, **284**, 569–577.

Carlier, I. V. E., Voerman, A. E. and Gersons, B. P. R. (2000). The influence of occupational debriefing on post-traumatic stress symptomatology in traumatized police officers. *British Journal of Medical Psychology*, **73**, 87–98.

Carr, V. J., Lewin, T. J., Webster, R. A., Kenardy, J. A., Hazell, P. L. and Carter, G. L. (1997). Psychological sequelae of the 1989 Newcastle earthquake: II. Exposure and morbidity profiles during the first 2 years post-disaster. *Psychological Medicine*, **27**, 167–178.

Catani, C., Kohiladevy, M., Ruf, M., Schauer, E., Elbert, T. and Neuner, F. (2009). Treating children traumatized by war and tsunami: A comparison between exposure therapy and meditation-relaxation in North-East Sri Lanka. *BMC Psychiatry*, **9**, 22.

Chae, E.-H., Tong Won, K., Rhee, S.-J. and Henderson, T. (2005). The impact of flooding on the mental health of affected people in South Korea. *Community Mental Health Journal*, **41**, 633–645.

Cloitre, M., Koenen, K. C., Cohen, L. R. and Han, H. (2002). Skills training in affective and interpersonal regulation followed by exposure: A phase-based treatment for PTSD related to childhood abuse. *Journal of Consulting and Clinical Psychology*, **70**, 1067–1074.

Conlon, L., Fahy, T. J. and Conroy, R. (1999). PTSD in ambulant RTA victims: A randomized controlled trial of debriefing. *Journal of Psychosomatic Research*, **46**, 37–44.

Connor, K. M., Sutherland, S. M., Tupler, L. A., Malik, M. L. and Davidson, J. R. (1999). Fluoxetine in post-traumatic stress disorder: Randomised, double-blind study. *The British Journal of Psychiatry*, **175**, 17–22.

Cosgrove-Mather, B. (June 10, 2002). *New York City Nine months later (Poll: Most New Yorkers worry about security in and around city)*. New York: CBSNEWS. Accessed on March 24, 2010 at http://www.cbsnews.com/stories/2002/06/10/opinion/polls/main511729.shtml

Davidson, J., Baldwin, D., Stein, D. J., Kuper, E., Benattia, I., Ahmed, S., Pedersen, R. and Musgnung, J. (2006a). Treatment of posttraumatic stress disorder with Venlafaxine extended release: A 6-month randomized controlled trial. *Archives of General Psychiatry*, **63**, 1158–1165.

Davidson, J., Pearlstein, T., Londborg, P., Brady, K. T., Rothbaum, B., Bell, J., Maddock, R., Hegel, M. T. and Farfel, G. (2001a). Efficacy of Sertraline in preventing relapse of posttraumatic stress disorder: Results of a 28-week double-blind, placebo-controlled study. *American Journal of Psychiatry*, **158**, 1974–1981.

Davidson, J., Rothbaum, B. O., Tucker, P., Asnis, G. M., Benattia, I. and Musgnung, J. (2006b). Venlafaxine extended release in posttraumatic stress disorder: A sertraline- and placebo-controlled study. *Journal of Clinical Psychopharmacology*, **26**, 259–267.

Davidson, J. R. T., Rothbaum, B. O., Van Der Kolk, B. A., Sikes, C. R. and Farfel, G. M. (2001b). Multicenter, double-blind comparison of sertraline and placebo in the treatment of posttraumatic stress disorder. *Archives of General Psychiatry*, **58**, 485–492.

Davidson, J. R. T., Weisler, R. H., Butterfield, M. I., Casat, C. D., Connor, K. M., Barnett, S. and Van Meter, S. (2003). Mirtazapine vs. placebo in posttraumatic stress disorder: A pilot trial. *Biological Psychiatry*, **53**, 188–191.

Davidson, P. R. and Parker, K. C. (2001). Eye movement desensitization and reprocessing (EMDR): A meta-analysis 2001. *Journal of Consulting and Clinical Psychology*, **69**, 305–316.

de Jong, J. T. V. M., Komproe, I. H., Van Ommeren, M., El Masri, M., Araya, M., Khaled, N., Van De Put, W. and Somasundaram, D. (2001). Lifetime events and posttraumatic stress disorder in 4 postconflict settings. *Journal of the American Medical Association*, **286**, 555–562.

Devilly, G. J. and Foa, E. B. (2001). The investigation of exposure and cognitive therapy: Comment on Tarrier et al. (1999). *Journal of Consulting and Clinical Psychology*, **69**, 114–116.

Ehlers, A., Clark, D. M., Hackmann, A., Mcmanus, F., Fennell, M., Herbert, C. and Mayou, R. (2003). A randomized controlled trial of cognitive therapy, a self-help booklet, and repeated assessments as early interventions for posttraumatic stress disorder. *Archives of General Psychiatry*, **60**, 1024–1032.

Foa, E. B., Dancu, C. V., Hembree, E. A., Jaycox, L. H., Meadows, E. A. and Street, G. P. (1999). A comparison of exposure therapy, stress inoculation training, and their combination for reducing posttraumatic stress disorder in female assault victims. *Journal of Consulting and Clinical Psychology*, **67**, 194–200.

Foa, E. B., Hearstikeda, D. and Perry, K. J. (1995). Evaluation of a brief cognitive-behavioral program for the prevention of chronic PTSD in recent assault victims. *Journal of Consulting and Clinical Psychology*, **63**, 948–955.

Foa, E. B., Hembree, E. A., Cahill, S. P., Rauch, S. A. M., Riggs, D. S., Feeny, N. C. and Yadin, E. (2005). Randomized trial of prolonged exposure for posttraumatic stress disorder with and without cognitive restructuring: Outcome at academic and community clinics. *Journal of Consulting and Clinical Psychology*, **73**, 953–964.

Foa, E. B. and Rauch, S. A. M. (2004). Cognitive changes during prolonged exposure versus prolonged exposure plus cognitive restructuring in female assault survivors with posttraumatic stress disorder. *Journal of Consulting and Clinical Psychology*, **72**, 879–884.

Foa, E. B., Rothbaum, B. O., Riggs, D. S. and Murdock, T. (1991). Treatment of posttraumatic stress disorder in rape victims: A comparison between cognitive-behavioral procedures and counseling. *Journal of Consulting and Clinical Psychology*, **59**, 715–723.

Friedman, M. J. and Davidson, J. R. T. (2007). Pharmacotherapy for PTSD. In *Handbook of PTSD: Science and Practice*, ed. M. J. Friedman, T. M. Keane and P. A. Resick. New York: Guilford Press, 376–405.

Friedman, M. J., Davidson, J. R. T., Mellman, T. A. and Southwick, S. M. (2000). Pharmacotherapy. In *Effective Treatments for PTSD*, ed. E. B. Foa, T. M. Keane and M. J. Friedman. New York: Guilford Press, 84–105.

Friedman, M. J., Marmar, C. R., Baker, D. G., Sikes, C. R. and Farfel, G. M. (2007). Randomized, double-blind comparison of sertraline and placebo for posttraumatic stress disorder in a Department of Veterans Affairs setting. *Journal of Clinical Psychiatry*, **68**, 711–720.

Ganesan, M. (2006). Psychosocial response to disasters: Some concerns. *International Review of Psychiatry*, **18**, 241–247.

Glynn, S. M., Eth, S., Randolph, E. T., Foy, D. W., Urbaitis, M., Boxer, L., Paz, G. G., Leong, G. B., Firman, G., Salk, J. D., Katzman, J. W. and Crothers, J. (1999). A test of behavioral family therapy to augment exposure for combat-related posttraumatic stress disorder. *Journal of Consulting and Clinical Psychology*, **67**, 243–251.

Goenjian, A. K., Najarian, L. M., Pynoos, R. S., Steinberg, A. M., Manoukian, G., Tavosian, A. and Fairbanks, L. A. (1994). Posttraumatic stress disorder in elderly and younger adults after the 1988 earthquake in Armenia. *American Journal of Psychiatry*, **151**, 895–901.

Gorst-Unsworth, C. and Goldenberg, E. (1998). Psychological sequelae of torture and organised violence suffered by refugees from Iraq: Trauma-related factors compared with social factors in exile. *British Journal of Psychiatry*, **172**, 90–94.

Hamner, M. B., Faldowski, R. A., Ulmer, H. G., Frueh, B. C., Huber, M. G. and Arana, G. W. (2003). Adjunctive risperidone treatment in post-traumatic stress disorder: A preliminary controlled trial of effects on comorbid psychotic symptoms. *International Clinical Psychopharmacology*, **18**, 1–8.

Handley, R. V., Salkovskis, P. M., Scragg, P. and Ehlers, A. (2009). Clinically significant avoidance of public transport following the London bombings: Travel phobia or subthreshold posttraumatic stress disorder? *Journal of Anxiety Disorders*, **23**, 1170–1176.

Hobbs, M., Mayou, R., Harrison, B. and Warlock, P. (1996). A randomized trial of psychological debriefing for victims of road traffic accidents. *British Medical Journal*, **313**, 1438–1439.

Hobfoll, S. E., Watson, P., Bell, C. C., Bryant, R. A., Brymer, M. J., Friedman, M. J., Friedman, M., Gersons, B. P. R., de Jong, J. T. V. M., Layne, C. M., Maguen, S., Neria, Y., Norwood, A. E., Pynoos, R. S., Reissman, D., Ruzek, J. I., Shalev, A. Y., Solomon, Z., Steinberg, A. M. and Ursano, R. J. (2007). Five essential elements of immediate and mid-term mass trauma intervention: Empirical evidence. *Psychiatry*, **70**, 283–315.

Kaminer, D., Stein, D. J., Mbanga, I. and Zungu-Dirwayi, N. (2001). The Truth and Reconciliation Commission in South Africa: Relation to psychiatric status and forgiveness among survivors of human rights abuses. *The British Journal of Psychiatry*, **178**, 373–377.

Keane, T. M., Fairbank, J. A., Caddell, J. M. and Zimering, R. T. (1989). Implosive (flooding) therapy reduces symptoms of PTSD in Vietnam combat veterans. *Behavior Therapy*, **20**, 245–260.

King, D. W., Leskin, G. A., King, L. A. and Weathers, F. W. (1998). Confirmatory factor analysis of the Clinician-Administered PTSD Scale: Evidence for the dimensionality of posttraumatic stress disorder. *Psychological Assessment*, **10**, 90–96.

Kirsch, I., Deacon, B. J., Huedo-Medina, T. B., Scoboria, A., Moore, T. J. and Johnson, B. T. (2008). Initial severity and antidepressant benefits: A meta-analysis of data submitted to the food and drug administration. *PLoS Medicine*, **5**(2), e45. doi:10.1371/journal. pmed.0050045.

Lee, C., Gavriel, H., Drummond, P., Richards, J. and Greenwald, R. (2002). Treatment of PTSD: Stress inoculation training with prolonged exposure compared to EMDR. *Journal of Clinical Psychology*, **58**, 1071–1089.

Livanou, M., Başoğlu, M., Şalcıoğlu, E. and Kalender, D. (2002). Traumatic stress responses in treatment-seeking earthquake survivors in Turkey. *Journal of Nervous and Mental Disease*, **190**, 816–823.

Livanou, M., Kasvikis, Y., Başoğlu, M., Mytskidou, P., Sotiropoulou, V., Spanea, E., Mitsopoulou, T. and Voutsa, N. (2005). Earthquake-related psychological distress and associated factors 4 years after the Parnitha earthquake in Greece. *European Psychiatry*, **20**, 137–144.

Marks, I. and Dar, R. (2000). Fear reduction by psychotherapies: Recent findings, future directions. *The British Journal of Psychiatry*, **176**, 507–511.

Marks, I. M., Lovell, K., Noshirvani, H. and Livanou, M. (1998). Treatment of posttraumatic stress disorder by exposure and/or cognitive restructuring: A controlled study. *Archives of General Psychiatry*, **55**, 317–325.

Marshall, M. D., Bryant, R. A., Amsel, L., Suh, E. J., Cook, J. M. and Neria, Y. (2007a). The psychology of ongoing threat: Relative risk appraisal, the September 11 attacks, and terrorism-related fears. *American Psychologist*, **62**, 304–316.

Marshall, R. D., Beebe, K. L., Oldham, M. and Zaninelli, R. (2001). Efficacy and safety of paroxetine treatment for chronic PTSD: A fixed-dose, placebo-controlled study. *American Journal of Psychiatry*, **158**, 1982–1988.

Marshall, R. D., Lewis-Fernandez, R., Blanco, C., Simpson, H. B., Lin, S. H., Vermes, D., Garcia, W., Schneier, F., Neria, Y., Sanchez-Lacay, A. and Liebowitz, M. R. (2007b). A controlled trial of paroxetine for chronic PTSD, dissociation, and interpersonal problems in mostly minority adults. *Depression and Anxiety*, **24**, 77–84.

Martenyi, F., Brown, E. B. and Caldwell, C. D. (2007). Failed efficacy of fluoxetine in the treatment of posttraumatic stress disorder. *Journal of Clinical Psychopharmacology*, **27**, 166–170.

Martenyi, F., Brown, E. B., Zhang, H., Koke, S. C. and Prakash, A. (2002a). Fluoxetine v. placebo in prevention of relapse in post-traumatic stress disorder. *The British Journal of Psychiatry*, **181**, 315–320.

Martenyi, F., Brown, E. B., Zhang, H., Prakash, A. and Koke, S. C. (2002b). Fluoxetine versus placebo in posttraumatic stress disorder. *Journal of Clinical Psychiatry*, **63**, 199–206.

McMillen, C. J., North, C. S. and Smith, E. M. (2000). What parts of PTSD are normal: Intrusion, avoidance, or arousal? Data from the Northridge, California, earthquake. *Journal of Traumatic Stress*, **13**, 57–75.

Mineka, S. and Sutton, J. (2006). Contemporary Learning Theory Perspectives on the Etiology of Fears and Phobias. In *Fear and Learning: From Basic Principles to Clinical Implications*, ed. M. G. Craske, D. Hermans and D. Vansteenwegen. Washington, DC: American Psychological Association, 75–97.

Mollica, R. F., Sarajlic, N., Chernoff, M., Lavelle, J., Vukovic, I. S. and Massagli, M. P. (2001). Longitudinal study of psychiatric symptoms, disability, mortality, and emigration among Bosnian refugees. *Journal of the American Medical Association*, **286**, 546–554.

Neria, Y., Gross, R., Litz, B., Maguen, S., Insel, B., Seirmarco, G., Rosenfeld, H., Suh, E. J., Kishon, R., Cook, J. M. and Marshall, R. D. (2007). Prevalence and psychological corrolates of complicated grief among bereaved adults 2.5–3.5 years after September 11th attacks. *Journal of Traumatic Stress*, **20**, 251–262.

Neuner, F., Onyut, P. L., Ertl, V., Odenwald, V., Schauer, E. and Elbert, T. (2008). Treatment of posttraumatic stress disorder by trained lay counselors in an African refugee settlement: A randomized controlled trial. *Journal of Consulting and Clinical Psychology*, **76**, 686–694.

Neuner, F., Schauer, M., Klaschik, C., Karunakara, U. and Elbert, T. (2004). A comparison of narrative exposure therapy, supportive counseling, and psychoeducation for treating posttraumatic stress disorder in an African refugee settlement. *Journal of Consulting and Clinical Psychology*, **72**, 579–587.

Norris, F. H., Murphy, A. D., Baker, C. K. and Perilla, J. L. (2004). Postdisaster PTSD over four waves of a panel study of Mexico's 1999 flood. *Journal of Traumatic Stress*, **17**, 283–292.

Otto, M. W., Hinton, D., Korbly, N. B., Chea, A., Ba, P., Gershuny, B. S. and Pollack, M. H. (2003). Treatment of pharmacotherapy-refractory posttraumatic stress disorder among Cambodian refugees: A pilot study of combination treatment with cognitive-behavior therapy vs sertraline alone. *Behaviour Research and Therapy*, **41**, 1271–1276.

Palmieri, P. A., Weathers, F. W., Difede, J. and King, D. W. (2007). Confirmatory factor analysis of the PTSD Checklist and the Clinician-Administered PTSD Scale in disaster workers exposed to the World Trade Center ground zero. *Journal of Abnormal Psychology*, **116**, 329–341.

Paunovic, N. and Öst, L.-G. (2001). Cognitive-behavior therapy vs exposure therapy in the treatment of PTSD in refugees. *Behaviour Research and Therapy*, **39**, 1183–1197.

Pfefferbaum, B., Doughty, D., Reddy, C., Patel, N., Gurwitch, R., Nixon, S. and Tivis, R. (2002). Exposure and peritraumatic response as predictors of posttraumatic stress in children following the 1995 Oklahoma City bombing. *Journal of Urban Health*, **79**, 354–363.

Pham, P. N., Weinstein, H. M. and Longman, T. (2004). Trauma and PTSD symptoms in Rwanda: Implications for attitudes toward justice and reconciliation. *Journal of the American Medical Association*, **292**, 602–612.

Ramsay, R., Gorst-Unsworth, C. and Turner, S. (1993). Psychiatric morbidity in survivors of organised state violence including torture. A retrospective series. *British Journal of Psychiatry*, **162**, 55–59.

Rapaport, M. H., Endicott, J. and Clary, C. M. (2002). Posttraumatic stress disorder and quality of life: Results across 64 weeks of sertraline treatment. *Journal of Clinical Psychiatry*, **63**, 59–65.

Reich, D. B., Winternitz, S., Hennen, J., Watts, T. and Stanculescu, C. (2004). A preliminary study of risperidone in the treatment of posttraumatic stress disorder related to childhood abuse in women. *Journal of Clinical Psychiatry*, **65**, 1601–1606.

Resick, P. A., Nishith, P., Weaver, T. L., Astin, M. C. and Feuer, C. A. (2002). A comparison of cognitive-processing therapy with prolonged exposure and a waiting condition for the treatment of chronic posttraumatic stress disorder in female rape victims. *Journal of Consulting and Clinical Psychology*, **70**, 867–879.

Rose, S., Brewin, C. R., Andrews, B. and Kirk, M. (1999). A randomized controlled trial of individual psychological debriefing for victims of violent crime. *Psychological Medicine*, **29**, 793–799.

Rothbaum, B. O., Cahill, S. P., Foa, E. B., Davidson, J. R. T., Compton, J., Connor, K. M., Astin, M. C. and Hahn, C.-G. (2006). Augmentation of sertraline with prolonged exposure in the treatment of posttraumatic stress disorder. *Journal of Traumatic Stress*, **19**, 625–638.

Rothbaum, B. O., Killeen, T. K., Davidson, J. R. T., Brady, K. T., Connor, K. M. and Heekin, M. H. (2008). Placebo-controlled trial of risperidone augmentation for selective serotonin reuptake inhibitor-resistant civilian posttraumatic stress disorder. *Journal of Clinical Psychiatry*, **69**, 520–525.

Rubin, G. J., Brewin, C. R., Greenberg, N., Hughes, J. H., Simpson, J. and Wessely, S. (2007). Enduring consequences of terrorism: 7-month follow-up survey of reactions to the bombings in London on 7 July 2005. *British Journal of Psychiatry*, **190**, 350–356.

Şalcıoğlu, E. (2004). *The effect of beliefs, attribution of responsibility, redress and compensation on posttraumatic stress disorder in earthquake survivors in Turkey*. PhD Dissertation. Institute of Psychiatry, King's College London, London.

Şalcıoğlu, E. and Başoğlu, M. (2009). Treatment of Posttraumatic Stress Disorder. In *International Encyclopedia of Rehabilitation*, ed. M. Boulin and J. Stone. Quebec: Center for International Rehabilitation Research Information and Exchange (CRRIE) and L'Institut de Réadaptation en Déficience Physique de Québec. Available online at http://cirrie.buffalo.edu/encyclopedia/article.php?id=106andlanguage=en.

Şalcıoğlu, E., Başoğlu, M. and Livanou, M. (2003). Long-term psychological outcome for non-treatment-seeking earthquake survivors in Turkey. *Journal of Nervous and Mental Disease*, **191**, 154–160.

Şalcıoğlu, E., Başoğlu, M. and Livanou, M. (2007a). Effects of live exposure on symptoms of posttraumatic stress disorder: The role of reduced behavioral avoidance in improvement. *Behaviour Research and Therapy*, **45**, 2268–2279.

Şalcıoğlu, E., Başoğlu, M. and Livanou, M. (2007b). Post-traumatic stress disorder and comorbid depression among survivors of the 1999 earthquake in Turkey. *Disasters*, **31**, 115–129.

Saxena, S., Van Ommeren, M. and Saraceno, B. (2006). Mental health assistance to populations affected by disasters: World Health Organization's role. *International Review of Psychiatry*, **18**, 199–204.

Schlenger, W. E., Caddell, J. M., Ebert, L., Jordan, B. K., Rourke, K. M., Wilson, D., Thalji, L., Dennis, J. M., Fairbank, J. A. and Kulka, R. A. (2002). Psychological reactions to terrorist attacks: Findings from the national study of Americans' reactions to September 11. *Journal of the American Medical Association*, **288**, 581–588.

Scholes, C., Turpin, G. and Mason, S. (2007). A randomised controlled trial to assess the effectiveness of providing self-help information to people with symptoms of acute stress disorder following a traumatic injury. *Behaviour Research and Therapy*, **45**, 2527–2536.

Schwarz, J. (September 5, 2002) Americans adapt to life after terrorist attacks. *The Associated Press*. Accessed on March 24, 2010 at the Associated Press Archive: http://nl.newsbank.com/sites/apab.

Sharan, P., Chaudhary, G., Kavathekar, S. A. and Saxena, S. (1996). Preliminary report of psychiatric disorders in survivors of a severe earthquake. *American Journal of Psychiatry*, **153**, 556–558.

Silver, R. C., Holman, E. A., Mcintosh, D. N., Poulin, M. and Gil-Rivas, V. (2002). Nationwide longitudinal study of psychological responses to September 11. *Journal of the American Medical Association*, **288**, 1235–1244.

Simms, L. J., Watson, D. and Doebbeling, B. N. (2002). Confirmatory factor analyses of posttraumatic stress symptoms in deployed and nondeployed veterans of the Gulf War. *Journal of Abnormal Psychology*, **111**, 637–647.

Simon, N. M., Connor, K. M., Lang, A. J., Rauch, S., Krulewicz, S., Lebeau, R. T., Davidson, J. R. T., Stein, M. B., Otto, M. W., Foa, E. B. and Pollack, M. H. (2008). Paroxetine CR augmentation for posttraumatic stress disorder refractory to prolonged exposure therapy. *Journal of Clinical Psychiatry*, **69**, 400–405.

Tarrier, N., Pilgrim, H., Sommerfield, C., Faragher, B., Reynolds, M., Graham, E. and Barrowclough, C. (1999). A randomized trial of cognitive therapy and imaginal exposure in the treatment of chronic posttraumatic stress disorder. *Journal of Consulting and Clinical Psychology*, **67**, 13–18.

Taylor, S., Kuch, K., Koch, W. J., Crockett, D. J. and Passey, G. (1998). The structure of posttraumatic stress symptoms. *Journal of Abnormal Psychology*, **107**, 154–160.

Thienkrua, W., Cardozo, B. L., Chakkraband, M. L. S., Guadamuz, T. E., Pengjuntr, W., Tantipiwatanaskul, P., Sakornsatian, S., Ekassawin, S., Panyayong, B., Varangrat, A., Tappero, J. W., Schreiber, M., Van Griensven, F. and For the Thailand Post-Tsunami Mental Health Study Group (2006). Symptoms of posttraumatic stress disorder and depression among children in tsunami-affected areas in southern Thailand. *Journal of the American Medical Association*, **296**, 549–559.

Tucker, P., Zaninelli, R., Yehuda, R., Ruggiero, L., Dillingham, K. and Pitts, C. D. (2001). Paroxetine in the treatment of chronic posttraumatic stress disorder: Results of a placebo-controlled, flexible dosage trial. *Journal of Clinical Psychiatry*, **62**, 860–868.

US Geological Survey (November 22, 1999). *Implications for earthquake risk reduction in the United States from Kocaeli, Turkey earthquake of August 17, 1999. US Geological Survey Circular 1193*. United States Government Printing Office.

Van Der Kolk, B. A., Dryfuss, D., Michaels, M. J., Shera, D., Berkowitz, R., Fisler, R. and Saxe, G. (1994). Fluoxetine in post-traumatic stress disorder. *Journal of Clinical Psychiatry*, **55**, 517–522.

Van Der Kolk, B. A., Spinazzola, J., Blaustein, M. E., Hopper, J. W., Hopper, E. K., Korn, D. L. and Simpson, W. B. (2007). A randomized clinical trial of eye movement desensitization and reprocessing (EMDR), fluoxetine, and pill placebo in the treatment of posttraumatic stress disorder: Treatment effects and long term maintenance. *Journal of Clinical Psychiatry*, **68**, 37–46.

Van Etten, M. L. and Taylor, S. (1998). Comparative efficacy of treatments for post-traumatic stress disorder: A meta-analysis. *Clinical Psychology and Psychotherapy*, **5**, 126–144.

Van Ommeren, M., Saxena, S. and Saraceno, B. (2005a). Aid after disasters. *British Medical Journal*, **330**, 1160–1161.

Van Ommeren, M., Saxena, S. and Saraceno, B. (2005b). Mental and social health during and after acute emergencies: Emerging consensus? *Bulletin of the World Health Organization*, **83**, 71–75.

Wang, X., Gao, L., Shinfuku, N., Zhang, H., Zhao, C. and Shen, Y. (2000). Longitudinal study of earthquake-related PTSD in a randomly selected community sample in North China. *American Journal of Psychiatry*, **157**, 1260–1266.

World Health Organization (2003). *Mental Health in Emergencies: Psychological and Social Aspects of Health of Populations Exposed to Extreme Stressors*. Geneva: World Health Organization. Accessed on June 07, 2010 at www.who.int/mental_health/media/en/640.pdf.

Zohar, J., Amital, D., Miodownik, C., Kotler, M., Bleich, A., Lane, R. M. and Austin, C. (2002). Double-blind placebo-controlled pilot study of sertraline in military veterans with posttraumatic stress disorder. *Journal of Clinical Psychopharmacology*, **22**, 190–195.

Issues in rehabilitation of war and torture survivors

While many of the issues in care of mass trauma survivors reviewed in Chapter 8 also pertain to rehabilitation of war and torture survivors, certain issues that are rather characteristic of the field of torture rehabilitation deserve special attention. In 1988 we had published an editorial in the British Medical Journal pointing to the fact that torture rehabilitation programs lacked any evidence of effectiveness (Başoğlu and Marks, 1988). Another editorial (Başoğlu, 2006) nearly two decades later pointed to the lack of progress in torture rehabilitation and reviewed advances in trauma treatment suggesting that relatively brief and effective treatment of torture survivors is possible. The responses to this editorial and the debate (British Medical Journal, 2006) that ensued were quite informative with respect to the rationale behind lengthy rehabilitation programs. Such programs were defended on the grounds that tortured refugees are more difficult to treat than natural disaster survivors, mainly because of the cognitive effects of torture and additional psychosocial stressors associated with asylum-seeking or refugee status. Such beliefs characterize much of the current thinking in the human rights field, despite lack of any evidence in support of them. In this chapter we first review some evidence that highlights the state of the art in torture rehabilitation. As there are no comparative studies of war, torture, and natural disaster trauma, we present evidence from our studies that might shed some light on this issue. We also present two recent case studies, which suggest that traumatized asylum-seekers with war and torture experiences are just as responsive to brief behavioral treatment as earthquake survivors. Finally, we review some of the reasons that may account for lack of progress in this field and make some recommendations for future work.

State of the art in torture rehabilitation

Work in the torture rehabilitation area was largely pioneered by the International Rehabilitation Council for Torture Victims (IRCT) in Denmark, leading to the establishment of more than 200 torture rehabilitation centers around the world (van Willigen, 2007). In 2003, the European Commission (EC) was financially supporting 48 rehabilitation projects, many of which were part of the IRCT network (van Willigen, 2007). In recent years the EC commissioned several projects to evaluate the work of seven rehabilitation centers in Europe and elsewhere, including *Primo Levi* in France, the *Medical Foundation for the Care of Victims of Torture* in the United Kingdom, *Centre Medico-Psychosocial pour des Personnes Exiles et pour des Victims de Torture* (EXIL) in Belgium, *Medical Rehabilitation Centre for Torture Victims* in Greece, the *Centre for Victims of Torture in Nepal* (CVICT), *Centro de Atencion Psicosocial* in Peru, and the *Human Rights Foundation* in Turkey. The expert reports (Guillet et al., 2005; van Willigen, 2007; van Willigen et al., 2003) based on these evaluations revealed little convincing evidence with respect to the impact of these centers, either in prevention of torture or rehabilitation of survivors. In their report on four centers in Europe, Guillet et al (2005) concluded that the projects "*lack objectively verifiable indicators to monitor the work undertaken ... there is some reluctance and / or lack of knowledge on how to identify evaluation tools and indicators to measure and assess the impact of the work*" (pp. 5) "*... the impact on patients is difficult to assess in quantitative terms*" (pp. 4) and that "*... in most cases the centers have very little impact on primary prevention* [of torture]" (pp. 6). The concerns expressed about torture rehabilitation programs in our 1988 editorial (Başoğlu and Marks, 1988) were further supported by recent outcome evaluation studies conducted at the Rehabilitation and Research Centre for Torture Victims in Denmark, which showed that their 9-month-long rehabilitation program was ineffective not only in reducing chronic traumatic stress problems (Carlsson et al., 2005) but also torture-related chronic pain in parts of the body (Olsen, 2006).

Considering the costly nature of rehabilitation programs, these results raise serious questions about the justification for such projects. According to the Rehabilitation and Research Centre for Torture Victims 2007 annual report (2008) rehabilitation of 129 cases in 2007 cost about 2.44 million USD, which constituted 22% of their total budget of 11 million USD. This yields a cost of about $18 900 per case. In 2008 about 2.8 million USD (23% of the total budget of about 12.1 million USD) was spent on rehabilitation (Rehabilitation and Research Centre for Torture Victims, 2009); the total number of treated cases was not indicated in their report. In the same year 5.3 million USD was spent on Torture and Organized Violence and development projects in various countries, presumably to assist local professionals in torture prevention and rehabilitation efforts. The usefulness of these projects is also uncertain in the light of the EC commissioned evaluations of similar projects. A further 2.9 million USD was spent on research and documentation. Indeed, the Rehabilitation and Research Centre for Torture Victims states one of its objectives as "*to develop clinical diagnoses and treatment methods of torture survivors on the basis of systematic examinations of the torture survivors and research into torture and organized violence*" (Rehabilitation and Research Centre for Torture Victims, 2010). Yet, none of the projects listed under rehabilitation or publications in their 2009 report included research on alternative evidence-based treatments, despite findings pointing to the ineffectiveness of their rehabilitation program.

Natural disaster versus human-made trauma: are they different?

Because of their similar methodologies, our studies of war, torture, and earthquake survivors provided a unique opportunity for direct comparisons between different survivor samples. To test the hypothesis that human-made trauma is different from natural disasters we compared samples from four studies summarized in Table 1 in the Introduction. These samples included 202 torture survivors in Turkey (Study 1), 230 torture survivors in former Yugoslavia (Study 2), 1079 non-tortured war survivors in former Yugoslavia (Study 3), and 188 earthquake survivors in Turkey (Study 4). The treatment-seeking survivors were excluded from the Study 4 sample. Thus, all four samples involved non-treatment-seeking community subjects accessed through outreach programs or snowballing. In these studies we assessed post-trauma psychiatric conditions using the same structured interviews. The samples were compared on several parameters, including duration and severity of trauma, mechanisms of traumatic stress, the nature, prevalence, and severity of mental health outcomes, and response to effective interventions.

Duration and severity of trauma

A common misconception is that earthquake trauma differs from war and torture in being a single traumatic event. Earthquake trauma is not limited to the impact of the initial major shock. The prolonged nature of earthquake trauma involving a wide range of stressor events, including unpredictable and uncontrollable aftershocks that continue for many months, was detailed in Chapter 1. In Study 4 the earthquake survivors reported mean 16 (SD = 8) traumatic stressors during the earthquake and the early days of the disaster (data based on Exposure to Earthquake Stressors Scale). The torture survivors in Study 1 and Study 2 reported mean 22 (SD = 8) and mean 20 (SD = 8) stressors events during their torture experience, respectively (data based on Exposure to Torture Scale). The respective figure for war survivors in Study 3 (based on Exposure to War Stressors Scale) was 10 (SD = 6). These figures show that earthquakes, like war and torture trauma, involve a wide range of traumatic stressors. It is worth noting that the Exposure to Earthquake Stressors Scale underestimates the number of earthquake-related stressor events, because it does not include events in the long term (e.g. displacement, relocation, loss of resources, continuing aftershocks, etc.). In any event, the subjective impact of trauma is a more important predictor of post-trauma outcome than the mere count of stressor events (evidence reviewed in Part 1).

Immediate and long-term psychological impact of trauma

In all four studies the survivors rated their perceived distress in relation to each reported stressor event on a 0–4 scale (0 = no distress / fear, 4 = extreme distress / fear). These ratings were averaged across events to obtain a Mean Distress Score. The torture survivors in former Yugoslavia countries had the highest mean distress scores (mean = 3.1, SD = 0.6), followed by the earthquake survivors (mean = 2.8, SD = 0.9), war survivors (mean = 2.7, SD = 0.6), and torture survivors in

Table 9.1 Rates of psychiatric diagnoses[a]

	Torture		War	Earthquake	
	Study 1 (n = 202)	Study 2 (n = 230)	Study 3 (n = 1079)	Study 4 (n = 188)	χ^2
Current PTSD	37	56	13	30	221.1***
Current Major Depressive Episode	13	17	7	21	48.0***
Other anxiety disorders	11	15	13	25	19.2***
Any other Axis-I disorder[b]	11	20	17	16	6.5

*** $p < 0.001$.
[a] Based on Structured Clinical Interview for DSM-III-R / DSM-IV Axis I Disorders (First et al., 1996).
[b] Mood disorders other than depression, substance abuse / dependence disorders, somatization disorders, eating disorders, and adjustment disorder.

Turkey (mean = 2.4, SD = 0.7)(F = 45.4, p < 0.001; all pairwise comparisons significant at p < 0.05 level).

With respect to the long-term mental health outcomes of trauma, Table 9.1 shows the rates of psychiatric disorders in the study samples. Several findings deserve attention here. The high distress scores and rates of PTSD among the torture survivors in former Yugoslavia countries might reflect greater perceived threat to life associated with being held captive by the enemy in detention camps under extremely precarious conditions. In Chapter 2 we discussed the role of resilience and captivity context factors that explain the differences in response to torture in the different socio-political settings of Turkey and former Yugoslavia countries. These findings once again suggest that the impact of torture is mediated by individual and contextual factors and thus does not invariably lead to more severe distress and PTSD than do other traumas. This is supported by the fact that the differences in Mean Distress Scores and the rates of PTSD in torture versus earthquake survivors in Turkey (Study 1 versus Study 4 samples) were not substantial. That these differences were statistically significant may not mean much, as even small differences may turn out to be significant in relatively large samples (Kazdin, 2003, pp. 440). Furthermore, the rates of depression, anxiety disorders other than PTSD, and other DSM-IV Axis-I disorders (American Psychiatric Association, 1994) in earthquake survivors were not lower than those in war and torture survivors.

All these findings imply that a resilient person subjected to extremely severe torture in objective terms (i.e. the nature and number of torture events endured) might present with relatively mild mental health problems, whereas a less resilient natural disaster survivor exposed to relatively milder trauma might present with severe psychiatric problems. Clinically, the latter case would be more difficult to treat. It is worth noting in this connection that the common misconception that torture is more difficult to treat than natural disaster trauma largely arises from a failure to take into account the fact that it is the subjective rather than the objective severity of the trauma that mediates traumatic stress.

Severity of mental health outcomes

An important factor that might be expected to determine response to treatment is the severity of PTSD and psychiatric conditions comorbid with PTSD. The severity of PTSD was measured using the Clinician Administered PTSD Scale (CAPS; Blake et al., 1990) in all participants of the four studies (except 55 cases in Study 1). A CAPS score range of 40–59 indicates moderately severe PTSD, while scores from 60 to 79 indicate severe PTSD (Weathers et al., 2001). The four study samples did not significantly differ in mean total CAPS scores (respectively, mean = 64, SD = 15; mean = 66, SD = 18; mean = 61, SD = 17; mean = 68, SD = 17; F = 2.42, p = 0.07). Table 9.2 shows the rates of depression, anxiety disorders, and other psychiatric conditions in cases with PTSD in the four studies (all diagnoses established with Structured Clinical Interview for DSM-IV Axis I Disorders – SCID). The data show no distinct pattern suggesting that war- and torture-induced PTSD is more commonly associated with other comorbid

Table 9.2 Rates of psychiatric conditions comorbid with PTSD[a]

	Torture		War	Earthquake	
	Study 1 (n = 202)	Study 2 (n = 230)	Study 3 (n = 1079)	Study 4 (n = 188)	χ^2
Current depression	28	30	33	42	3.6
Other anxiety disorders	12	19	32	42	22.0***
Other SCID diagnoses[b]	12	29	27	25	8.1*

* $p < 0.05$, *** $p < 0.001$.
[a] Based on Structured Clinical Interview for DSM-III-R / DSM-IV Axis I Disorders (First et al., 1996).
[b] Mood disorders other than depression, substance abuse / dependence disorders, somatization disorders, eating disorders, and adjustment disorder.

psychiatric conditions than earthquake-related PTSD. If anything, earthquake survivors had a substantially higher rate of other anxiety disorders comorbid with PTSD than did both groups of torture survivors.

Attributions of blame and appraisal of impunity

In all studies but the study of torture survivors in Turkey we also used a *Redress for Trauma Survivors Questionnaire* (RTSQ) to assess attributions of responsibility for trauma and levels of dissatisfaction associated with perceived impunity for those held responsible for trauma (see Chapter 2 for details). All war and torture survivors in former Yugoslavia attributed responsibility for their trauma to other people, as would be expected. Interestingly, however, a similarly high percentage (97%) of the earthquake survivors in Turkey also blamed other people for their trauma (Şalcıoğlu, 2004). Most commonly they blamed building contractors for having constructed sub-standard buildings and government authorities for having allowed this to happen. The government authorities were also blamed for their delayed and inadequate rescue and relief efforts. Some survivors regarded the earthquake as a punishment for the sins of 'morally depraved' people in society. Only about 1% of the survivors attributed the disaster to natural causes and thought no one was to blame. These findings show that natural disaster survivors perceive a strong element of human involvement in their trauma.

Eighty-seven percent of both war and torture survivors in former Yugoslavia countries and 80% of the earthquake survivors reported that those they thought were responsible for their trauma were not brought to justice. These survivors were asked to rate their dissatisfaction in relation to this issue on a 1–7 scale (1 = very much dissatisfied, 4 = no effect / don't know, 7 = very much satisfied). Those survivors who reported that those they held responsible for their trauma were brought to justice were asked to rate their satisfaction with the outcome of this process on the same scale. The mean scores for torture, war, and earthquake survivors were 1.7 (SD = 1.4), 2.1 (SD = 1.5), and 1.7 (SD = 1.1), respectively (F = 13.1, $p < 0.001$). Pairwise comparisons indicated that war survivors were significantly less dissatisfied than both torture and earthquake survivors and that the latter two groups did not significantly differ in their mean scores. These findings suggest that sense of injustice arising from perceived impunity for those held responsible for trauma may be as strong in earthquake survivors as in torture survivors.

The *Emotions and Beliefs after War* (EBAW) and *Emotions and Beliefs after Trauma* (EBAT) questionnaires (see Chapter 3) were used in measuring the intensity of emotional responses to perceived impunity for those held responsible for trauma. Of the 11 items that measured these emotional responses, nine were common to all studies. Table 9.3 shows the mean item scores in cases with PTSD in the four studies (excluding 89 survivors from Study 1 on whom EBAW data were not available). Significant differences were noted in five items. Earthquake survivors did not significantly differ from war and torture survivors in feelings of anger / rage, demoralization, sense of injustice, and desire for punishment with own hands. The pairwise comparisons did not reveal consistent findings in support of the hypothesis that war and torture

Table 9.3 Emotional responses to perceived impunity for those held responsible for trauma in torture, war, and earthquake survivors with PTSD

	Torture		War	Earthquake		
	Study 1	Study 2	Study 3	Study 4		
	n = 50 M (SD)	n = 128 M (SD)	n = 141 M (SD)	n = 59 M (SD)	p	Pairwise comparisons
Feelings of anger / rage	7.0 (1.5)	7.1 (1.7)	6.8 (1.9)	6.4 (2.3)	0.11	
Feeling distressed	6.5 (1.9)	6.7 (1.9)	6.6 (2.0)	5.3 (2.9)	0.001	4 < 1, 2, 3
Feelings of demoralization	5.9 (2.4)	6.5 (2.0)	5.8 (2.3)	5.6 (2.8)	0.06	
Sense of injustice	7.1 (1.4)	7.2 (1.6)	7.0 (1.9)	6.7 (2.2)	0.32	
Feelings of helplessness	4.1 (3.0)	6.1 (2.1)	5.6 (2.5)	5.2 (2.6)	0.001	1 < 2, 3, 4; 4 < 2
Feeling pessimistic about the future	4.4 (3.1)	6.2 (2.1)	5.7 (2.4)	6.1 (2.4)	0.001	1 < 2, 3, 4
Desire for punishment with own hands	5.3 (2.9)	4.5 (3.1)	4.5 (3.3)	4.0 (3.5)	0.23	
Dreams about acts of revenge	3.3 (2.9)	3.3 (2.9)	2.9 (2.9)	1.7 (2.5)	0.01	4 < 1, 2, 3
Daydreams about revenge	4.5 (3.1)	3.0 (2.8)	2.8 (2.8)	2.3 (3.1)	0.001	2, 3, 4 < 1

have stronger emotional effects than earthquake trauma. War and torture survivors in both Turkey and former Yugoslavia scored higher than earthquake survivors only on items relating to distress and revenge dreams. Earthquake survivors, on the other hand, scored higher on items relating to pessimism and helplessness than did torture survivors in Turkey. As in comparisons of other trauma impact reviewed earlier, contextual factors appeared to play a role in emotional responses to perceived impunity. On the basis of these findings it is difficult to conclude that traumas of human design invariably lead to more attributions of blame to others and stronger emotional responses to impunity than do natural disasters.

Mechanisms of traumatic stress

Does greater cognitive impact of trauma imply more severe post-traumatic stress? In Chapter 2 we reviewed the results of a regression analysis examining the contribution of trauma-altered beliefs on PTSD. Helplessness associated with appraisal of ongoing threat to safety was a much stronger predictor of PTSD than helplessness related to perceived impunity for those held responsible for trauma and sense of defeat and loss of belief in war cause. A similar analysis with 387 earthquake survivors (including Study 4 sample) yielded essentially the same results (Şalcıoğlu,

2004). These findings suggest that PTSD is most strongly associated with fear-induced helplessness responses and not with the impact of trauma on beliefs about justice or trust. The fact that war, torture, and earthquake trauma share the same mechanisms of traumatic stress implies that they are likely to respond similarly to effective interventions that can reverse the traumatic process.

Response to treatment

Available evidence shows that exposure-based treatments are effective in reducing PTSD in survivors of human-made traumas, such as combat (Keane et al., 1989; Schnurr et al., 2007), war and torture (Paunovic and Öst, 2001), and rape (Foa et al., 1999; Foa et al., 2005), as well as in survivors of natural disasters (Başoğlu et al., 2003a; Başoğlu et al., 2003b; Başoğlu et al., 2005; Başoğlu et al., 2007b). Evidence from a study (Marks et al., 1998) also shows that survivors of 'personal' traumas (e.g. physical assaults, rape, etc.) do not respond less to exposure treatment than those with 'impersonal' traumas (e.g. road traffic accidents, etc.), which suggests that cognitive effects of human-made trauma do not necessarily impede improvement. It is indeed such consistent evidence across different types of trauma that has led to a consensus on exposure-based treatments being the treatment of choice in trauma survivors (National Institute of Clinical Excellence, 2005).

Psychosocial problems experienced by tortured refugees or asylum-seekers in a host country are often thought to be a complicating factor in treatment. In a case study (Başoğlu et al., 2004) involving an asylum-seeker in Sweden, we demonstrated that exposure treatment achieves substantial improvement, despite the uncertainties involved in being an asylum-seeker in a host country. The anxiety associated with risk of repatriation to home country and further threat to safety does not necessarily impede improvement with a treatment that enhances resilience against traumatic stressors. This was demonstrated in another case study (Başoğlu and Aker, 1996) involving a torture survivor who improved with exposure treatment, despite further threat of re-arrest and torture in her country. These cases were treated before we developed Control-Focused Behavioral Treatment (CFBT), using a traditional habituation-based exposure approach combined with cognitive interventions. Recently, we tested CFBT in two case studies involving two asylum-seekers in Turkey. We present these cases in some detail below for further discussion, as they are quite informative with respect to various issues in treatment. These were the first two cases referred to us by a refugee care organization in Istanbul when we decided to test CFBT with asylum-seekers and refugees. Some details are modified to protect the identity of these cases.

Case vignette #1

Alain was an 18-year-old, male, single, French-speaking asylum-seeker from an African country. He had been in Turkey for 16 months and his refugee claim was under consideration by the United Nations High Commissioner for Refugees (UNHCR). He was living in a church dormitory with other refugees. He reported multiple trauma experiences arising from the armed conflict in his country, including witnessing three incidents of mass killings, killing of his parents by armed forces, destruction of his home, witnessing rape of his sisters, going into hiding to avoid capture by the military, and imprisonment and death of his siblings. He was also detained for several weeks and subjected to beating and other ill-treatment. He managed to leave his country with the help of his relatives.

After his arrival in Turkey, Alain received psychiatric treatment, including antidepressant (citalopram 20 mg/day) and antipsychotic (olanzapine 5 mg/day)

medication and weekly therapy sessions for about 6 months, with no benefit. In psychiatric examination he had full-blown PTSD (assessment based on the CAPS; Blake et al., 1990) and major depression (assessment based on the SCID; First et al., 1996). He had suicidal ideas. His CAPS score was 82, which indicates 'extremely severe PTSD' according to the severity score ranges proposed by Weathers and colleagues (2001). He scored 50 on a self-rated PTSD Checklist (PCL; Ventureyra et al., 2002; Weathers et al., 1993) and 36 on the Beck Depression Inventory (BDI; Beck et al., 1985; Cottraux, 1985), indicating severe depression. Treatment started after a baseline assessment and involved weekly or twice-weekly sessions. Further assessments were at week 4, week 6, and week 8 (post-treatment). Assessment and treatment sessions were conducted by the second author with the help of an interpreter.

During the first session Alain was helped to understand how avoidance of trauma reminders maintained his PTSD symptoms. His avoidance behaviors included talking about his traumatic experiences, watching and reading news about violence and war, talking about or listening to people talking about the circumstances in his country, meeting his compatriots and listening to their trauma stories, watching movies depicting war or political violence, sleeping alone or in the dark, and walking alone in empty streets. He also avoided social interactions and had difficulty in establishing stable relationships with people because he thought that at some point they would ask him about his trauma story. He was then given an explanation about the treatment and its rationale. Systematic cognitive restructuring, imaginal exposure, and anxiety management techniques were not used.

Exposure treatment was first initiated on a self-administered basis, starting with the least anxiety-evoking situation (i.e. walking alone on empty streets during the day). At the second session the patient reported that he could not conduct self-exposure because he found it too difficult. The therapist decided to continue treatment with therapist-aided exposure. The subsequent sessions involved reading documents about the ongoing violence in the patient's country, watching movies depicting violence, and documentaries on human rights violations in Africa. While these sessions often ended with a reduction in his distress, occasionally high levels of distress were maintained throughout the session. As CFBT does not require detailed probing into the trauma story, Alain was never asked to relate his trauma story in detail. However, as exposure sessions reduced cognitive and behavioral avoidance, on several occasions he spontaneously volunteered various aspects of his trauma story that he had not told anyone.

After each session Alain was given self-exposure exercises, such as reading the documents about the ongoing violence in his country, talking to his friends about his trauma story, resuming contact with friends whom he stopped seeing because they asked questions about this past, and not avoiding trauma-related thoughts as they came to his mind. He was generally compliant with these exercises, despite occasional difficulties. Treatment also involved other interventions designed to enhance his sense of control over his life. As he spent much of his time during the day sleeping or sitting idly, he was asked to conduct various behavioral activation exercises to help him restructure his daily routines and take control of his life. He was asked to cut down his sleeping time from 12 to 8 hours, do some physical exercise, read a book, spend more time learning Turkish and English, and improve his computer skills. About halfway through treatment he decided to take up humanitarian work and receive some training in this regard. He also mentioned his plan to organize a project to help refugees. He was told that this would be an effective way of fighting back his trauma and provided strong support and encouragement in this direction.

At the eighth session, Alain stated that for the first time since he came to Turkey he had started thinking and worrying about his future. This meant that for the first time he was able to think about the future instead of the past, reflecting a reduction in intrusive thoughts about his trauma. After the tenth session he received news that his brother had been killed in prison. At the next session he expressed some natural grief reactions, such as anger, guilt, sadness, and demoralization but showed no signs of relapse. The session was spent providing emotional support and discussing ways of overcoming possible disabling effects of grief. He was asked to share the news with friends and other people in his life. He was encouraged to move on with his life and reminded that surrendering to despair and grief would mean surrendering to the people who killed his brother. He agreed and expressed a resolve to continue to fight and win the battle. His response to the loss of his brother was noteworthy, considering that earlier in treatment he had said that he would kill himself if he found out that his brother was dead.

At the 12th and last session he was advised to organize a symbolic funeral ceremony at the church where he resided with a view to facilitating resolution of his grief through exposure to cues that trigger grief reactions. Such a ceremony was indeed held during the same week as part of the Sunday mass, which was also attended by Alain's friends and his therapist. The speech he made at the ceremony is provided below, as it highlights some of the cognitive changes during treatment. This ceremony was meant to represent closure for his grief, while also marking the end of treatment.

> Lord, I return to your hands my brother as well as the other members of my family who are not here today. May their souls rest in peace … Being strong believers, my parents liked a lot to pray and devoted their life to others, to the poorest. As a sentence decorating our living room in my country and my father used to remind us daily: One can go far in life if one first does something for someone else. My brother … took the path of my father and we all have, in one way or the other, tried to follow this path. Lord, forgive those who hurt my family and help me forgive them one day. Lord, may peace reign in my country … where corpses are being collected every day, but also in all regions of the world where people suffer. Lord, for us who don't understand, comfort us in our faith and hope in you. You know the reasons for everything. Amen.

On the night of this event, Alain sent the following SMS to his therapist in English:

> Ebru, do you know how much I am happy today. It is my first time in Turkey to be happy like this and thank you very much for being there. You make me very happy today and don't forget you are very important for my life. Now I understand that you help me very much I cannot say – Seeing you helped me very much. I feel a change because I can do things that I have never been able to do before, thank you.

Alain's treatment lasted a total of 8 weeks involving 12 sessions, seven of which involved therapist-aided exposure. The total time spent in sessions was 22.7 hours (i.e. mean 1.9 hours per session). By week 4 assessment Alain had had only one session of therapist-aided live exposure (listening to the news articles about his country) and self-exposure to two previously avoided situations (sleeping alone in the dark and talking about the events in his country with strangers). This resulted in 32% reduction in self-rated PTSD symptoms and 53% reduction in depression scores. Between week 4 and week 6 he was given four sessions of therapist-aided exposure and he continued not avoiding trauma reminders (e.g. sleeping alone in the dark, telling his trauma story to others, reading news documents about the war and violence in his country). At week 6 there was 74% reduction in his self-rated PTSD Checklist score and 83% reduction in his depression score. By week 8, he was given two more sessions of therapist-aided exposure and he continued live exposure exercises in daily life. He also focused on restructuring his life in line with newly acquired aims, which also necessitated further exposure to previously avoided situations. At post-treatment assessment he showed 96% reduction in his self-rated PTSD symptoms (79% according to the CAPS) and 86% reduction in his depression. Global improvement was assessed using the Clinician's Global Impression-Improvement Scale (Guy, 1976) and the Patient's Global Impression-Improvement scale (Guy, 1976), both of which involve a single 1–7 scale assessing improvement relative to baseline psychological status (1 = *Very much improved*, 4 = *No change*, 7 = *Very much worse*). The ratings on these scales were, respectively, '*very much improved*' and '*much improved.*' Improvement was maintained at 1- and 3-month follow-up with 96% reduction in CAPS score, 98% reduction in PCL score, and 100% reduction in BDI score at last follow-up. Before his 1-month follow-up assessment he suffered two racist physical assaults (stabbing attempts) from several young men but survived both without any injury. He nevertheless maintained his improvement without any signs of relapse.

The improvement in Alain's case is unlikely to reflect non-specific time or therapist contact effects for several reasons. The fact that he had shown minimal and transient improvement in response to a previous 6-month-long treatment, including drugs, attests to the chronic and treatment-resistant nature of his problems. In addition, we know from our previous studies (Başoğlu et al., 2005; Başoğlu et al., 2007b) and those of others (Ehlers et al., 2005; Foa et al., 1999; Foa et al., 2005) that non-specific treatment effects do not account for more than 15–20% improvement in PTSD symptoms during a waiting period. Furthermore, repeated assessments during the treatment and follow-up period pointed to the progressive and stable nature of treatment gains. Although the stability of treatment effects needs to be confirmed by longer-term follow-up, Alain is likely to maintain his improvement in the long term, considering that early treatment response in the first weeks of behavioral treatment is the most important predictor of long-term outcome (Marks et al., 1988; Marks et al., 1993).

Certain changes in Alain's psychological status reflected improvement in his functional impairment. For example, with improvement in PTSD and depression, he began to distance himself from his distressing trauma memories and focus on his plans for the future. Together with this development, his determination to take up humanitarian work is an indication of increased sense of control over his life. Behavioral activation exercises and restructuring of his daily activities helped him reorganize his social life, make contact with his old friends, spend less time sleeping or sitting idly, and making more effort in learning English and improving his computer skills. The change in his attitudes towards life observed during the recovery process is an indication of how important it is to focus on traumatic stress as a matter of priority in asylum-seekers and refugees. Considering the various forms of social support Alain received from various sources since his arrival in Turkey, his case demonstrates that social support alone without specific interventions for PTSD is not sufficient in rehabilitation of asylum-seekers and refugees.

In Alain's treatment we did not use any systematic cognitive restructuring to correct faulty forms of thinking. Any cognitive intervention during treatment was aimed at enhancing his sense of control over his trauma and his life. Yet, improvement in PTSD and depression led to substantial change in his cognitions, particularly those relating to his purpose in life and plans for the future. His decision to take up humanitarian work reflects such cognitive change. Furthermore, his plea to God in his speech at the symbolic funeral ceremony about forgiving those who hurt his family is an entirely 'spontaneous' response, given that we never focused on issues relating to anger, sense of injustice, or forgiveness. Such a plea would have been inconceivable in his psychological state before treatment, a point which he also acknowledged at the end of his treatment. His response to the funeral ceremony (expressed in his SMS message to his therapist) illustrated the positive impact of the event.

Case vignette #2

Chantal was a 17-year-old, female, single asylum-seeker from a French-speaking African country. At the time of assessment she had been in Turkey for 5 months and her refugee claim was under consideration by the UNHCR. She was living in an orphanage run by the State. She was kidnapped in her home country by some men and kept in a barrack in the woods for several days. She was subjected to torture, including beating, burning of parts of the body, pulling by hair, sexual advances, forced fellatio, threats of death, verbal abuse, forced stress positions, restriction of movement, threats against her family, food and water deprivation, sleep deprivation, prevention of urination and defecation, prevention of personal hygiene, denial of privacy, and exposure to infested surroundings. She managed to escape and leave the country with the help of her relatives. She had not heard from her parents and siblings since the day she was kidnapped. After her arrival in Turkey she was diagnosed with PTSD and major depression. She received psychiatric treatment including antidepressant medication (sertraline 100 mg/day and mianserin 10 mg/day) and weekly psychotherapy sessions. Four months after this treatment she stated that only mianserin helped her sleep but reported no improvement in other traumatic stress symptoms.

Chantal was assessed twice in 3 weeks before treatment was started. At the first assessment, her CAPS score was 101 (Weathers et al., 2001), which indicated 'extremely severe PTSD' according to the proposed severity score ranges. She scored 48 on the self-rated PCL (Ventureyra et al., 2002; Weathers et al., 1993) and 32 on the BDI (Beck et al., 1985; Cottraux, 1985), indicating severe depression. At the second baseline assessment she scored 99 on the CAPS, 46 on the PCL, and 28 on the BDI, indicating no clinically significant change, despite therapist contact and assessment. She reported severe distress and functional impairment due to traumatic stress symptoms. She was not on good terms with the other girls at the orphanage because of her irritability and inability to attend social activities due to her fear and avoidance of trauma reminders. These reminders included watching movies depicting violence, sitting or standing next to men, talking to or physical contact with men, sleeping alone, and sleeping in the dark. She also avoided people who smoked and sight of cigarettes, because her kidnappers were smokers. She had nightmares 3–4 times a week, during which she often woke up to find herself screaming and crying. This posed a problem at the orphanage, because she was sharing a room with other girls. She had

problems reading and learning Turkish because of her intrusive memories and flashbacks. She was considering suicide and said that if she had access to her medicines (supplied daily by the orphanage administration) she would take them all at once.

Treatment was started after the second baseline assessment and involved twice-weekly sessions. A total of eight sessions were conducted, which altogether lasted about 14 hours. Further assessments were conducted mid-treatment (week 2), post-treatment (week 4), and 1 and 2 months post-treatment. Treatment and assessment sessions were conducted by the second author with the help of an interpreter. The first session was spent explaining the treatment rationale. Subsequent treatment sessions consisted of therapist-aided live exposure to distress-evoking trauma reminders. After each session she was given self-exposure homework exercises. Exposure involved watching a documentary about rape survivors in Africa, movies depicting violence, taking public transport and sitting next to men, initiating conversations with male classmates at the language course she was attending and the male caretakers at the orphanage, not avoiding situations where people smoked, dining in a restaurant alone, and going to a male hairdresser. The latter was a powerful trauma reminder as it involved physical contact with a man and also she was pulled by her hair during torture.

Chantal's medications were gradually tapered off during the first 3 weeks of treatment for several reasons. First, literature evidence (reviewed in Chapter 8) points to the limited efficacy of antidepressant treatment in PTSD as well as depression. Indeed, Chantal reported no benefit from drug treatment. Second, evidence (US Food and Drug Administration, 2007; US Food and Drug Administration, 2004) shows that treatment with antidepressants may increase the likelihood of suicidal acts in children or adolescents. Furthermore, our experience shows that depression and suicidal ideas disappear together with improvement in traumatic stress. This was indeed corroborated by her progress.

Two weeks into the therapy there was 59% reduction in Chantal's self-reported PTSD symptoms and 75% reduction in depression symptoms. During this period she had nightmares only twice. At post-treatment assessment (week 4) PTSD symptoms had reduced by 94% according to PCL and 90% according to CAPS and depression symptoms by 100%. Her suicidal ideas had completely disappeared. She was able to sleep without medication and had no nightmares. With such improvement her relationship with her room-mates improved and she was able to focus on learning Turkish and English. Improvement was maintained at 2-month follow-up.

These case studies support the findings of a previous case study (Başoğlu et al., 2004) in demonstrating once again that effective treatment of asylum-seekers is possible, despite various factors that might make recovery difficult. First, both survivors' trauma stories involve a wide range of intensely traumatic events, including loss of close ones, exposure to various atrocities typical of armed conflict settings in Africa, and a personal experience of captivity and torture. Second, both had severe PTSD complicated by severe depression with suicidal ideas, which normally poses a challenge for any treatment. Third, the uncertainty in their situation in Turkey as asylum-seekers, constant worries about family members in their home country, and inability to make plans for their future further complicated their psychological status. Yet, they showed remarkable recovery against all these odds. The dramatic improvement in their (drug-resistant) depression without any change in their life circumstances and without any specific intervention for depression suggests that the latter was largely secondary to the disabling (hopelessness) effects of PTSD. These findings imply that the most common psychiatric outcomes of trauma (i.e. PTSD and depression) can be independent of adverse environmental circumstances in a host country, at least to a sufficient extent to allow substantial recovery in the

absence of any significant change in these circumstances. Such recovery in turn enables the survivors to engage in active problem-solving behaviors vis-à-vis other current life problems that may or may not be related to the trauma.

It is worth comparing these two cases' treatment response with the average improvement rates in two treatment studies (Başoğlu et al., 2005; Başoğlu et al., 2007b) with earthquake survivors. The first study (EQ Study 1; n = 51) involved a single session of self-exposure instructions with no therapist involvement in exposure exercises, whereas the second study (EQ Study 2; n = 25) involved a single session of therapist-delivered exposure (using an earthquake simulator) combined with self-exposure instructions. The mean pre-treatment CAPS scores in these studies were 65 (range 21–105) and 61 (range 36–91), respectively. Alain's and Chantal's CAPS scores (82 and 99, respectively) were thus well above the group means in these studies. The mean pre-treatment BDI scores in the two studies of earthquake survivors were 20 (range 1–48) and 24 (range 11–45), respectively, and Alain's and Chantal's pre-treatment BDI scores (36 and 28, respectively) were above these sample means.

Figure 9.1a and Figure 9.1b compare Alain's and Chantal's treatment response with that of earthquake survivors in terms of percentage of improvement in scale scores. Post-treatment assessment was conducted at week 6 in EQ Study 1, at week 8 in EQ Study 2, at week 4 with Chantal, and at week 8 with Alain. Subsequent assessment points indicate treatment-free follow-up.

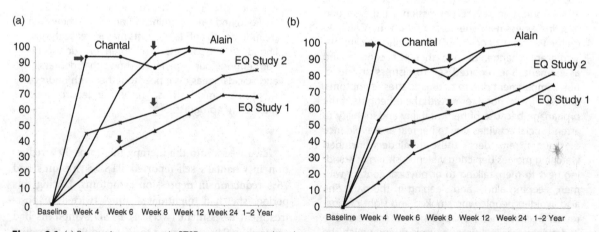

Figure 9.1 (a) Percent improvement in PTSD symptoms in earthquake survivors and traumatized refugees treated with Control-Focused Behavioral Treatment. Arrows indicate post-treatment assessment points. (b) Percent improvement in depression symptoms in earthquake survivors and traumatized refugees treated with Control-Focused Behavioral Treatment. Arrows indicate post-treatment assessment points.

In both cases improvement in PTSD at post-treatment was above the average post-treatment improvement rate in EQ Study 1 and EQ Study 2. A comparison of improvement rates across assessment points does not support the view that asylum-seekers respond less or more slowly to treatment. Treatment could have continued on an entirely self-help basis with no further therapist involvement beyond week 2 in Chantal's case and week 6 in Alain's case. We nevertheless continued with therapist-aided exposure sessions because we wanted to explore the time frame for maximum improvement with intensive treatment. A good early treatment response in these cases suggests that the prospect of brief treatment for asylum-seekers and refugees is not inconceivable. It is also worth noting that such early improvement is comparable to post-treatment outcome achieved by 9- or 10-session exposure protocols used in other studies (Foa et al., 2005; Marks et al., 1998).

Conclusions

The results of between-sample comparisons do not support the view that war, torture, and earthquake traumas differ substantially in their subjective impact, cognitive effects, mechanisms of traumatic stress, and the nature, prevalence, and severity of their mental health outcomes. Having said this, we acknowledge the fact that, unlike natural disasters, torture by definition involves deliberate strategies to remove control from the person and may thus be more traumatic in certain circumstances where such strategies are highly effective. The contextual factors may also contribute to this process. However, even if we assume for a moment that torture is generally a more traumatic event, this does not necessarily mean that it is a difficult trauma to treat, provided that the right treatment is chosen. Indeed, the case studies above illustrate this point. This might be explained by our findings, which imply that (a) PTSD can be effectively treated with an intervention specifically designed to enhance sense of control over traumatic stressors and (b) trauma-altered beliefs do not need to be specifically targeted in treatment. There is also other evidence showing that a treatment focus on trauma-altered beliefs (e.g. cognitive restructuring) confers no additional benefit in exposure treatment (Foa et al., 2005; Marks et al., 1998; Paunovic and Öst, 2001) and that beliefs change with exposure treatment alone (Foa and Rauch, 2004; Paunovic and Öst, 2001). These case studies also demonstrate that recovery from trauma is possible without a change in adverse environmental circumstances associated with asylum-seeker or refugee status or in external socio-political realities that define a culture of impunity.

Reasons for lack of progress in torture prevention and rehabilitation

Most torture rehabilitation centers around the world quite rightly concern themselves with primary prevention of torture as well as rehabilitation of survivors. As noted earlier, an EC commissioned evaluation of four centers in Europe (Guillet et al., 2005) concluded that these centers have very little impact on primary prevention. Although this conclusion cannot be generalized to all other centers, in view of lack of any published evidence to the contrary, it would be only fair to conclude that there is as yet no evidence to show that these centers serve a useful function in primary prevention of torture. Having said this, we should also note in all fairness that research in this area is difficult for obvious reasons and requires a fairly sophisticated methodology that is certainly not easy to develop. However, we get the impression from the EU commissioned evaluation reports cited earlier that these centers do not have the will or knowledge to undertake such work.

The reasons for lack of progress in torture prevention and rehabilitation are quite complex and a comprehensive analysis of this issue is not possible in this chapter. Nevertheless, drawing from our experience and observations in the field, we will examine some of the reasons that may account for lack of progress in both prevention of torture and rehabilitation of survivors.

Lack of scientific approach to the problem

Although prevention of torture and rehabilitation of survivors may appear to require different lines of work, such as political action and medical / psychological care of survivors, both lines of work require a good understanding of what constitutes torture and how various torture events exert their impact on individuals. In the last 30 years an understanding of torture has not progressed much beyond simplistic views such as *an act designed to break the will of the person and destroy his/her personality.* This is partly due to the fact that current theories of psychological trauma have not been able to provide sufficient guidance in achieving a sound theory-based formulation of torture trauma that can be empirically tested. Although learning theory and experimental animal work on the role of unpredictable and uncontrollable stressors as causal processes in anxiety offered much prospect in this regard, the applicability of such work to human behavior under duress was uncertain.

Advocacy and political action against torture has traditionally been conceived as lobbying with governments, media and public campaigning, and helping survivors seek redress for their trauma. Little attention has been paid to the need for scientific work that is essential in both political and rehabilitation work. This problem arises in part from an ideological opposition to a medical, psychiatric, or psychological approach to the problem of torture, which is dismissed by some as *reductionist medicalising* of a political issue. We pointed to this issue many years ago (Başoğlu, 1992b; Başoğlu, 1993; Başoğlu and Marks, 1988) arguing for the need for an integrated approach to the problem involving both scientific research and political action. In the introduction to the book on *Torture and Its Consequences: Current Treatment Approaches* (Başoğlu, 1992b), the first author noted:

> Study of torture and care of tortured individuals is not merely a humanitarian concern; it is also an effective political statement against the most abhorrent form of human rights violation. Such political statements are essential in preserving hard-earned human rights in democratic societies. Torture is not a problem confined to a remote dictatorship or a totalitarian regime but one that concerns the very moral fabric of the democratic societies in which we live ... as international pressure on torturers grows, more and more sophisticated methods of torture, mainly of a psychological nature, are being developed to avoid leaving physical scars on the tortured individuals. We need a better understanding of these methods and their psychological effects ... The emergence of a new science in this field could make significant contributions to the political struggle against torture. The knowledge generated by this science could be used as a powerful instrument in increasing public awareness of the problem and in directing this awareness to bring pressure upon governments and international organizations such as the United Nations to take more effective measures against the practice of torture.
>
> (pp. 3–4).

Unfortunately, time proved these predictions right. The developments in the post-9/11 world indeed made it amply clear that torture is not confined to remote dictatorships and confronted us with the issue of preserving hard-earned human rights in democratic societies.

The human rights abuses in Guantanamo, Iraq, and Afghanistan following the 9/11 events, the infamous images from the Abu Ghraib prison, the US government memorandum on torture in 2004 (US Justice Department, 2004) limiting definition of torture to treatments that cause 'severe physical pain,' academic arguments (Dershowitz, 2002) in favor of 'light torture' in certain exceptional circumstances (e.g. 'the ticking bomb' scenario), and, most importantly, the endorsement of the US definition of torture by 46% of the American public (Pew Research Center for the People and the Press, 2005) are indeed signs of erosion that crept into the very moral fabric of our societies. More and more sophisticated methods of torture were indeed developed (e.g. waterboarding among others). Pointing to the role of some psychologists in designing the CIA's 'enhanced interrogation' techniques, Jane Meyer reported in her book *The Dark Side* (Meyer, 2008) that the central idea was the psychological concept of learned helplessness. She noted that

> The apparent leader of the CIA team was a former military psychologist named James Mitchell, whom the intelligence agency had hired on a contract (pp. 156) ... Central to Mitchell's thinking, the associates said, was the work of one of America's best known and most successful psychologists, Martin Seligman, the former president of the American Psychological association and an esteemed professor in the Department of Psychology at the University of Pennsylvania. It was Seligman's experiments with dogs to which Mitchell had referred when defending his approaches to the FBI. (pp. 163) ... In the spring of 2002 ... Seligman was invited by the CIA to speak at the Navy' SERE [Survival, Evasion, Resistance, and Escape] school in San Diego. Among the organizers was Kirk Hubbard, Director of Behavioral Sciences research at the CIA until 2005. Neither Hubbard nor Seligman would comment on the special briefing. But in an email Seligman acknowledged that he spoke for three hours. Seligman emphasized that his talk was aimed at helping American soldiers "resist torture," not inflict it. But whether Seligman wanted his discoveries applied as they were or not, Mitchell cited the uses of Learned Helplessness in handling human detainees. According to Steve Kleinman, a reserve Air Force colonel and an experienced interrogator who has known Mitchell professionally for years, "Learned

Helplessness was his whole paradigm." Mitchell, he said, "draws a diagram showing what he says is the whole cycle. It starts with isolation. Then they eliminate the prisoner's ability to forecast the future – when their next meal is – when they can go to the bathroom. It creates dread and dependency. It was the KGB model. But the KGB model used it to turn people who had turned against the state to confess falsely. The KGB wasn't after intelligence." Kleinman had been a SERE instructor himself, as in his view, the reverse-engineering of the science was morally, legally, and tactically wrong. He described the CIA's reliance on Mitchell as "surreal."

Asked about his theories, Mitchell noted that Seligman was "a brilliant man" and his experiments were "good science." But through a lawyer, he disputed that Learned Helplessness was the model he used for the CIA interrogation program. Nevertheless, soon after he arrived in the CIA's black site in Thailand, Abu Zubayda [America's first "high value detainee" (pp. 140)] found himself naked in a small cage, like a dog. (pp. 164)

It is rather ironical that our efforts over the last 20 years to develop more effective torture treatment methods using the principles of learned helplessness theory were paralleled by efforts to develop more effective torture methods using the very same principles. It is rather sobering to see designers of torture using scientific knowledge in developing more effective torture techniques, when the human rights community in general (some exceptions aside) has failed to recognize the importance of scientific knowledge in the struggle against torture. It is also worth noting in this connection that the first author had to face intense criticism and condemnation and at times outright hostility and insults from certain sectors of the human rights community in the 1990s for conducting scientific research with torture survivors. Among many anecdotes to this effect, one is particularly worth mentioning. In the early 1990s we embarked on a finding from our first study of torture trauma (Başoğlu et al., 1994) suggesting that asphyxiation is among the most traumatic torture methods in terms of its immediate and long-term effects. Unfortunately, we could not publish this finding because of intense pressures from certain circles of the human rights community on grounds that such knowledge would be abused by torturers. Had it been published, such knowledge would have been quite useful in countering the arguments that waterboarding does not constitute torture because it does not involve severe physical pain.

In our view the developments in the aftermath of 9/11 put the human rights cause against torture back 100 years. We now find ourselves having to engage in debates over issues that were previously regarded as unquestionable, such as whether waterboarding is torture or whether 'light' torture is acceptable in certain circumstances. Worse still, despite the fact that any form of torture or cruel, inhuman, and degrading treatment (CIDT) is categorically prohibited by international law, there are efforts to argue that torture is not effective as an interrogation method, as if it would be acceptable in the name of national security if it were effective. All this is very confusing for an already fearful public, particularly in view of the fact there is no evidence to prove the point one way or the other.

In the post-9/11 world of today, the human rights community is unfortunately facing the consequences of neglect of and ideologically driven resistance to scientific research. Judging from the requests for information from the first author over the years, human rights campaigners, lawyers, and a large part of the world media appear to be in desperate search for scientific evidence relevant to the debate on what constitutes torture. Scientific evidence turned out to be indeed critically important in this debate in view of the fact that the arguments for a narrow definition of torture in the US Justice Department memorandum of 2004 were based in part on a 'review' of the literature evidence on the effects of torture. Furthermore, such evidence appears to play a critically important role in trials of terrorism suspects (Deutsch and Thompson, 2008a; Deutsch and Thompson, 2008b) in the USA and elsewhere. It is indeed sad to see that, after more than 30 years of work in the field of torture prevention and rehabilitation, there has not been a single publication of credible research evidence that sheds some light on this issue. Available evidence (reviewed by Başoğlu et al., 2001; see also more recent reviews by Campbell, 2007; Johnson and Thompson, 2008; Steel et al., 2009) concerns mainly mental health effects of torture and no study explored how individual forms of torture exert their impact on individuals. This is in part due to the fact that such research requires a sound theory and a rather sophisticated methodology, neither of which was developed in the course of 30 years.

We conducted studies of torture trauma in the 1990s, well before the 9/11 events, which turned out to be relevant to the current debate on definition of torture. These studies involved a methodology that allowed us to obtain detailed information on commonly used torture methods and their immediate and long-term psychological effects. When the controversy on this issue broke out, we first published evidence from our study (Başoğlu et al., 2007a) of 279 torture survivors in former Yugoslavia showing that there is no distinction between torture and CIDT in terms of their immediate psychological impact and long-term mental health effects. Then, based on a larger sample of 432 torture survivors, we published a second article (Başoğlu, 2009) reporting evidence to show that CIDT is more traumatic than physical torture in terms of associated distress and their long-term mental health effects. The extent of media coverage of these articles and their impact were well beyond our expectations. Below we provide an example that highlights the usefulness of research evidence for the human rights cause. This concerns the case of Binyam Mohamed presented on *The Torture Report*, an initiative of the American Civil Liberties Union aiming to give the full account of the Bush administration's torture program.

> At the center of the story is Binyam Mohamed, an Ethiopian émigré living in the UK who was arrested in Pakistan in April 2002, taken into US custody, flown to Morocco, where he was tortured for 18 months, then flown to a secret CIA prison in Afghanistan where he was again tortured, and finally delivered, in September 2004, to Guantánamo, where he remained until he was released last year. Binyam Mohamed, who today is a free man living in London ...
>
> One of the remarkable documents ... is the November 17, 2009 ruling of Federal District Judge Gladys Kessler in the habeas corpus petition of another Guantánamo detainee, Farhi Saeed Bin Mohammed. The government's case that Farhi Saeed Bin Mohammed was an enemy combatant hinged on information Binyam Mohamed had provided that they had spent time together at an al-Qaeda training camp in Afghanistan. That information was likely the fruit of torture, Judge Kessler found, and ordered the government "to take all necessary and appropriate diplomatic steps to facilitate [Farhi Saeed Bin Mohammed's] release forthwith."
>
> In one particularly striking passage in her opinion, Judge Kessler rejects the government's assertion that because Binyam made the allegations about Farhi Saeed Bin Mohammed during relatively benign interrogations after arriving at Guantánamo, rather than during his earlier torture in Morocco and Afghanistan, the information

should be admissible in the habeas corpus proceeding. Citing new studies on the neurological and psychological impact of abusive interrogations, she writes:

> *Torture and "enhanced interrogation techniques" employed by the government during the War on Terror have been shown to be "geared toward creating anxiety or fear in the detainee while at the same time removing any form of control from the person to create a state of total helplessness." Metin Basoglu, M. D., PhD., et al., Torture vs. Other Cruel, Inhuman, and Degrading Treatment: Is the Distinction Real or Apparent? 64 Archives of Gen. Psychiatry 277, 283 (2007). Indeed, rates of Post-Traumatic Stress Disorder ("PTSD") in torture survivors far exceed the rate among the general population. Physicians for Human Rights, Leave No Marks: Enhanced Interrogation Techniques and the Risk of Criminality, 43–44; 43 n. 337 (Aug. 2007) ...*
>
> (Siems, January 2010, see also Kessler, November 2009).

Turning to the issue of torture rehabilitation, lack of appropriate research also accounts in large part for the stagnation in rehabilitation work. A good understanding of torture and its psychological effects is also important for development of effective treatment methods. There have been some advances in treatment of trauma in general, particularly with the use of evidence-based treatments, such as cognitive-behavioral treatment, but the field of torture rehabilitation has lagged behind such progress. In the sections below we review some of the possible reasons.

Lack of evidence-based thinking

Torture is a highly emotional issue, given the abhorrent nature of the act and the strong human element in it. An emotional appraisal of torture often leads to preconceived notions about its traumatic impact. Our experiences in this field have shown that such preconceived notions can be so entrenched that they can be impervious even to empirical evidence to the contrary. For example, in the debate (British Medical Journal, 2006) that followed the 2006 editorial (Başoğlu, 2006), the first author pointed to a lack of studies comparing torture with natural disaster trauma and noted that available evidence does not support the view that torture is a generally more severe and therefore more difficult trauma to treat. Some of the evidence reviewed above, a product of nearly 20 years of work, was briefly summarized in support of this point. Some of the responses to the evidence presented in this debate are rather sobering in their implications:

> PTSD among refugees is too serious a matter to be entrusted [to] psychiatrists only. It is surprising, indeed disrespectful to compare victims of natural disasters like earthquake and victims of torture ...
> I don't see where is the "strong human element" of the trauma linked to earthquake, other than the symptoms of PTSD.

Durieux-Paillard, S. Re: Facts and myths about torture trauma – II. British Medical Journal, 13 January 2007

> In times of evidence-based medicine it has become very easy to advance a position in a medical debate and to refute another. One has to put forth his/her empirical evidence and then claim for the opponents' evidence. Like in a boxing match, the points are added up finally and the one who scores more points is the winner. While the loser has to remain silent henceforth. Owing to this type of argument, more and more medical debates are in danger to degenerate into cockfights, especially when predominantly based on auto quotations ...

Maier T. Treatment of torture survivors: Some observations on the current debate. British Medical Journal, 24 February 2007.

While lack of evidence-based thinking in this field may be attributable in part to care providers' orientation in psychotherapy, it may also reflect their own emotional responses to horrific stories of human-made trauma in their daily practice (e.g. anxiety, distress, anger, outrage, sense of injustice, etc.), which may cloud rational thinking. In view of the emotional nature of this issue, it may indeed be difficult to maintain an evidence-based perspective on this issue, particularly without sufficient clinical and research experience with different survivor populations. While such emotional responses on the part of care providers are understandable to a certain extent, their consequences in work with war and torture survivors are unfortunately too serious to ignore.

Reinforcement of helplessness: 'secondary victimization'

Evidence reviewed throughout this book strongly suggests that helplessness is the mediating process in traumatic stress and that treatment is effective to the extent that it reduces helplessness. In view of the close

association between avoidance and helplessness, staff attitudes that perpetuate or reinforce avoidance are tantamount to 'secondary victimization' in the sense that they may not only block natural recovery processes but also aggravate traumatic stress problems. In a discussion of potentially therapeutic and anti-therapeutic aspects of rehabilitation programs for torture survivors (Başoğlu, 1992a), the first author had noted that an understanding among the rehabilitation staff such as 'whatever you do, do not remind the survivor of his/her trauma experiences' is likely to reinforce avoidance behaviors (and hence helplessness responses) in survivors and thus perpetuate their victim role. Such attitudes may also block various therapeutic elements inherent in certain rehabilitation procedures. For example, physiotherapy sessions with torture survivors (e.g. when conducted semi-naked in a pool in the presence of authority figures often dressed in white uniform) often trigger memories of the torture and evoke considerable anxiety or even panic. These sessions provide valuable opportunities for exposure to trauma reminders and might be expected to produce some therapeutic effects, even inadvertently when not conducted as part of a concurrent exposure treatment program. Yet, such potentially therapeutic effects of exposure are likely to be neutralized by avoidant and consequently avoidance-reinforcing attitudes among rehabilitation staff. There are many other aspects of rehabilitation programs (e.g. interviews with clients, psychological assessments, medical investigations and treatments, social support interventions, etc.) with similar exposure elements, the therapeutic effects of which may be blocked by anti-exposure attitudes or the 'avoidance culture' that often prevails among the staff. We know from experience with waitlist control groups in treatment studies of PTSD that detailed assessment of psychological status alone, a process that involves elements of imaginal exposure, leads to about 20% improvement in PTSD (Başoğlu et al., 2005; Başoğlu et al., 2007b; Ehlers et al., 2003; Foa et al., 1999; Foa et al., 2005). We also observed that some survivors, when asked questions about avoidance behaviors at initial assessment, recognized their avoidance as a problem and instigated self-exposure and improved during a 6 to 8 weeks waiting period before we had a chance to initiate treatment. The fact that an outcome study (Carlsson et al., 2005) of a 9-month-long torture rehabilitation program failed to demonstrate even limited improvement in tortured refugees might well be due to anti-therapeutic elements of the program. Indeed, evidence (Marks et al., 1988) shows that reinforcement of avoidance behaviors (e.g. by anti-exposure instructions) can even block the therapeutic effects of certain antidepressants in anxiety disorders.

A further related anti-therapeutic aspect of rehabilitation programs concerns the view of torture survivors as 'victims' who need unconditional attention and social / emotional support to recover from trauma. The perception of a torture survivor as a fragile being that needs strong support and protection from further adversity and stress is particularly prevalent in western countries. Such an approach in rehabilitation essentially amounts to an overprotective parental role on the part of care providers and deprives the survivors of much needed opportunities to learn effective ways of dealing with their own problems and to regain control over their life. We know from our own experience that many torture survivors, particularly political activists, resent being treated like victims and find the label rather demeaning or even offensive. Unconditional social or emotional support is likely to perpetuate helplessness responses and thus the victim role if the survivor is not encouraged to take an active role in dealing with their psychological and social problems. This may be a particularly serious problem in view of the long duration of some rehabilitation programs, which last nearly a year or more. Such a lengthy process means more exposure to helplessness-reinforcing elements in the rehabilitation program. Survivors need to take an active role in treatment and efforts in this direction need to be rewarded verbally and emotionally and reinforced in every way possible. Any failure to make sufficient effort to overcome problems, on the other hand, needs to be discouraged by withholding verbal rewards. Moreover, treatment needs to be time-limited and conditional on the survivor's compliance with and progress in treatment (see Chapter 4). This is a simple but highly effective behavioral technique in reducing helplessness. An environment of unconditional support makes such therapeutic techniques impossible to administer.

Resistance to exposure treatments

We have observed considerable resistance in the field of torture rehabilitation to exposure-based treatments arising in part from the fact these interventions may evoke considerable anxiety and distress in both the client and the therapist. This phenomenon is not unique to this field, given that exposure-based treatments, despite their well-established efficacy, are among the least commonly used interventions in treatment of trauma survivors in general (Becker et al., 2004). Exposure treatment may pose even greater emotional difficulty for therapists involved in care of torture survivors, because of the intensely disturbing nature of torture trauma. Indeed, some therapists may even be vicariously traumatized by just listening to such trauma stories. Thus, training of therapists in behavioral treatment may require helping them overcome their own emotional vulnerabilities by using the same behavioral treatment techniques. Indeed, during our work with earthquake survivors some of our team members developed traumatic stress problems, which they effectively overcame by using self-exposure strategies. It is also worth noting in this connection that although CFBT is an exposure-based intervention, it does not involve detailed probing into the trauma story, as a focus on avoidance behaviors is often sufficient for improvement.

Limitations of evidence-based treatments

Lack of progress in torture rehabilitation also arises from the limitations of evidence-based treatments, some of which were reviewed in Chapter 8. Most importantly, their focus on anxiety reduction rather than on anxiety tolerance and control and lack of focus on live exposure as the most critical process in enhancing resilience against traumatic stressors are likely to limit their efficacy. Furthermore, these treatments, often involving a mixed bag of interventions, were developed for use in western cultures and convincing evidence as to their practicability and usefulness in people from developing countries is relatively scarce. Effective delivery of cognitive restructuring, for example, requires a certain degree of cognitive differentiation and psychological sophistication and an adequate capacity for introspection on the part of the client. This poses a serious problem, particularly with war survivors of lower socio-educational status in developing countries. Behavioral interventions, on the other hand, are easier to administer in such cases, as they are generally more compliant with self-exposure instructions than those with higher educational status (Başoğlu et al., 2005). In addition, when treatment needs to be delivered through an interpreter, this poses communication problems that are often difficult to overcome. Indeed, we have observed in our work with refugees that much gets lost in translation in the delivery of even a relatively simple treatment such as CFBT. We had to overcome this problem by training and involving interpreters in treatment as lay co-therapists.

Resistance to idea of brief treatments

Thinking in this field is also generally characterized by resistance to the idea of brief treatment, which is sometimes dismissed as a 'quick fix' approach to the problems of torture survivors. Such thinking arises largely from lack of recourse to a sound theory in understanding trauma and various misconceptions that stem from an inadequate understanding of the mechanisms of traumatic stress in torture trauma. It is worth emphasizing once again that the improvement achieved by CFBT does not entirely occur in one or two sessions. Rather, when delivered in one or two sessions, it initiates a self-help process that takes about 3 months to yield maximum effects. It should also be evident from this book that CFBT is not merely a form of psychotherapy limited to a few weekly sessions. It entails a behavioral approach in all aspects of rehabilitation aiming at empowerment of survivors.

Resistance to change in this field arises in part from institutionalization of rehabilitation services in the form of torture or refugee treatment centers in western countries and international organizations that support the formation of similar centers in developing countries. Indeed, institutionalized interventions of any kind can be quite resistant to evidence pointing to their ineffectiveness, as the case of psychological debriefing has demonstrated. In the case of torture rehabilitation, there are also other factors at play. These institutions often enjoy non-negligible funding support from western governments or other funding organizations in western countries, as well as considerable media and public support. Their activities are also regarded as enhancing the international image of the country in which they are based. Moreover, lengthy rehabilitation programs are consonant with media and public perception of torture as an extreme form of trauma likely to leave deep scars in a person. In view of such socio-political and cultural background, it is not difficult to understand how these institutions managed to maintain the status quo in this field for so long, despite lack of evidence for the usefulness of their rehabilitation programs, and what the idea of brief treatment might imply for them.

Needless to say, war and torture trauma may indeed lead to complex psychosocial problems, particularly in those survivors who have to face the additional problems of uprooting and re-settlement in a host country. It is worth bearing in mind, however, that complex problems do not necessarily require complex solutions, as the case studies presented earlier demonstrate. Considering that the majority of war and torture survivors worldwide do not have access to rehabilitation centers, outright dismissal of the idea of brief self-help treatments as a quick fix is certainly not in the interest of survivors.

Role of funding organizations

Funding organizations have unfortunately played an important role in maintaining the status quo in the field of torture rehabilitation by providing unquestioning support for essentially ineffective rehabilitation programs. The possible reasons for such support are beyond the scope of this chapter but suffice it to say that political considerations have always overridden scientific ones. This has contributed to the problem by not only encouraging a non-evidence-based approach but also discouraging scientific research in the field. Indeed, we pointed to this problem many years ago (Başoğlu, 1993), emphasizing the need for research for progress in torture rehabilitation. The fact that there has not been a single randomized controlled treatment study in this field since it came into existence in the 1970s is not a coincidence. Lack of attention to the need for treatment research in this field has led to a bizarre situation where projects that propose to provide essentially ineffective rehabilitation services stand a better chance of obtaining funding than those that propose research to develop effective treatments. This is a curious phenomenon, considering that there is no lack of awareness in western countries of the importance of scientific research for development of effective treatments for other medical conditions. This could be explained in part by the fact that research in this field has fallen between two stools. The organizations that fund medical research tend to view torture as a political or human rights problem and those that fund humanitarian assistance or rehabilitation projects are generally not interested in scientific research. The latter is even reflected in the mandate of international organizations established with the specific aim of helping torture survivors, such as the United Nations Fund for Victims of Torture, which explicitly states that "*Priority in allocating grants is given to projects providing direct medical, psychological, social, economic, legal, humanitarian, educational or other forms of assistance, to torture victims and members of their family … Activities such as investigations, studies, research, and publication of newsletters or similar activities are ineligible for funding from the Fund"* (United Nations Office of the High Commissioner for Human Rights, 2010). This is indeed another curious phenomenon in view of the ineffectiveness of current psychological rehabilitation approaches and the fact that effective treatments can only be developed through scientific research.

Funding organizations, including governments, also need to be aware of the fact that scientific research of high quality requires substantial expertise and laborious work that often takes many years to complete. Our work with earthquake survivors, for example, took 6 years to complete and cost more than 3 million USD. Research is thus a costly endeavor that requires substantially more funding than usual direct assistance projects. While such projects may come across as too costly, research is the only way of avoiding waste of valuable resources on ineffective rehabilitation programs. Moreover, research is the most cost-effective approach to trauma-induced mental health problems in a society, given that the enormous economic costs of social and occupational disability arising from these problems can only be prevented by effective interventions developed through research.

Potential problems in using evidence-based treatments in rehabilitation

Having said all this, we should acknowledge the fact that there is growing awareness in some torture rehabilitation centers of the need for an evidence-based approach in rehabilitation of torture survivors. Indeed, Sjölund, Kastrup, Montgomery, and Persson (2009) have recently pointed to the urgent need for evaluation of rehabilitation outcomes and noted that evidence-based interventions, such as cognitive-behavioral treatment (CBT), should be a component of rehabilitation programs. We also know that CBT is already being used in certain rehabilitation centers, such as the Rehabilitation and Research Centre for Torture Victims. While we regard this as a positive development, we also foresee various problems with incorporating evidence-based treatments into multi-disciplinary rehabilitation programs in their current state. First of all, in view of the various limitations of these treatments reviewed in Chapter 8, their usefulness with refugees is uncertain. Cognitive interventions are likely to pose practical problems with refugees, while habituation-focused exposure interventions are likely to have only partial effects at best (see Chapter 6 for discussion of possible reasons). Most importantly, in view of the anti-therapeutic elements inherent in an existing ineffective rehabilitation program, the mere addition of a potentially effective treatment is unlikely to achieve the desired outcomes without a restructuring of the entire program along behavioral lines. This means getting rid of all anti-therapeutic elements in the program, including the cultural milieu that promotes the victim role and avoidance-reinforcing attitudes. Such a radical paradigm shift would require extensive re-training of existing staff involved in all aspects of rehabilitation, including even the receptionist at the front door. In view of the many misconceptions about behavioral treatment and potential resistance to the idea of brief treatments, this is obviously not an easy task.

In closing this chapter, it is worth briefly commenting on recent attempts to evaluate the outcome of current rehabilitation programs using the World Health Organization (WHO) International Classification of Functioning, Disability and Health (ICF)(World Health Organization, 2002), which involves an assessment of physical, mental, and social well-being. Although this is a commendable effort, it is not immediately apparent to us how the ICF section on assessment of mental functions effectively guides the assessor in capturing vital information on functional impairment caused by fear- or distress-induced helplessness / avoidance responses in trauma survivors, unless the assessor is well aware of the mechanisms of traumatic stress reviewed in Part 1 and has sufficient experience in behavioral assessment. Furthermore, outcome measures relating to the most common outcomes of traumatic stress (e.g. PTSD and depression) are critical in assessment of treatment effects, as these outcomes are the most important factors that have a direct impact not only on mental and physical health status but also on life functioning. In addition, physical disability (e.g. loss of a limb) arising from a traumatic event may result in social disability not only because of objective loss of functionality related to a particular organ, but also because of its subjective psychological impact, such as helplessness responses exacerbated or sustained by the loss and its additional impact as a constant trauma reminder. Treatment outcome evaluation based primarily on a measure of disability in trauma survivors without an adequate understanding of mechanisms of traumatic stress in trauma survivors is likely to lead to loss of important information in assessment and misguided interpretation of the data resulting in unwarranted conclusions.

Conclusions and recommendations

The evidence in support of learning theory of traumatic stress and its applications in clinical and field practice generally support the view that empowerment of trauma survivors is essential in recovery from trauma. Our work simply takes this understanding one step further in demonstrating how such empowerment can be achieved in an effective fashion. The mental healthcare model proposed in Chapter 7 has important implications regarding where the focus needs to be in rehabilitation of mass trauma survivors. Figure 7.2 in that chapter implies that only a small minority of survivors are likely to need more intensive mental healthcare. In view of the fact that the majority of survivors will never have access to specialized rehabilitation services, a paradigm shift in survivor care is essential in meeting their needs. This can only be achieved by using outreach programs and delivering psychological care through brief interventions and / or self-help tools. Our work with earthquake survivors suggests that this is a useful and cost-effective approach.

On a final note in ending this book, we are well aware of the fact that the implications of the material covered in this book go against mainstream thinking in the field of psychological trauma. There will most probably be challenges to the evidence presented or disagreements with our conclusions or recommendations and all this is natural in the field of science. Some might argue that the evidence on effectiveness of CFBT presented in this book is limited to a few studies and needs replication by others in other settings. It is important to bear in mind that CFBT, despite its important differences from exposure treatment (reviewed in Chapter 6), is essentially an exposure-based intervention and there is already substantial evidence attesting to the efficacy of such interventions in PTSD related to a wide range of traumas. Our work could thus well be regarded as simply advancing the knowledge on an already well-established treatment with a robust evidence base (American Psychiatric Association, 2004; Bradley et al., 2005; National Institute of Clinical Excellence, 2005) by suggesting that its efficacy can be enhanced by certain theoretical

and practical modifications. The evidence from our treatment studies also needs to be interpreted in the broader context of all other evidence presented in support of the learning theory formulation of traumatic stress. This theoretical approach to trauma, with its focus on possibly evolutionarily determined human potential for recovery from trauma, points to certain previously inconceivable prospects in the care of mass trauma survivors. It is certainly true that much more work needs to be done to develop further the mental healthcare model presented in Chapter 7 in mass trauma survivors and we hope that this book will pave the way for concerted efforts in this direction.

References

American Psychiatric Association (1994). *Diagnostic and Statistical Manual of Mental Disorders (4th Edition)*. Washington, DC: American Psychiatric Association.

American Psychiatric Association (2004). *Practice Guideline for the Treatment of Patients with Acute Stress Disorder and Posttraumatic Stress Disorder*. Arlington, VA: American Psychiatric Association Practice Guidelines.

Başoğlu, M. (1992a). Behavioural and cognitive treatment of PTSD in torture survivors. In *Torture and Its Consequences: Current Treatment Approaches*, ed. M. Başoğlu. Cambridge: Cambridge University Press, 402–429.

Başoğlu, M. (1992b). Introduction. In *Torture and Its Consequences: Current Treatment Approaches*, ed. M. Başoğlu. Cambridge: Cambridge University Press, 1–8.

Başoğlu, M. (1993). Prevention of torture and care of survivors: An integrated approach. *Journal of the American Medical Association*, **270**, 606–611.

Başoğlu, M. (2006). Rehabilitation of traumatised refugees and survivors of torture: After almost two decades we are still not using evidence based treatments. *British Medical Journal*, **333**, 1230–1231.

Başoğlu, M. (2009). A multivariate contextual analysis of torture and cruel, inhuman, and degrading treatments: Implications for an evidence-based definition of torture. *American Journal of Orthopsychiatry*, **79**, 135–145.

Başoğlu, M. and Aker, T. (1996). Cognitive-behavioural treatment of torture survivors: A case study. *Torture*, **6**, 61–65.

Başoğlu, M., Ekblad, S., Bäärnhielm, S. and Livanou, M. (2004). Cognitive-behavioral treatment of tortured asylum seekers: A case study. *Journal of Anxiety Disorders*, **18**, 357–369.

Başoğlu, M., Jaranson, J. M., Mollica, R. F. and Kastrup, M. (2001). Torture and mental health: A research overview.

In *The Mental Health Consequences of Torture*, ed. E. Gerrity, T. M. Keane and F. Tuma. Kluwer Academic / Plenum Publishers, 35–62.

Başoğlu, M., Livanou, M. and Crnobarić, C. (2007a). Torture vs other cruel, inhuman, and degrading treatment: Is the distinction real or apparent? *Archives of General Psychiatry*, **64**, 277–285.

Başoğlu, M., Livanou, M. and Şalcıoğlu, E. (2003a). A single session with an earthquake simulator for traumatic stress in earthquake survivors. *American Journal of Psychiatry*, **160**, 788–790.

Başoğlu, M., Livanou, M., Şalcıoğlu, E. and Kalender, D. (2003b). A brief behavioural treatment of chronic post-traumatic stress disorder in earthquake survivors: Results from an open clinical trial. *Psychological Medicine*, **33**, 647–654.

Başoğlu, M. and Marks, I. (1988). Torture. *British Medical Journal*, **297**, 1423–1424.

Başoğlu, M., Paker, M., Paker, O., Özmen, E., Marks, I., İncesu, C., Şahin, D. and Sarımurat, N. (1994). Psychological effects of torture: A comparison of tortured with nontortured political activists in Turkey. *American Journal of Psychiatry*, **151**, 76–81.

Başoğlu, M., Şalcıoğlu, E. and Livanou, M. (2007b). A randomized controlled study of single-session behavioural treatment of earthquake-related post-traumatic stress disorder using an earthquake simulator. *Psychological Medicine*, **37**, 203–213.

Başoğlu, M., Şalcıoğlu, E., Livanou, M., Kalender, D. and Acar, G. (2005). Single-session behavioral treatment of earthquake-related posttraumatic stress disorder: A randomized waiting list controlled trial. *Journal of Traumatic Stress*, **18**, 1–11.

Beck, A. T., Emery, G. and Greenberg, R. (1985). *Anxiety Disorders and Phobias: A Cognitive Perspective*. New York: Basic Books.

Becker, C. B., Zayfert, C. and Anderson, E. (2004). A survey of psychologists' attitudes towards and utilization of exposure therapy for PTSD. *Behaviour Research and Therapy*, **42**, 277–292.

Blake, D. D., Weathers, F. W., Nagy, L. M., Kaloupek, D. G., Charney, D. S. and Keane, T. M. (1990). *Clinician-Administered PTSD Scale (CAPS): Current and Lifetime Diagnostic Version*. Boston: National Center for Posttraumatic Stress Disorder, Behavioral Science Division.

Bradley, R., Greene, J., Russ, E., Dutra, L. and Westen, D. (2005). A multidimensional meta-analysis of psychotherapy for PTSD. *American Journal of Psychiatry*, **162**, 214–227.

British Medical Journal (2006). Rapid Responses to Metin Basoglu, Rehabilitation of traumatised refugees and survivors of torture, British Medical Journal 2006; 333: 1230–1231. Published at http://www.bmj.com/cgi/eletters/333/7581/1230

Campbell, T. A. (2007). Psychological assessment, diagnosis, and treatment of torture survivors: A review. *Clinical Psychology Review*, **27**, 628–641.

Carlsson, J. M., Mortensen, E. L. and Kastrup, M. (2005). A follow-up study of mental health and health-related quality of life in tortured refugees in multidisciplinary treatment. *Journal of Nervous and Mental Disease*, **193**, 651–657.

Cottraux, J. (1985). Evaluation clinique et psychométrique des états dépressifs. *Collection Scientifique Survector*, p. 75.

Dershowitz, A. M. (2002). *Why Terrorism Works: Understanding the Threat, Responding to the Challenge*. New Haven, CT: Yale University Press.

Deutsch, M. E. and Thompson, E. (2008a). Secret and lies: The persecution of Muhammed Salah (Part I). *Journal of Palestine Studies*, **37**, 38–57.

Deutsch, M. E. and Thompson, E. (2008b). Secret and lies: The persecution of Muhammed Salah (Part II). *Journal of Palestine Studies*, **38**, 25–53.

Ehlers, A., Clark, D. M., Hackmann, A., Mcmanus, F. and Fennell, M. (2005). Cognitive therapy for post-traumatic stress disorder: Development and evaluation. *Behaviour Research and Therapy*, **43**, 413–431.

Ehlers, A., Clark, D. M., Hackmann, A., Mcmanus, F., Fennell, M., Herbert, C. and Mayou, R. (2003). A randomized controlled trial of cognitive therapy, a self-help booklet, and repeated assessments as early interventions for posttraumatic stress disorder. *Archives of General Psychiatry*, **60**, 1024–1032.

First, M. B., Spitzer, R. L., Gibbon, M. and Williams, J. B. W. (1996). *Structured Clinical Interview for DSM-IV Axis I Disorders: Non-patient Edition (SCID-I/NP, Version 2)*. New York: Biometrics Research Department, New York State Psychiatric Institute.

Foa, E. B., Dancu, C. V., Hembree, E. A., Jaycox, L. H., Meadows, E. A. and Street, G. P. (1999). A comparison of exposure therapy, stress inoculation training, and their combination for reducing posttraumatic stress disorder in female assault victims. *Journal of Consulting and Clinical Psychology*, **67**, 194–200.

Foa, E. B., Hembree, E. A., Cahill, S. P., Rauch, S. A. M., Riggs, D. S., Feeny, N. C. and Yadin, E. (2005). Randomized trial of prolonged exposure for posttraumatic stress disorder with and without cognitive restructuring: Outcome at academic and community clinics. *Journal of Consulting and Clinical Psychology*, **73**, 953–964.

Foa, E. B. and Rauch, S. A. M. (2004). Cognitive changes during prolonged exposure versus prolonged exposure plus cognitive restructuring in female assault survivors with posttraumatic stress disorder. *Journal of Consulting and Clinical Psychology*, **72**, 879–884.

Guillet, S., Perren-Klingler, G. and Agger, I. (2005). *Torture Rehabilitation Centres Europe*. Human European Consultancy in partnership with the Netherlands Humanist Committee on Human Rights and the Danish Institute for Human Rights. Accessed on May 5, 2010 at http://www.humanconsultancy.com/Torture%20Rehabilitation%20Europe.pdf

Guy, W. (1976). *ECDEU Assessment Manual for Psychopharmacology: Publication ADM 76–338* (DHEW Publ No ADM 76–338). National Institute of Mental Health, US Department of Health, Education, and Welfare, 218–222.

Johnson, H. and Thompson, A. (2008). The development and maintenance of post-traumatic stress disorder (PTSD) in civilian adult survivors of war trauma and torture: A review. *Clinical Psychology Review*, **28**, 36–47.

Kazdin, A. E. (2003). Statistical methods of data evaluation. In *Research Design in Clinical Psychology*. Boston: Allyn and Bacon, 436–470.

Keane, T. M., Fairbank, J. A., Caddell, J. M. and Zimering, R. T. (1989). Implosive (flooding) therapy reduces symptoms of PTSD in Vietnam combat veterans. *Behavior Therapy*, **20**, 245–260.

Kessler, G. (2009). *Farhi Saeed Bin Mohamed, et al. v. Barrack H. Obama et al: Memorandum opinion of Federal District Judge Gladys Kessler*. Accessed on May 9, 2010 at http://www.aclu.org/files/assets/12170928jECF.pdf

Marks, I. M., Lelliott, P., Başoğlu, M., Noshirvani, H., Monteiro, W., Cohen, D. and Kasvikis, Y. (1988). Clomipramine, self-exposure and therapist-aided exposure for obsessive- compulsive rituals. *British Journal of Psychiatry*, **152**, 522–534.

Marks, I. M., Lovell, K., Noshirvani, H. and Livanou, M. (1998). Treatment of posttraumatic stress disorder by exposure and/or cognitive restructuring: A controlled study. *Archives of General Psychiatry*, **55**, 317–325.

Marks, I. M., Swinson, R. P., Başoğlu, M., Kuch, K., Noshirvani, H., O'Sullivan, G., Lelliott, P. T., Kirby, M., Mcnamee, G. and Şengün, S. (1993). Alprazolam and exposure alone and combined in panic disorder with agoraphobia: A controlled study in London and Toronto. *British Journal of Psychiatry*, **162**, 776–787.

Meyer, J. (2008). *The Dark Side*. New York: Anchor Books.

National Institute of Clinical Excellence (NICE) (2005). *Posttraumatic Stress Disorder (PTSD): The Management of PTSD in Adults and Children in Primary and Secondary Care*. London: Gaskel and the British Psychological Society.

Olsen, D. R. (2006). *Prevalent pain in refugees previously exposed to torture*. PhD Dissertation. University of Aaarhus.

Paunovic, N. and Öst, L.-G. (2001). Cognitive-behavior therapy vs exposure therapy in the treatment of PTSD in refugees. *Behaviour Research and Therapy*, **39**, 1183–1197.

Pew Research Center for the People and the Press (2005). *America's place in the world 2005: An investigation of the attitudes of American opinion leaders and the American public about international affairs*. Accessed on May 9, 2010 at http://people-press.org/reports/pdf/263.pdf

Rehabilitation and Research Centre for Torture Victims (2008). *Annual Report 2007*. Accessed on May 5, 2010 at http://www.rct.dk/About_RCT/Material/~/media/0DE45EFA1D714698A083974822AD3299.ashx

Rehabilitation and Research Centre for Torture Victims (2009). *Annual Report 2008*. Accessed on May 5, 2010 at http://www.uk.rct.dk/About_RCT/Material/~/media/FDAB02E3FE3A4B4B998B8B0A4D411828.ashx

Rehabilitation and Research Centre for Torture Victims (2010). Vision and objectives. Available online at http://www.uk.rct.dk/About_RCT/Vision.aspx

Şalcıoğlu, E. (2004). *The effect of beliefs, attribution of responsibility, redress and compensation on posttraumatic stress disorder in earthquake survivors in Turkey*. PhD Dissertation. Institute of Psychiatry, King's College London, London.

Schnurr, P. P., Friedman, M. J., Engel, C. C., Foa, E. B., Shea, M. T., Chow, B. K., Resick, P. A., Thurston, V., Orsillo, S. M., Haug, R., Turner, C. and Bernardy, N. (2007). Cognitive behavioral therapy for posttraumatic stress disorder in women: A randomized controlled trial. *Journal of the American Medical Association*, **297**, 820–830.

Siems, L. (January 2010). *The Fruits of Torture*. Published on The Torture Report website of the American Civil Liberties Union and the ACLU Foundation. Accessed on May 9, 2010 at http://www.thetorturereport.org/diary/fruits-torture.

Sjölund, B. H., Kastrup, M., Montgomery, E. and Persson, A. L. (2009). Rehabilitating torture survivors. *Journal of Rehabilitation Medicine*, **41**, 689–696.

Steel, Z., Chey, T., Silove, D., Marnane, C., Bryant, R. A. and Van Ommeren, M. (2009). Association of torture and other potentially traumatic events with mental health outcomes among populations exposed to mass conflict and displacement: A systematic review and meta-analysis. *Journal of the American Medical Association*, **302**, 537–549.

197

US Food and Drug Administration (2004). FDA launches a multi-pronged strategy to strengthen safeguards for children treated with antidepressant medication. *FDA Press Announcements*, October 15, 2004. Accessed on April 7, 2010 at http://www.fda.gov/NewsEvents/Newsroom/PressAnnouncements/2004/ucm108363.htm

US Food and Drug Administration (2007). FDA proposes new warnings about suicidal thinking, behavior in young adults who take antidepressant medications. *FDA Press Announcements*, May 2, 2007. Accessed on April 7, 2010 at http://www.fda.gov/downloads/Drugs/DrugSafety/InformationbyDrugClass/ucm100211.pdf

US Justice Department (2004). *Memorandum for James B. Comey Deputy Attorney General Re: Legal standards applicable under 18 U.S.C. §§ 2340–2340A*. December 30, 2004. Accessed on April 30, 2010 at http://www.justice.gov/olc/18usc23402340a2.htm

United Nations Office of the High Commissioner for Human Rights (2010). *UN Voluntary Fund for Victims of Torture: Guidelines of the Fund*. Available online at http://www.ohchr.org/EN/Issues/Pages/TortureFundGuidelines.aspx#9

Van Willigen, L. H. M. (2007). *The torture rehabilitation system in Turkey, including an assessment of the torture rehabilitation centres established and operated by the Human Rights Foundation of Turkey and other related EC financial assistance*. Accessed on May 5, 2010 at http://www.avrupa.info.tr/Files/Torture-Rehabilitation-ATOS.pdf

Van Willigen, L. H. M., Agger, I., Barandiarán, T. and Khanal, P. (2003). *Evaluations EIDHR: Torture Rehabilitation Centres*. MEDE European Consultancy in partnership with the Netherlands Humanist Committee on Human Rights and the Danish Institute for Human Rights, November 2003. Accessed on May 5, 2010 at http://www.humanconsultancy.com/Torture%20web.pdf

Ventureyra, V. A. G., Yao, S.-N., Cottraux, J., Note, I. and De Mey-Guillard, C. (2002). The validation of the Posttraumatic Stress Disorder Checklist scale in posttraumatic stress disorder and nonclinical subjects. *Psychotherapy and Psychosomatics*, **71**, 47–53.

Weathers, F. W., Keane, T. M. and Davidson, J. R. T. (2001). Clinician-administered PTSD scale: A review of the first ten years of research. *Depression and Anxiety*, **13**, 132–156.

Weathers, F. W., Litz, B. T., Herman, D. S., Huska, J. A. and Keane, T. M. (1993). *The PTSD checklist: Reliability, validity and diagnostic utility*. Paper presented at the Annual Meeting of the International Society for Traumatic Stress Studies, October, 1993, San Antonio.

World Health Organization (2002). *Towards a common language for functioning, disability and health. The International Classification of Functioning, Disability and Health*. Geneva: World Health Organization. Accessed on April 10, 2010 at http://www.who.int/classifications/icf/site/beginners/bg.pdf

Appendix A: Questionnaires

Screening Instrument for Traumatic Stress in Earthquake Survivors (SITSES)

Part I: Survivor Information Form

1. *Name:* _____

2. *Age:* _____

3. *Gender:*   1 = Male   2 = Female

4. *Education:*   1 = None   2 = Literate   3 = Primary   4 = Secondary   5 = High school   6 = University
   7 = Post-graduate

5. *Occupation:* _____

6. *Marital status:*   1 = Married / Cohabiting   2 = Single   3 = Widowed   4 = Separated

7. *Your address:* _____

8. *Telephone number:* _____

9. *How close were you to the epicenter during the earthquake?*
   1 = Within 50 kms   2 = 50 to 100 kms   3 = More than 100 kms

10. *Did you experience the tremors?*   0 = No   1 = Yes

11. *Where were you during the earthquake?*
    1 = In a building   2 = On the street   3 = In a transport vehicle   4 = Other_____

12. *Were you trapped under rubble?*   0 = No   1 = Yes

13. *Did anyone close to you die in the earthquake?*   0 = No   1 = Yes (If yes) Who?_____

14. *Have you participated in rescue work after the earthquake?*   0 = No   1 = Yes

15. *Have you had any serious property or financial loss as a result of the earthquake?*   0 = No   1 = Yes

16. *What is the current state of your house?*
    1 = Undamaged   2 = Slightly damaged   3 = Moderately damaged   4 = Severely damaged
    5 = Collapsed   6 = Demolished after the earthquake   7 = Don't know

17. *Where are you living at present?*
    1 = My usual house   2 = A new house   3 = A tent   4 = Temporary shelter   5 = Other_____

18. *Did you have any psychiatric illness requiring treatment before the earthquake?*   0 = No   1 = Yes

19. *Using the scale below, how would you rate the intensity of your fear during the earthquake?*
    0 = No fear at all   1 = Slight fear   2 = Marked fear   3 = Severe fear   4 = Extremely severe fear

20. *How anxious / fearful have you been lately thinking about possible earthquakes in the near future?*
    0 = Not anxious / fearful at all   1 = Slightly   2 = Markedly   3 = Severely   4 = Extremely anxious / fearful

21. *How much control do you have over your life at present?*
    0 = Not at all in control / Feeling very helpless   1 = Slightly in control   2 = Markedly in control
    3 = Completely in control / Not feeling helpless at all

Part II – Traumatic Stress Symptom Cheklist (TSSC-E)

Below is a list of problems some people experience after earthquakes. Please indicate how much you were bothered by these problems within the LAST WEEK by putting X under the appropriate column.

	Not at all bothered	Slightly	Fairly	Very much bothered
1. I cannot help thinking about certain memories / images related to the earthquake.				
2. Sometimes all of a sudden past events pass before my eyes like a movie and I feel as if I am re-living the events.				
3. I frequently have nightmares.				
4. I cannot do certain things easily for fear of an earthquake (e.g. entering undamaged houses, taking a shower, being alone or sleeping in the dark).				
5. I have lost interest in things.				
6. I feel distant and estranged from people.				
7. I feel as if my feelings are dead.				
8. I have sleeping difficulty.				
9. I lose my temper more easily.				
10. I have difficulty remembering things or concentrating on what I am doing.				
11. I am on edge all the time for fear of an earthquake.				
12. I get startled when there is a sudden noise or movement.				
13. I feel upset when something reminds me of my experiences during the earthquake.				
14. I try to get rid of thoughts and feelings about my experiences during the earthquake.				
15. I have difficulty remembering certain parts of my experiences during the earthquake.				
16. Making long-term plans seems meaningless to me because the earthquake made me realize I may die anytime.				
17. I have physical symptoms such as palpitations, sweating, dizziness, and tension in my body when something reminds me of my experiences during the earthquake.				
18. I feel guilty.				
19. I feel depressed.				
20. I cannot enjoy life as I used to.				
21. I feel hopeless about the future.				
22. I have thoughts of killing myself from time to time.				
23. I have less energy for my daily activities.				

Part III: Severity of Disability Scale (SDS)

1. How distressed / bothered are you by the problems listed above?

    0 = Not at all   1 = Slightly   2 = Fairly   3 = Extremely

2. How impaired is your work, family life, and relationships with others because of the problems above?

    0 = No impairment. I can lead my daily life.

    1 = Slight impairment. I can lead my daily life with a little effort.

    2 = Marked impairment. There is marked disruption in my daily life.

    3 = Severe impairment. I cannot do most of the things in my daily life.

3. Would you like to have help from a psychiatrist or psychologist for your problems?

    0 = No   1 = Yes   2 = Not sure / don't know

Screening Instrument for Traumatic Stress in Earthquake Survivors-Child Version (SITSES-C)

Part I: Survivor Information Form

Please put X in the box next to the correct answer.

1. Your name and surname?_____

2. Your age? _____

3. Your gender? ☐ Male ☐ Female

4. Your grade? 1. ☐ 2. ☐ 3. ☐ 4. ☐ 5. ☐ 6. ☐ 7. ☐ 8. ☐

5. In which village, town, or city were you living during the earthquake?_____

6. Where do you live now?

    ☐ 1. Our usual house ☐ 2. A new house ☐ 3. Temporary shelter (camp)

    ☐ 4. Own built shelter (makeshift barrack, tent) ☐ 5. Another place (Indicate

    where_____)

7. Your current address?_____

8. Home telephone number (if any)?_____

9. Did the building where you were staying during the earthquake collapse? ☐ 0. No ☐ 1. Yes

10. Were you trapped under rubble? ☐ 0. No ☐ 1. Yes

11. Did any of your close ones die in the earthquake?

    ☐ 0. No ☐ 1. My mother ☐ 2. My father ☐ 3. Some of my brothers / sisters

    ☐ 4. Some of my relatives ☐ 5. Some of my friends ☐ 6. Some of our neighbors

12. How much damage did the earthquake cause in your house?

    ☐ 1. No damage ☐ 2. Minimal damage ☐ 3. Moderate damage ☐ 4. Severe damage

    ☐ 5. Collapsed ☐ 6. Demolished after the earthquake ☐ 7. Don't know

13. Which of the events below did you experience before the earthquake?

    ☐ 0. No event ☐ 1. Flood ☐ 2. Fire ☐ 3. Traffic accident ☐ 4. Physical injury

    ☐ 5. Physical assault ☐ 6. Falling from a high place ☐ 7. Burglary

    ☐ 8. Other such events (Indicate which_____)

14. How frightened were you during the earthquake?

    ☐ 0. Not at all ☐ 1. A little ☐ 2. Much ☐ 3. Very much

15. How much fear have you had lately thinking about new earthquakes?

    ☐ 0. Not at all ☐ 1. A little ☐ 2. Much ☐ 3. Very much

Part II – Traumatic Stress Symptom Checklist – Child Version (TSSC-C)

Below are some questions about the problems some people have after earthquakes. Please answer these questions by putting X under the appropriate column.

	No	A little	Fairly	Very much
1. Do you keep thinking about what happened during the earthquake even when you do not want to?				
2. Do you suddenly feel like the same events are happening all over again and feel scared?				
3. Do you try to keep away from situations that remind you of the earthquake?				
4. Do you have frightening dreams?				
5. Have you lost interest in doing things you used to like?				
6. Do you have difficulty sleeping?				
7. Do you feel like other people do not understand what you have been through during the earthquake?				
8. Do you have difficulty remembering any events that happened during the earthquake?				
9. Do you find yourself unable to feel emotions like joy or sadness as you used to?				
10. Do you feel you will not live as long as you used to think?				
11. Do you get startled by sudden noises or movements?				
12. Do you feel on edge thinking there might be an earthquake anytime?				
13. Do you feel bad when something reminds you of the earthquake?				
14. Do you find yourself trying not to think about the earthquake?				
15. Do you have difficulty remembering things or concentrating on something?				
16. Do you have racing of the heart, sweating, trembling, dizziness, headaches, or stomach aches when something reminds you of the earthquake?				
17. Are you more snappy than usual?				
18. Are you afraid of doing certain things for fear of earthquakes (like going into safe buildings, taking a shower, staying at home alone, or sleeping in the dark)?				
19. Have you been feeling sad and tearful lately?				
20. Do you find yourself feeling guilty about something at times?				
21. Do you ever find yourself wishing you were dead?				
22. Do you have less appetite than usual?				
23. Do you get more easily tired than usual?				
24. Do you feel restless or fidgety?				

PART III – Functional Impairment Scale

Please place "X" next to the appropriate answer.

1. How bothered are you by the problems listed above?

   0. Not bothered at all

   1. Slightly

   2. Fairly

   3. Very much bothered

2. How much do these problems interfere with your daily activities, such as going to school, attending classes, doing homework, helping with housework, playing, or meeting your friends?

   0. I can do everything as usual.

   1. I cannot do some of the things I used to do.

   2. I cannot do most of the things I used to do.

   3. I cannot do any of the things I used to do.

Fear and Avoidance Questionnaire

Below is a list of activities that may cause anxiety, fear, or distress in people who have experienced an earthquake. Please indicate by putting X under the appropriate column how much difficulty you have in carrying out these activities because of associated anxiety, fear, or distress.

NONE = Not difficult at all / I can do it easily.
SLIGHTLY = Slightly difficult / Sometimes cannot do it.
FAIRLY = Fairly difficult / Cannot do it most of the time.
EXTREMELY = Extremely difficult / Cannot do it at all.

	None	Slightly	Fairly	Extremely
1. Going into safe buildings by day.				
2. Going into safe buildings at night.				
3. Staying in safe buildings at night.				
4. Staying alone in safe buildings by day.				
5. Staying alone in safe buildings at night.				
6. Sleeping alone in safe buildings at night.				
7. Sleeping alone in a room at night.				
8. Sleeping before the time that the earthquake occurred.				
9. Sleeping at home with no one else awake.				
10. Being in the dark.				
11. Sleeping in the dark.				
12. Taking a bath in a safe house with other people there.				
13. Taking a bath in a safe house alone.				
14. Taking as long in the bathroom as before.				
15. Getting undressed (into pyjamas / nightdress) before going to bed.				
16. Closing or locking the doors when sleeping in a safe house at night.				
17. Watching news about the earthquake on television.				
18. Reading news about the earthquake in the newspapers.				
19. Joining in conversations about the earthquake.				
20. Talking about earthquake experiences.				
21. Being in confined spaces.				
22. Going anywhere high up.				
23. Using an elevator.				
24. Going to the upper floors of safe buildings.				
25. Going to the lower floors of safe buildings.				
26. Going shopping.				
27. Going out alone.				
28. Travelling alone on public transport.				
29. Going past collapsed buildings.				
30. Going close to collapsed buildings.				
31. Looking at damaged buildings.				

Fear and Avoidance Questionnaire (cont.)

	None	Slightly	Fairly	Extremely
32. Looking at pictures of acquaintances that died in the earthquake.				
33. Visiting the graves of acquaintances that died in the earthquake.				
34. Looking at things that make you think there could be an earthquake (e.g. the sky, the sea, animals, etc.).				
35. Thinking about things that happened during or after the earthquake.				
Other feared activities (please indicate below)				
36.				
37.				
38.				

Depression Rating Scale

Below are statements about how you might be feeling. Please consider whether you had these problems IN THE LAST WEEK and indicate how much you were bothered by them by putting X under the appropriate column.

	Not at all	Slightly	Fairly	Very much
1. I lose my temper easily.				
2. I feel fidgety and restless.				
3. I have difficulty in making decisions in my daily life.				
4. I feel guilty.				
5. I feel hopeless about the future.				
6. There has been slowing in my speech or bodily movements.				
7. I feel worthless.				
8. I have thoughts of killing myself.				
9. I lost (or gained) weight against my will.				
10. I have difficulty thinking or concentrating.				
11. I cry easily.				
12. I feel tired and lacking in energy.				
13. I feel depressed.				
14. I have difficulty doing my daily work.				
15. I have difficulty sleeping.				
16. I have bodily complaints (e.g. headaches, pains and aches in the body, stomach complaints, shortness of breath, palpitations, sweating, feeling faint, etc.).				
17. I have less interest in sex.				
18. I have decreased (or increased) appetite.				
19. I have lost pleasure in life.				

Screening Instrument for Traumatic Stress in Survivors of War (SITSOW)

Part I: Survivor Information Form

1. *Name:* _____

2. *Age:* _____

3. *Gender:*   1 = Male   2 = Female

4. *Education:*   1 = None   2 = Literate   3 = Primary   4 = Secondary   5 = High school   6 = University
   7 = Post-graduate

5. *Occupation:* _____

6. *Marital status:*   1 = Married-co-habiting   2 = Single   3 = Widowed   4 = Separated

7. *Your address:* _____

8. *Telephone number:* _____

9. *Did you ever have active involvement in a combat or armed conflict as a soldier or fighter?*
   0 = No   1 = Yes

10. *Did you ever have any captivity experience during a war or armed conflict?*
    0 = No   1 = Yes

11. *Did you ever have to leave home and seek refuge elsewhere?*   0 = No   1 = Yes

12. *Did anyone close to you get killed during the war?*   0 = No   1 = Yes
    (If yes) Who?_____

13. *Have you had any serious property or financial loss as a result of war or armed conflict?*
    0 = No   1 = Yes

14. *Did you have any psychiatric illness requiring treatment before the war?*
    0 = No   1 = Yes

15. *Using the scale below, how would you rate the intensity of the fear or terror you experienced during the most distressing event you experienced during the war?*
    0 = No fear at all   1 = Slight   2 = Marked   3 = Severe   4 = Extremely severe fear / terror

16. *How anxious / fearful have you been lately thinking about similar events occurring in the future?*
    0 = Not anxious / fearful at all   1 = Slightly   2 = Markedly   3 = Severely
    4 = Extremely anxious / fearful

17. *How much control do you have over your life at present?*
    0 = Not at all in control / Feeling very helpless   1 = Slightly in control   2 = Markedly in control
    3 = Completely in control / Not feeling helpless at all

Part II: Traumatic Stress Symptom Checklist (TSSC-W)

Below is a list of problems some people experience after traumatic events. Please consider the most distressing events you have experienced during the war and indicate how much you were bothered by these problems within the last month by putting X under the appropriate column.

Please specify most distressing events during the war:

. . . .

	Not at all bothered	Slightly	Fairly	Very much bothered
1. I cannot help thinking about certain memories/images related to the events.				
2. Sometimes all of a sudden the event passes before my eyes like a movie and I feel as if I am re-living the events.				
3. I have nightmares about the events.				
4. I cannot do certain things easily for fear of situations that remind me of the events.				
5. I have lost interest in things.				
6. I feel distant and estranged from people.				
7. I feel as if my feelings have gone numb.				
8. I have sleeping difficulty.				
9. I lose my temper more easily.				
10. I have difficulty remembering things or concentrating on what I am doing.				
11. I feel fidgety or on edge.				
12. I get startled when there is a sudden noise or movement.				
13. I feel upset when something reminds me of the events.				
14. I try to get rid of thoughts and feelings about the events.				
15. I have difficulty remembering certain parts of my experiences during the events.				
16. Making long-term plans seems meaningless to me because I feel my life has been shortened.				
17. I have physical symptoms such as palpitations, sweating, dizziness, and tension in my body when something reminds me of the events.				

Part III: Severity of Disability Scale (SDS)

1. How distressed / bothered are you by the problems listed above?

    0 = Not at all   1 = Slightly   2 = Fairly   3 = Extremely

2. How impaired is your work, family life, and relationships with others because of the problems above?

    0 = No impairment. I can lead my daily life.

    1 = Slight impairment. I can lead my daily life with a little effort.

    2 = Marked impairment. There is marked disruption in my daily life.

    3 = Severe impairment. I cannot do most of the things in my daily life.

3. Would you like to have help from a psychiatrist or psychologist for your problems?

    0 = No   1 = Yes   2 = Not sure / don't know

Global Improvement Scale – Self (GIS-S)

Please indicate on the scale below how much improvement has occurred in the problems for which you received treatment? In rating your improvement please make sure you compare your present situation with how you were BEFORE treatment.

0 = No change
1 = Slightly improved (less than 20%)
2 = Moderately improved (20%-60%)
3 = Much improved (60%-80%)
4 = Very much improved (more than 80%)

Global Improvement Scale – Assessor (GIS-A)

Indicate on the scale below how much improvement has occurred in the patient's problems compared with pre-treatment.

0 = No change
1 = Slightly improved (less than 20%)
2 = Moderately improved (20%-60%)
3 = Much improved (60%-80%)
4 = Very much improved (more than 80%)

Work / Social Adjustment Scale (self-rated)

In previous questionnaires you indicated the nature and severity of the problems you experienced since the traumatic event. Please answer the questions below by bearing in mind how these problems affect your daily life. Circle the number on each scale that best answers the question.

1. How much difficulty do you have working in or managing the home (for example, doing housework, taking care of children, shopping, etc.) because of your problems?

   0 ----------------- 1 ----------------- 2 ----------------- 3 ----------------- 4
   No difficulty at all   slight   moderate   much   very much / I cannot work

2. How much difficulty do you have with your social life (for example, going out, visiting friends / relatives, etc.) because of your problems?

   0 ----------------- 1 ----------------- 2 ----------------- 3 ----------------- 4
   No difficulty at all   slight   moderate   much   very much / no social life

3. How much difficulty do you have doing things that you enjoy doing by yourself (for example, watching TV, listening to music, knitting, sports, hobbies, etc.)?

   0 ----------------- 1 ----------------- 2 ----------------- 3 ----------------- 4
   No difficulty at all   slight   moderate   much   very much / cannot do anything

4. How impaired are your family relationships because of your problems?

   0 ----------------- 1 ----------------- 2 ----------------- 3 ----------------- 4
   No impairment at all   slight   moderate   much   very much

Work / Social Adjustment Scale (assessor-rated)

Circle a number that best describes the extent of impairment in each life domain as a result of post-traumatic stress reactions.

1. How much difficulty does the client have working in or managing the home (e.g. doing housework, taking care of children, shopping, etc.) because of his/her problems?

0 ---------------- 1 ---------------- 2 ---------------- 3 ---------------- 4
No difficulty at all   slight   moderate   much   very much / cannot work

2. How much difficulty does the client have with social life (e.g. going out, visiting friends / relatives, etc.) because of his/her problems?

0 ---------------- 1 ---------------- 2 ---------------- 3 ---------------- 4
No difficulty at all   slight   moderate   much   very much / no social life

3. How much difficulty does the client have doing things that he/she enjoys doing in private (e.g. watching TV, listening to music, knitting, sports, hobbies, etc.)?

0 ---------------- 1 ---------------- 2 ---------------- 3 ---------------- 4
No difficulty at all   slight   moderate   much   very much / cannot do anything

4. How impaired are the client's family relationships because of his/her problems?

0 ---------------- 1 ---------------- 2 ---------------- 3 ---------------- 4
No impairment at all   slight   moderate   much   very much

Sense of Control Scale

You have learned so far in treatment how you can handle situations that cause anxiety, fear, or distress. We would now like to understand how the treatment affected your feelings and thoughts about your fears. Please answer the following questions in relation to fear-evoking or distressing situations that you have selected as targets in treatment.

AFTER WHAT YOU HAVE LEARNED SO FAR, HAS THERE BEEN ANY CHANGE IN YOUR:

1. Fear or distress?
   0 = No change / increase
   1 = Slight decrease
   2 = Marked decrease
   3 = Very much decrease

2. Sense of control over feared or distressing situations?
   0 = No change / decrease
   1 = Slight increase
   2 = Marked increase
   3 = Very much increase

3. Courage in confronting feared or distressing situations?
   0 = No change / decrease
   1 = Slight increase
   2 = Marked increase
   3 = Very much increase

4. Self-confidence in confronting feared or distressing situations?
   0 = No change / decrease
   1 = Slight increase
   2 = Marked increase
   3 = Very much increase

5. Belief in your ability to cope with your fear or distress?
   0 = No change / decrease
   1 = Slight increase
   2 = Marked increase
   3 = Very much increase

Grief Assessment Scale

Below are statements that describe feelings and thoughts that some people have after the loss of a close one. Please indicate how frequently you have experienced these feelings and thoughts IN THE LAST MONTH by putting a cross (X) under the appropriate column.

	Never	Sometimes	Often	Always
1. I feel bitter for having lost him / her.				
2. I go to places that he / she used to go in the hope that I might find him / her there.				
3. I feel detached / estranged from others after his / her death.				
4. I feel that a future without him / her will always be empty and pointless.				
5. His / her death makes me feel like a part of me has died.				
6. I cry when I think about him / her.				
7. I cannot accept the fact that he / she is dead.				
8. I have lost trust in people because of his / her death.				
9. I feel lonely without him / her.				
10. I do things that remind me of him / her in day to day life (for example, keeping his / her pictures or belongings out in the open, thinking or talking about him / her, visiting his / her grave, etc.)				
11. I feel that life is empty or meaningless without him / her.				
12. I feel guilty when I enjoy myself.				
13. I acquired some of his / her harmful habits or behaviors (e.g. smoking or drinking).				
14. I yearn for him / her.				
15. I have physical complaints (e.g. headaches, pains, etc.) that started after his / her death.				
16. I see him / her stand before me.				
17. I feel as if my feelings have died after his / her death.				
18. I feel I have no control over my life.				
19. I cannot stop thinking about him / her.				
20. I feel helpless without him / her.				
21. I have physical complaints that he / she used to have when he / she was alive.				
22. I cannot do things that remind me of him / her in day to day life (for example, looking at his / her pictures, visiting his / her grave, talking about him / her, etc.).				
23. I hear his / her voice.				
24. I cannot believe that he / she is dead.				
25. I blame myself for not having tried hard enough to save him / her.				
26. I feel angry with him / her because he / she left me.				
27. I have dreams of him / her.				
28. I feel envious of people who have not lost their loved ones.				
29. I feel angry for having lost him / her.				
30. I feel insecure because of his / her death.				

Behavior Checklist for Grief

After the loss of a close one some people feel the urge to do certain things to keep the memory of the lost one alive all the time. Others have difficulty with certain activities that bring back distressing memories of the lost one. Below are some statements that describe such activities. Please indicate how much they apply to you IN THE LAST WEEK by putting a cross (X) under the appropriate column. If you have lost more than one close person, you may consider each statement in relation to any of them.

	Not at all	Slightly	Fairly	Very much
I feel like seeing his / her belongings out in the open.				
I have difficulty looking at his / her pictures.				
I avoid going to the place where he / she died.				
I feel like seeing his / her pictures out in the open.				
I feel like going to the places where we used to go together.				
I have difficulty mentioning his / her name.				
I avoid meeting his / her friends.				
I have difficulty cooking / eating the meals that he / she used to like.				
I avoid visiting his / her grave.				
I have difficulty listening to the music he / she liked.				
I feel like talking about him / her.				
I have difficulty going to the places where we used to go together.				
I avoid talking about him / her.				
I have difficulty looking at his / her belongings.				
I feel like visiting his / her grave.				

Appendix B: Helping people recover from earthquake trauma

Control-focused behavioral treatment delivery manual

Metin Başoğlu and Ebru Şalcıoğlu
Trauma Studies, Department of Psychological Medicine, Institute of Psychiatry,
King's College London & Istanbul Center for Behavior Research and Therapy

About the Authors

Professor Metin Başoğlu and Associate Professor Ebru Şalcıoğlu are currently the directors of the Istanbul Centre for Behavior Research and Therapy (ICBRT / DABATEM) in Istanbul. They are also affiliated with the Institute of Psychiatry, King's College London, where Prof. Başoğlu is head of Trauma Studies. Prof. Başoğlu has published extensively on behavioral treatment of anxiety disorders, including post-traumatic stress disorder. He is internationally recognized for his extensive research on war, torture, and earthquake trauma and their treatment. After the 1999 earthquakes in Turkey the authors developed brief behavioral interventions designed to facilitate recovery from earthquake trauma. Cognizant of the urgent need for cost-effective methods of treatment dissemination to mass trauma survivors around the world, particularly in low-income countries, they developed a mental healthcare model that utilizes various treatment dissemination methods, including an outreach care delivery program, treatment delivery manuals for professional and lay therapists, and self-help tools. They presented this work in a book on '*A Mental Healthcare Model for Mass Trauma Survivors: Control-Focused Behavioral Treatment of Earthquake, War, and Torture Trauma*' published by Cambridge University Press. More information on the authors' work can be found at http://www.dabatem.org.

Introduction

Large-scale devastating earthquakes often cause widespread psychological problems in millions of people, thus necessitating effective psychological care delivery through all means possible. This booklet is designed to assist health professionals (mental healthcare providers, general practitioners, nurses, social workers, etc.), as well as lay people with an adequate educational background in delivering psychological care to survivors. It is based on *Control-Focused Behavioral Treatment*, which is a fairly simple intervention that facilitates recovery from traumatic stress by helping survivors overcome their anxiety, fear, or distress caused by earthquakes. This intervention has been developed through work with more than 6000 earthquake survivors in Turkey and demonstrated to be highly effective in scientific studies (Başoğlu et al., 2003a; Başoğlu et al., 2003b; Başoğlu et al., 2005; Başoğlu et al., 2007). The manual consists of seven sections. Section 1 provides brief information about common psychological problems after major earthquakes. Section 2 will help you assess survivors' psychological problems and determine their need for treatment. Section 3 details the procedures of the first treatment session. Section 4 is about monitoring progress in subsequent weeks and dealing with problems in treatment. Section 5 concerns treatment of children. Section 6 will help you deliver the treatment in a single session when the need arises. Finally, Section 7 will guide you in helping bereaved survivors with unresolved grief problems.

If you are not previously trained in psychological treatment, you may be wondering whether you can be of any help to people. There are several reasons why we think you can. First of all, the treatment is fairly simple and easy to deliver. The manual will guide you through the process almost step by step. Furthermore, you will see various WARNINGS that will help you recognize various psychological problems that may need attention by a mental health specialist. If you come across these problems, all you need to do is to refer the person you are helping to a specialist, which is by itself an important form of help. Therefore, provided that you pay close attention to these warnings, you would be working only with people whom you can help. In any event, do not worry if you cannot help everyone, as this is not possible even for professional therapists. Bear in mind that you will be trying to help people who may otherwise never have an opportunity to receive any form of effective care.

Together with this manual, you may have been given a self-help manual designed for use by earthquake survivors. It is quite similar to the present manual in its content. A study has shown that most survivors who read and utilize the self-help manual benefit from it (Başoğlu et al., 2009). You may consider giving a copy to a person you are intending to help, if you think they would be willing and able to utilize it on their own. You could still help them by using the present manual, as some people may need support, encouragement, and guidance during treatment. Alternatively, you may first give the person a chance with the self-help manual and consider helping them only if they fail to administer treatment on their own for some reason.

When using these manuals, you may contact us by email (dabatem@dabatem.org) with any questions, comments, or suggestions you might have. Your feedback could be very useful in future editions of these manuals. Good luck with your work!

References

Başoğlu, M., Livanou, M., Şalcıoğlu, E., et al. (2003a). A brief behavioural treatment of chronic post-traumatic stress disorder in earthquake survivors: Results from an open clinical trial. *Psychological Medicine*, **33**, 647–654.

Başoğlu, M., Livanou, M., Şalcıoğlu, E. (2003b). A single session with an earthquake simulator for traumatic stress in earthquake survivors. *American Journal of Psychiatry*, **160**, 788–790.

Başoğlu, M., Şalcıoğlu, E., Livanou, M., et al. (2005). Single-session behavioral treatment of earthquake-related posttraumatic stress disorder: A randomized waiting list controlled trial. *Journal of Traumatic Stress*, **18**, 1–11.

Başoğlu, M., Şalcıoğlu, E., Livanou, M. (2007). A randomized controlled study of single-session behavioural treatment of earthquake-related post-traumatic stress disorder using an earthquake simulator. *Psychological Medicine*, **37**, 203–213.

Başoğlu, M., Şalcıoğlu, E., Livanou, M. (2009). Single-case experimental studies of a self-help manual for traumatic stress in earthquake survivors. *Journal of Behavior Therapy and Experimental Psychiatry*, **40**, 50–58.

Section 1: Understanding traumatic stress

Trauma events, such as earthquakes and other natural disasters, road traffic accidents, fires, rape, war violence, torture, physical assault, serious injury, and other similar events may cause intense distress, fear, terror, and helplessness in people. These emotional reactions – termed **traumatic stress** – may lead to chronic and debilitating psychological problems in some people, if left untreated. In this section you will find a brief description of some traumatic stress problems that people commonly experience after earthquakes. This information will help you understand better the problems of people you want to help.

Re-experiencing of trauma events

Most earthquake survivors re-experience the trauma in various ways. They may not be able to stop thinking about the trauma events they experienced, no matter how hard they try. Their daily routine may be upset by such distressing thoughts and they may have difficulty concentrating on what they are doing. They may have **flashbacks** or the feeling **as if they are re-living** the traumatic events of the earthquake. Flashbacks generally last for a few seconds or minutes but in exceptional cases they may last for as long as 10–15 minutes. When it happens, a person may feel like **they are watching a filmstrip of the trauma events**. They may see what they saw during the earthquake, hear the sounds that they heard, feel the objects they touched, or smell the smells they smelled all over again. They may also experience the fear and terror they experienced before with the same intensity. Because they think they are in the same situation all over again, they may rush outside, begin screaming, cry for help or think that their family is in danger and try to rescue them. For the duration of the flashback they may not be aware of what is going on around them. If someone speaks to them, for example, they may not be able to hear them. Once the flashback is over, they may not remember what has happened. Flashbacks are generally triggered by something that recalls the traumatic event. This could be an image, a sound, a smell, a feeling, or a thought. People who experience the symptom may worry that they are '*losing their mind*' or '*going mad.*'

Some people have **nightmares** about the trauma events. Nightmares may sometimes be so powerful as to wake a person up terrified. Having woken up, they may have trouble getting back to sleep, or not want to go back to sleep at all for fear of further nightmares. Others may feel anxious or distressed when something reminds them of the trauma. This could be television news or press stories about the earthquake, something someone says, a conversation about the earthquake, the sight of collapsed or damaged buildings in the area, or an image, sound, or object that reminds them of where they were at the time of the earthquake. As there are a lot of things around that remind them of the trauma, they may find themselves frequently feeling distressed.

Avoidance

Survivors often avoid trauma reminders, because they make them feel frightened, anxious, or distressed. They may, for example, avoid going into safe buildings, going into their home or staying there overnight (even when it is safe or only minimally damaged), staying or sleeping in the dark, going shopping, going anywhere where they can see collapsed buildings, looking at damaged buildings, sleeping alone, taking a bath, getting into bed undressed, being in places where people are talking about the earthquake, or following news of the earthquake on television or in the press. These are called **avoidance behaviors**. Although avoidance may seem like a normal response, it is one of the problems that most affects and limits a person's life. Avoidance may also take on another form. When thoughts of the traumatic events enter a person's mind, they may try to banish them because they cause distress. Most of the time, these thoughts enter their mind no matter how hard they try to block them.

Some people lose interest in things they used to like doing. They may not get the same enjoyment or pleasure from these activities. These activities may include housework, handicrafts, sewing, watching popular television programs, reading, and going out or to the cinema, sports, games, or special interests. Others may experience a reduction in their capacity to experience certain emotions compared with before the earthquake. Depending on the circumstances, people normally experience emotions like feeling pleased or upset, loving, laughing, crying, feeling happy or unhappy, hating, feeling compassion, feeling close to family and friends, getting annoyed, getting angry or feeling depressed. Survivors may find themselves unable to feel happy in a situation where they should be happy or unable to feel sad when they should be sad. They may be unable to feel close to their family for no reason. Their emotions may seem to be 'numbed'. If they have children, they may not be able to feel the love

219

and affection for them that they should. People with this symptom feel 'different' or that they have 'changed.' Close friends and family will also be aware of the situation given that there is often a numbing in that person's emotional responses to them.

Some survivors may feel alienated and distant from people. Often, the reason for this is the thought that family and friends who did not have the same experience do not understand what they are going through. When they look at the things that occupy people in their everyday lives, or the trivial matters that they make problems out of, they may react against this, thinking: "*How can anyone get caught up in such unnecessary, meaningless details when there are people like me who are going through all this?*" They may also find themselves affected by the way they have seen some people act after the earthquake. For example, they may be struck by the way some people did not help others or made no effort to rescue people from the rubble or acted selfishly or insensitively. Incidences of this kind may have left them disillusioned about people or without respect for them. They may think: "*How could anyone do that?*" Such emotions may lead them to avoid people. As family and friends try to coax them back to a 'normal' life, they may get annoyed and do their best to avoid being with them. Sometimes being physically close to people or having physical contact can also be distressing. When, for instance, someone from the family wants to hug them, they may feel distinctly unenthusiastic.

Some survivors describe a feeling that they will not live as long as they used to think. Having witnessed many people dying in the earthquake, perhaps including some close ones, they may think that something could happen to them any minute, leaving them dead. Their life may seem to have been shortened. So making plans for the future may seem meaningless. They may have lost their home in the earthquake, or the property they spent their whole life striving to acquire. To start all over again to build a new life may seem pointless. Particularly when they hear rumors of more earthquakes to come, they may think that starting life all over again is pointless.

Some people may have difficulty remembering some of the traumatic events they experienced during the earthquake. For example, someone who was pulled out from the rubble may not be able to remember some of the hours they spent there. Similarly, someone who tried to rescue members of their family from the rubble may not be able to remember a few hours of the experience. Generally, people with this symptom try to think through events as they happened and realize there is a gap in their memory. They cannot piece together what happened in the period between one incident and another or one situation and another. When they hear from other people what they did during that time, they realize that they cannot remember anything, no matter how hard they try.

Hyperarousal symptoms

Hypervigilance, a state of extreme alertness, is common after earthquakes. Survivors may find themselves constantly straining to hear noises outside, or repeatedly checking objects at home, like ceiling lights, which signal a tremor. They may feel that an earthquake is happening because of the vibrations caused by a passing lorry. If they are at home, they may sit near a door or other possible 'escape route.' They may even sleep there at night. A sudden noise or bang may startle them. Sleeping difficulties are common, most often due to fear of another earthquake. Some people will take it in turns to sleep at home. People who have had nightmares may sometimes find it difficult to get back to sleep. And some people may even avoid sleeping for fear of nightmares.

Some survivors have memory and concentration difficulties, because trauma memories constantly preoccupy them. They may find themselves having to read what they are reading over and over again because they cannot concentrate. They may have trouble following the topic of conversation or watching a program on television from beginning to end. They may not remember where they put things at home, or forget the food on the stove and burn it. They may forget some of the things they have to do during the day. They have trouble remembering names or memorizing them.

Irritability is another common symptom. Some people may get annoyed very easily or lose their temper. They may have less patience for annoying things that happen around them. Even if they never did it before, they may find themselves frequently upbraiding members of their family, getting angry or even violent with them (beating their children, smashing objects etc.). The symptom may lead to a breakdown in their relationships with family and friends, incompatibility, and antagonism.

Depression

Depression should not to be confused with the common feelings of sadness or feeling low in everyday life.

A person with depression feels intense anguish, unhappiness, or distress. They no longer enjoy life as they used to. They lose interest in a lot of activities they liked and enjoyed before. They feel helpless, pessimistic, and hopeless about the future. They sleep badly, find it difficult to sleep, and wake up at night and find themselves unable to get back to sleep for a long time. They feel tired, exhausted, enervated, and cannot muster up the strength to go about their everyday business. As a result, their everyday business may suffer. They have appetite problems; most of the time they eat very little, but more rarely may eat excessive amounts. Lack of appetite may lead to weight loss. During the day they often feel worried and cannot stop thinking about their problems. They may become forgetful or find it difficult to concentrate on what they are doing. There may also be physical symptoms like sweating, dizziness, numbing of the extremities or other parts of the body, palpitations, feeling faint, shortness of breath, or localized pains. A loss of sexual desire can be experienced. The person may sometimes wish to die as a means of relief. In more serious cases they may contemplate suicide, or even take this as far as a suicide attempt. A loss of self-confidence is common, as is a sense of uselessness and worthlessness. The person may feel guilty because they have trouble carrying out their everyday responsibilities. For example, women may feel guilty about not being able to do enough housework, or look after the children as they should, or take a sufficient interest in them.

The role of fear and avoidance in traumatic stress

An earthquake is an intensely frightening experience for most people. Aftershocks intensify people's fear, because they occur **unpredictably** and there is no way of controlling or avoiding them. People feel more helpless when they are exposed to life-threatening events over which they have no control and it is such **helplessness** that causes traumatic stress. People often tend to avoid earthquakes by avoiding a wide range of situations where they think they may be caught up in an earthquake. For example, they may not enter particular buildings, even when they are not damaged by the earthquake. They also tend to avoid various situations that bring back distressing memories of the earthquake. Although avoidance may provide some temporary relief from distress or fear, it

maintains traumatic stress, because it does not alleviate helplessness. Some people avoid so many different situations or activities that they are unable to conduct their daily activities in the usual way. You will see more examples of avoidance behaviors in the next section. Such fear and avoidance often make people feel even more **helpless** and many eventually get **depressed**.

The traumatic stress problems described earlier are directly related to distress or fear. For example, because of fear, they are constantly vigilant, watching out for signs of an impending earthquake. Consequently, they are easily startled by sudden noises or movements, lose their sleep, feel irritable, and have problems with their memory and concentration. Furthermore, fear and avoidance interfere with important responsibilities in their life and make it more difficult for them to cope with everyday problems, thereby causing additional stress for them.

Is fear of earthquakes normal?

Fear is a natural reaction that helps people to protect themselves in the face of real danger. It is therefore normal to be afraid of earthquakes. However, it is important to distinguish **irrational** from **rational** fears. Taking realistic safety measures against earthquakes, such as strengthening one's house and learning how to protect oneself during an earthquake, reflects normal fear. However, after a major earthquake some people fear earthquakes so much that they are unable to stay alone at home, sleep in the dark, take a bath as usual, or get undressed when going to bed. Some cannot sleep in the room where they experienced the earthquake. Many people stay in shelters under difficult conditions for a long time even when their house is undamaged and inhabitable. Some people can stay at home during the day but not at night. Such fears are not rational, given that they do not afford realistic protection from earthquakes. Beyond a few precautionary measures, there is not much one can do to avoid earthquakes and therefore one has to resume normal life as soon as it is possible to do so after a major earthquake. Trying to avoid earthquakes at all costs is like trying to avoid many other possible dangers we face in life. For example, we can be run over by a car when we go out on the street. Yet we do not live in daily fear of having a car accident. A flowerpot could fall on our head and kill us as we are walking along the road. Because we do not notice these risks in our everyday lives, we are not afraid of them.

But, whether we are afraid or not, the dangers still exist for us. We build these risks into our lives, because otherwise it would be impossible to carry on living normally.

What does treatment involve?

The main principle of treatment is to help reduce a person's helplessness by increasing their **anxiety tolerance** and **sense of control** over traumatic stress. You can achieve this by encouraging the person to confront situations and trauma memories that evoke fear or distress until they no longer feel the need to avoid them. For example, if a person is afraid of staying alone at home, you would encourage them to stay alone at home until they overcome their fear. If they are trying to keep distressing thoughts away from their mind, they would focus on these thoughts until they no longer feel the urge to avoid them.

Why make an effort not to avoid fear or distress?

To use an analogy, confronting fear or distress is like getting vaccinated against a virus. When a small dose of the virus is in one's system, the body can build up its defense against the virus. This is also called **immunization**. People can be immunized against traumatic stress by confronting fear or distress. Confronting fear or distress is also like practicing weight-lifting. The more one does it, the stronger one gets.

Many people experience traumatic events during earthquakes but recover after a while. The reason why the person you are helping has not recovered so far is because they have been avoiding their distress or fear, instead of confronting it and learning to tolerate and control it. Avoidance may provide some relief from anxiety but this relief comes with a high price. Avoidance not only perpetuates the problem and makes a person more helpless but also interferes with one's life functioning. As mentioned earlier, **it is impossible to live a normal life without taking any**

risks. Therefore, a more realistic approach after an earthquake is to take reasonable safety precautions as much as possible and continue with normal life. Treatment means helping people to understand that fear is their worst **enemy** and avoidance means **surrendering** to the enemy and letting it take control of their life. Hence, the most important message you will need to convey to them is as follows:

DISTRESS – FEAR – AVOIDANCE is your worst enemy.

At this point you are facing a critical choice in your life:
either you **BEAT** your fear
and **TAKE CONTROL** over your life
or
SURRENDER and live a life in distress, fear, and helplessness.

How do people cope with fear?

The treatment in this booklet might make more sense if you consider examples of how people cope with fear. After major earthquakes many people eventually realize that they have to confront and overcome their fear of buildings for the simple reason that they cannot live in shelters forever. Accordingly, they begin to enter buildings, staying there for a short period each time, and gradually increase the time they spend in a building as their confidence grows. If you have a look around, you can see such people among survivors.

Some people have phobic fears of animals (dogs, cats, spiders, snakes, etc.) or particular situations, such as enclosed spaces, heights, crowded places, etc. If you ask the people you know if they had such fears in the past and what they did to overcome them, some of them will tell you that they beat their fears by gradually confronting the feared objects or situation in much the same way as described in this booklet. If you had a similar experience yourself in the past, you should have no difficulty in understanding what this treatment is about.

Section 2: Assessing traumatic stress problems

This section will help you understand how you can assess someone's psychological status after an earthquake, whether they need treatment, and whether there are other problems that you need to rule out before treatment. You will do this by using two questionnaires and asking some additional questions. The first step in assessment is to understand the impact of the earthquake on the person. Below is a questionnaire that includes statements concerning various traumatic stress problems that people have after earthquakes. Ask the survivor to fill in the questionnaire by following the instructions. Make sure that they think about whether they had these symptoms in the LAST WEEK. Also make sure that they do not skip any statement. You will be administering this questionnaire weekly during treatment, so either use a copy or ask the person to mark their responses on a separate sheet of paper.

Traumatic Stress Symptom Checklist

Below is a list of problems some people experience after earthquakes. Please indicate how much you were bothered by these problems within the LAST WEEK by putting X under the appropriate column.

	0 Not at all bothered	1 Slightly	2 Fairly	3 Very much bothered
I cannot help thinking about certain memories / images related to the earthquake.				
Sometimes all of a sudden past events pass before my eyes like a movie and I feel as if I am re-living the events.				
I frequently have nightmares.				
I cannot do certain things easily for fear of an earthquake (e.g. entering undamaged houses, taking a shower, being alone or sleeping in the dark).				
I have lost interest in things.				
I feel distant and estranged from people.				
I feel as if my feelings are dead.				
I have sleeping difficulty.				
I lose my temper more easily.				
I have difficulty remembering things or concentrating on what I am doing.				
I am on edge all the time for fear of an earthquake.				
I get startled when there is a sudden noise or movement.				
I feel upset when something reminds me of my experiences during the earthquake.				
I try to get rid of thoughts and feelings about my experiences during the earthquake.				
I have difficulty remembering certain parts of my experiences during the earthquake.				
Making long-term plans seems meaningless to me because the earthquake made me realize I may die anytime.				
I have physical symptoms such as palpitations, sweating, dizziness, and tension in my body when something reminds me of my experiences during the earthquake.				
I feel guilty.				
I feel depressed.				

Traumatic Stress Symptom Checklist (cont.)

	0 Not at all bothered	1 Slightly	2 Fairly	3 Very much bothered
I cannot enjoy life as I used to.				
I feel hopeless about the future.				
I have thoughts of killing myself from time to time.				
I have less energy for my daily activities.				
TOTAL SCORE				

Now work out the total score on this questionnaire. Give 0 points for each X in the '*Not at all bothered*' column, 1 point for each X in the '*Slightly*' column, 2 for each X in the '*Fairly*' column, and 3 for each X in the '*Very much bothered*' column. Add up the scores to obtain a total **Traumatic Stress Score** and write it underneath the questionnaire next to Total Score. Now let us see what the *Traumatic Stress Score* indicates.

Score 34 or higher → There is an 80% chance that the person has traumatic stress problems requiring treatment.

Score 38 or higher → There is an 80% chance that the person also has mild to moderate depression.

Score higher than 50 → There is an 80% chance that the person has severe traumatic stress and depression.

Depression (see Section 1 for a description) occurs fairly commonly in people after major earthquakes, often as a result of intense fear and helplessness caused by unpredictably occurring aftershocks. It may also occur in response to loss of close ones, property, or occupation, and financial difficulties.

Assessing severity of fear and avoidance

Although the *Traumatic Stress Score* gives you an idea about the severity of traumatic stress problems, this is not the only indicator of a person's need for treatment. You will need additional information to make this decision. Most importantly, you will need to know how these problems affect the person's life. To get an idea of how fear and avoidance might be affecting the person's life, administer the second questionnaire below. You will be using this questionnaire weekly, so either use a copy or ask the person to mark their responses on a separate sheet of paper. This questionnaire is not a comprehensive list of all possible avoidance behaviors in earthquake survivors. If the person has avoidance behaviors that are not included in this questionnaire, make sure that they list these under 'Other Feared Activities.'

Fear and Avoidance Questionnaire

Below is a list of activities that may cause anxiety, fear, or distress in people who have experienced an earthquake. Please indicate by putting X under the appropriate column how much difficulty you have in carrying out these activities because of associated anxiety, fear, or distress.

NONE = Not difficult at all / I can do it easily
SLIGHTLY = Slightly difficult / Sometimes cannot do it
FAIRLY = Fairly difficult / Cannot do it most of the time
EXTREMELY = Extremely difficult / Cannot do it at all

	0 None	1 Slightly	2 Fairly	3 Extremely
Going into safe buildings by day				
Going into safe buildings at night				
Staying in safe buildings at night				

Fear and Avoidance Questionnaire (cont.)

	0 None	1 Slightly	2 Fairly	3 Extremely
Staying alone in safe buildings by day				
Staying alone in safe buildings at night				
Sleeping alone in safe buildings at night				
Sleeping alone in a room at night				
Sleeping before the time that the earthquake occurred				
Sleeping at home with no one else awake				
Being in the dark				
Sleeping in the dark				
Taking a bath in a safe house with other people there				
Taking a bath in a safe house alone				
Taking as long in the bathroom as before				
Getting undressed (into pyjamas / nightdress) before going to bed				
Closing or locking the doors when sleeping in a safe house at night				
Watching news about the earthquake on television				
Reading news about the earthquake in the newspapers				
Joining in conversations about the earthquake				
Talking about earthquake experiences				
Being in confined spaces				
Going anywhere high up				
Using an elevator				
Going to the upper floors of safe buildings				
Going to the lower floors of safe buildings				
Going shopping				
Going out alone				
Travelling alone on public transport				
Going past collapsed buildings				
Going close to collapsed buildings				
Looking at damaged buildings				
Looking at pictures of acquaintances who died in the earthquake				
Visiting the graves of acquaintances who died in the earthquake				
Looking at things that make you think there could be an earthquake (e.g. the sky, the sea, animals, etc.)				
Thinking about things that happened during or after the earthquake				
Other feared activities (please indicate below):				
TOTAL SCORE				

Now work out the total score. Give each item 0 points for '*None*,' 1 point for '*Slightly*,' 2 points for '*Fairly*,' and 3 points for '*Extremely*' responses. Then, add up the scores to obtain a total **Fear and Avoidance Score** and write it next to Total Score. People who have experienced a devastating earthquake in the epicenter region avoid an average of 10 activities in this questionnaire and obtain an average score of 32. These figures will give you some idea about how the person compares with other people in this respect.

Assessing impact of fear and avoidance on life

To understand how fear and avoidance might be affecting the person's life, go through the list activities marked as '*Fairly difficult*' or '*Extremely difficult*' in the questionnaire and ask the following questions: "***How much do these fears interfere with your (1) work, (2) social life, and (3) family life?***" Fear and avoidance may cause serious problems in these areas of life. For example:

- The person may be living in difficult or even dangerous conditions in a shelter, because they are afraid of going into buildings, even when they are undamaged.
- Because of their fear of buildings, they may not be able to go to work or undertake any important function in life that requires entering particular buildings, such as schools, shops, government offices, etc.
- If they cannot go shopping, this may make it hard for them to carry out their responsibilities at home.
- If they cannot stay at home alone or take a bath without anyone present at home, this may create problems within the family.
- Their social life may have suffered, if they are unable to visit friends or relatives or join them in various leisure activities, such as going to the cinema, restaurants, parties, weddings, or other social gatherings.
- They may be making much effort every day to avoid memories and reminders of their earthquake experience. They may have stopped reading newspapers, listening to TV news, or seeing friends who remind them of the earthquake.
- Problems such as memory and concentration difficulties, feeling alert and anxious all the time, reduced sleep, and tiredness may be causing serious impairment in their learning capacity and school, work, and social performance.
- Irritability and difficulty in controlling anger may have strained their relationships with family, friends, and colleagues at work.

Discussing these issues will help the person understand better how this problem is affecting their life and motivate them for treatment. You may also discuss with the person how realistic these fears are. For example, the survivor may be avoiding being in a building at night but not during the day. Does this really make them any safer, given that earthquakes may happen any time of the day? This may help them understand better the **irrational** nature of their fears and feel more motivated for treatment.

How to decide whether a person needs treatment?

At this point you have almost all the information you need for a decision about whether the person needs treatment, except for one: does the person feel the need for help? Thus, ask the person if they want help for their problems.

⇒ If the person feels a need for help, then **there is a need for treatment**, regardless of their scores in the above questionnaires. A person may have a *Traumatic Stress Score* of 15 or lower and still feel a need for help. This is because some earthquake survivors, despite such low scores, may need help with their fear and avoidance problems.

⇒ If the person does not feel a need for help, this does not necessarily mean they do not need treatment. They may simply not see the connection between their trauma and psychological problems. Or they may not regard their problems as a condition requiring treatment. If their *Traumatic Stress Score* is 34 or more, there is an 80% chance that they need treatment. The higher their score, the more they need treatment. In such cases, consider carefully how their stress problems affect their life. Because of their fear or distress they may be having difficulty doing many things in everyday life. Their problems might have adversely affected their work and social and family life. If this is true for the person you are intending to help, ask them to give themselves a chance by initiating the treatment and see how they feel. If they still refuse help, give them a copy of the self-help manual and advise them to utilize it.

Ruling out conditions that require attention by a specialist

Before starting treatment, you need to rule out possible psychiatric or medical conditions that may need attention by healthcare specialists. As traumatic stress often leads to depression, this is the first condition you need to consider as a potential problem in treatment. Consider the following questions.

⇒ *Is the person depressed?*

Check the *Traumatic Stress Score*. If it is higher than 38, there is an 80% chance that the person is depressed. The higher the score above 38, the greater the chances of depression are. Depression by itself does not pose a problem in treatment, unless there is a risk of suicide and some depressive symptoms are severe enough to impede treatment.

⇒ *Is there a risk of suicide?*

Check item #22 of the *Traumatic Stress Symptom Checklist* ("*I have thoughts of killing myself from time to time*"). If the person has marked **Slightly**, **Fairly**, or **Very much bothered**, ask the following questions:

1. *I can see from your questionnaire that you have been having some ideas about suicide. Have you recently considered suicide and made plans to this end?*
2. *Have you ever tried to put a plan like this into practice since the earthquake?*

WARNING

If the answer to any of the above questions is YES, there could be a risk of suicide.
Refer the person to a mental health specialist.

Some people may express depressive feelings such as "*I'd be better off dead*" or "*I wish I were dead.*" This does not necessarily indicate serious suicide risk. Suicide risk may be serious, however, if the person has been contemplating **actual suicide plans** or has already made a **suicide attempt**. Bear also in mind that suicidal ideas may occur without severe depression in earthquake survivors. Therefore, always check suicidal ideas, whether or not the person is depressed. Plan for treatment after the person recovers from suicidal ideas and other depression symptoms.

⇒ *Is depression likely to impede treatment?*

Depression often improves with the treatment in this booklet. However, some depressed people may have feelings of **hopelessness** and **despair**, which may lead them to think they will never get better, whatever treatment they get. In addition, symptoms like **apathy**, **enervation**, and **exhaustion** may make it difficult for them to take action against their problems. Such people may reject your help. Try to understand how the person feels about prospects of getting better with treatment. Are they hopeful about their chances of getting better? Are they sufficiently motivated for treatment? Are they prepared to make an effort to get better? If they are not, it may be worth telling them the following:

> *The sense of hopelessness and despair, the apathy, enervation and exhaustion you are experiencing are symptoms of the depression you are currently going through. Once you have overcome your distress and fears with the treatment I am recommending, these symptoms will disappear. However, you will have to make an effort. My advice to you is this: give yourself a chance and make an effort to get better.*

If the person still thinks that they will not be able to overcome their problems, refer them to a mental health-care specialist. Also, advise them to come back to you for treatment when they have recovered from depression.

Let us now turn to some other conditions you need to rule out before treatment. Ask the questions below and pay close attention to various recommendations about appropriate course of action.

⇒ *Since the earthquake are you having frequent uncontrollable anger outbursts during any of which you caused (or felt like causing) serious harm to yourself or others?*
  WARNING: If the answer is YES, refer the person to a mental healthcare provider. Note that 'serious harm' refers to events such as physical injury to self or others, engaging in fights with people, acts of violence, or getting oneself into dangerous situations (e.g. reckless driving, engaging in dangerous sports, etc.).

⇒ *Since the earthquake have you ever had any flashbacks during which you lost total awareness of your surroundings or did something to endanger yourself or others around you?* (See description of flashbacks in Section 1)
  WARNING: If the answer is YES, refer the person to a mental healthcare provider.

⇒ *Do you currently have a psychiatric condition for which you were admitted to a psychiatric hospital and received drug treatment in the past?*
  WARNING: If the answer is YES, ask the person to contact their doctor first. Once their psychiatric problem is brought under control, you may consider delivering the treatment in this booklet.

227

⇒ *Do you have any physical conditions (such as serious heart problems requiring treatment or pregnancy) that might be affected by heightened anxiety?*
WARNING: If the answer is YES, ask the person to consult with a doctor first and find out if their condition is likely to be affected by heightened anxiety that they may experience in feared or distressing situations. If it is, the person may need to receive this treatment under the supervision of a professional therapist.

⇒ *Do you currently consume substantial amounts of alcohol or sedative drugs on a regular basis?*
WARNING: If the answer is YES, refer the person to a mental health specialist. If they were using alcohol or drugs before the earthquake, they will need help for this problem first. If they started using these substances after the earthquake, they can receive the treatment in this booklet under the guidance of a professional therapist as they begin to reduce intake of these substances. The treatment may be helpful in coming off these substances.

Summary of assessment procedures

⇒ Administer questionnaires and work out total scores.

⇒ Determine need for treatment. At least one of the following is present:
- The person feels a need for help or requests help.
- Traumatic Stress Score is 34 or higher.
- Fear and avoidance problems significantly impair life functioning.

⇒ Determine suitability for treatment. All conditions below need to be met.
- There is no risk of suicide.
- Depression symptoms do not undermine motivation for treatment.
- Since the earthquake the person has not had any uncontrollable anger outbursts during which they caused (or felt like causing) serious harm to self or others.
- The person does not have long-lasting flashbacks during which they lose total awareness of surroundings or do something to endanger themselves or others.
- The person does not have a current psychiatric condition for which they were admitted to a psychiatric hospital and received drug or other treatment in the past.
- The person does not have a physical condition (such as serious heart problems or pregnancy) that might be affected by heightened anxiety.
- The person does not currently consume substantial amounts of alcohol or sedative drugs on a regular basis.

⇒ If any of the above conditions is not met, refer the person to a mental healthcare specialist.

⇒ If all of the above conditions are met, offer the person help. If they accept it, start treatment. If not, give them a copy of the self-help manual and advise them to read it.

Section 3: Beating fear and distress

Session 1

In this section you will see how you can help the person overcome the impact of the trauma. If you are in the very early days or weeks of the disaster your main goal is to help the person not to give in to fear or distress caused by recurring aftershocks and maintain normal life activities as much as possible under the post-disaster circumstances. If it has been some months since the earthquake and the person has already developed extensive avoidance problems, your main goal in treatment is to help them regain control over their life by not avoiding fear and distress. This means helping them to resume normal life activities. It is best to start this treatment as early as possible after an earthquake, so that chronic problems associated with pervasive fear and avoidance can be prevented before they emerge.

The treatment can be delivered in four sessions in most cases. You can see the person weekly or twice weekly, depending on the circumstances. In situations where this is not feasible, the treatment could be delivered in a single session (see Section 6). The first session (usually 60–90 minutes) is most important, because this is when you explain to the person how they should go about overcoming their problems. In subsequent sessions you will evaluate their progress and help them with difficulties they encounter in treatment.

Step 1: Explaining treatment

In explaining the treatment you will need to make sure that the person fully understands why they need treatment, what the treatment is about, and how it works. It is of critical importance that you present the treatment in a convincing way, because this will largely determine whether or not the person accepts it. In this section you will see explanations (*in italics*) regarding various issues. These are provided to give you an idea about what to say about treatment and how to say it. They are stated in general terms here but you can make them more specific to the person by using the information you have on their problems.

*OK, now that your assessment is completed I have some idea about how you are affected by the distressing events you experienced during the earthquake. Let us consider what can be done about this problem. You are distressed by memories of these events and have fears of similar events happening to you in the future. Such anxiety is responsible for many of your stress problems [such as being alert all the time, sleeping problems, memory / concentration difficulty, irritability, helplessness, and depressed mood]. Because you avoid distressing / feared situations, you are unable to do many things that are important in your life. This makes you even more helpless and depressed. Fear is your worst **enemy** here, considering how it affects your life. Instead of fighting and defeating the enemy, you have so far chosen to surrender to it, letting it take control of your life. If avoiding distress / fear maintains your stress problems, what is the logical thing to do here to overcome these problems? [Most survivors say 'to overcome my fears by not avoiding them']. Yes, confronting your anxiety is indeed the most effective way of dealing with your problem. You need to do this regularly until you learn to tolerate and control your anxiety. This means you will have to make an effort not to avoid situations or activities that make you anxious. You stand a good chance of recovery with this treatment. I will tell you more about what you need to do in treatment later.*

Some survivors, when they find out what treatment involves, may be reluctant to do things that will make them anxious or distressed. Some may even refuse the idea of not avoiding various situations (like being in buildings), saying "*What if an earthquake happens while I am there? Is it not normal to be afraid of earthquakes?*" In such situations, you can offer the following explanation:

You have to make a distinction between normal fear of earthquakes and irrational fears that serve no purpose. Fear is normal to the extent that it makes you take reasonable precautions to protect yourself against earthquakes. Earthquakes cause a lot of irrational fears in people. Let us just consider which fears serve a useful purpose. For example [give examples of some of the person's irrational fears], some people no longer sleep in the room where they experienced the earthquake. They do this because being in that room brings back their fear. Other than perhaps making them feel a bit better, does sleeping in another room make them any safer during an earthquake? Consider another example. Some people do not take a shower alone at home and they go to bed with their clothes on and sleep with lights on. Are these really reasonable precautions that make them any safer during an earthquake? Such fears are not rational, because they do not actually protect anyone from earthquakes. Moreover, they make it impossible to lead a normal life. You might perhaps think that avoiding buildings is realistic because being in a building during an earthquake is dangerous. This is true to a certain extent, but you cannot avoid all buildings forever and expect to lead a normal life. You will eventually have to enter buildings. The most you can do is to take reasonable precautions against injury during an earthquake and learn to live with the risk. Bear also in mind that there are many other hazards in the world, besides earthquakes, that can cause loss of life. For example, the chances of dying in a car accident are probably higher than dying in an earthquake. Yet we do not stop going out or using transport thinking that there might be an accident. Certain domestic chores, such as ironing or cooking may lead to fires in the house. Yet, we do not give up these activities because they involve a risk to life. Because we are not aware of these dangers in our everyday lives, we do not make an effort to avoid them. We learn to live with such risks, because otherwise it would be impossible to lead a normal life. At this point you need to decide whether you want to fight your fears and take control over your life or surrender to your fear and live your life in misery and helplessness. This is entirely your choice and you will need to take the responsibility for it. Which one will it be?

If the person does not agree with this explanation, avoid going into lengthy discussions. Tell them that treatment does not involve realistically dangerous situations, such as entering a building known to be structurally severely damaged. If this does not help, simply remind the survivor that whether or not they want to get better is entirely up to them.

Once the person agrees to treatment, you will need to explain how treatment works.

When you come across situations that make you distressed or anxious, you feel an urge to get away from them and you often surrender to this urge. When you get away, your anxiety diminishes and you feel relieved. This is obviously not an effective strategy, given that it has not helped you with your fear and stress problems. Instead, try confronting your anxiety by not avoiding distressing situations every time you come across one. This will give you an opportunity to learn how to tolerate and control anxiety. Once you manage to do this, your confidence in yourself will grow and you will find it easier to tackle other anxiety-evoking situations. As your resilience against anxiety increases, you will feel less helpless and this will lead to an improvement in your stress problems. To use an analogy, building up your resilience by allowing yourself to experience anxiety is like getting vaccinated against a virus.

You need a small dose of the virus in your system so that your body can build up its defense against the virus. This is also like practicing weight-lifting. The more you do it, the stronger you get and the more weight you can lift.

Note that this account emphasizes *tolerance* and *control* of fear or distress, rather than reducing these emotions. You may tell the person that their anxiety is most likely to reduce if they continue to stay in the situation but do not emphasize this as *the* treatment goal. Remember that distress or fear, although an unpleasant emotion, provides an opportunity to build up one's capacity to tolerate and control it. Therefore, even if it does not diminish much while in the situation, the important thing is that the person has been able to confront and control it without having to run away from the situation. This is what resilience is about.

Step 2: Giving anti-avoidance instructions

Once the person is ready for treatment, the next step is to tell the person what to do to overcome fear and distress. Below is a list of some instructions you may consider giving to the person, depending on which activities the person avoids (see avoidance behaviors marked as present in the *Fear and Avoidance Questionnaire*).

⇒ Take a bath as usual, making sure that you do not cut short your time in the bathroom for fear of earthquakes. If you have stopped taking a bath when you are alone at home, make an effort to do it.
⇒ At night get undressed before going to bed, turn the light off, close the bedroom door, and do not keep the TV or radio on until you sleep.
⇒ Do not avoid sleeping in the dark or when you are alone at home.
⇒ Do not keep someone in the family awake at night in case an earthquake happens.
⇒ If you are afraid of sleeping alone in the house, make a point of sleeping alone whenever you need to.
⇒ If you have stopped sleeping in the room where you experienced the earthquake, make a point of sleeping in that room.
⇒ Do not seek the company of someone in the house because it makes you feel safer. Make sure you can stay in the house all by yourself. Do not go out of your way to visit friends, relatives, or neighbors when you are in fear. Take every opportunity to overcome your fear of being alone in the house.

⇒ *Stop trying to avoid earthquakes by watching out for signs of an impending earthquake. For example, do not repeatedly check the ceiling lights or keep a glass of water on the table to detect signs of any movement. Do not keep listening to sounds of dogs or birds or keep watching the sky or the sea for any signs of an impending earthquake. Do not keep checking with your friends to see if they have heard any rumors about an earthquake in the near future.*

⇒ *If you have developed fear of various other situations that you did not have before the earthquake, make a point of not avoiding them. For example, confront and overcome any fear of confined spaces, heights, lifts, going out alone, swimming, or travelling in public transport.*

⇒ *Do not avoid sights of devastation or destroyed buildings simply because you feel distressed. If you need to pass by such locations in your everyday life, make sure that you do not take a different route. Look closely at these sights, examine them, and do not try to avoid any memories of the earthquake that may come to your mind. If necessary, make a point of going to these locations and stay there until you have complete control over your distress.*

⇒ *Do not avoid talking about things you experienced during the earthquake with friends, acquaintances, or others.*

⇒ *Take every opportunity to participate in conversations or discussions about earthquakes.*

⇒ *Do not avoid earthquake-related news in the media. Listen to such news on TV or radio or read them in the newspapers.*

⇒ *Do not avoid any other reminders of the earthquake. Make a point of looking at pictures of acquaintances that died in the earthquake, seeing particular people or visiting particular locations in the region that bring back your memories, and attending community meetings, ceremonies for the dead, anniversaries of the disaster and so on.*

⇒ *Whenever something reminds you of your earthquake experiences, do not try to avoid memories, thoughts, or images about your experiences by pushing them away from your mind. Do not try to divert your attention from these thoughts or prevent them from entering your mind by occupying yourself with other activities, such as keeping the radio on, reading something, or doing housework. Instead, focus your attention on these thoughts and go through the earthquake events as they happened over and over again until you no*

longer feel the need to avoid them in your mind. You will see that when you do not try to avoid such thoughts, they will come to your mind less frequently.

The *Fear and Avoidance Questionnaire* can be useful in guiding the survivor in treatment. So give the person a copy of their own ratings. Ask them to identify fears that they consider as causing most problems in daily life. Generally, avoidances that impair work, family, and social functioning are deemed as most troublesome by most people. You may advise the person to give priority to these avoidances in treatment.

Step 3: Giving homework exercises

Some survivors may have difficulty with certain situations or activities they find most distressing or frightening. They will usually tell you what these situations or activities are. Most people find situations where they experienced the trauma as the most distressing. Staying alone at home, for example, might pose the greatest difficulty in people who experienced the earthquake at home. Others who witnessed their close ones dying under rubble may have difficulty going to the location where this happened. Entering buildings poses difficulty for many people, particularly in the early weeks or months of the disaster. In such cases it would be useful to give specific homework exercises to overcome distress or fear associated with a difficult task and describe in detail how to manage this task. Successful completion of such a difficult task increases the person's self-confidence and makes subsequent tasks easier to tackle.

To illustrate how you can do this, let us take the example of a person who has been living in a shelter for fear of earthquakes and who wants to overcome their fear of buildings so that they can go back home. Let us assume that the person thinks they would be unable to do this because they tried it before and failed. In such cases, ask the person to break the task into easier steps and tackle it one at a time. For example:

STEP 1: *Go near the building and stand near the door.*
STEP 2: *Go into the building, have a look around and then leave.*
STEP 3: *Go into your home, have a cup of coffee and then leave.*
STEP 4: *Go back home, tidy up the place and then leave.*
STEP 5: *Spend the whole day at home and leave in the evening.*

STEP 6: *Spend the day and the evening at home and leave late at night.*
STEP 7: *Start spending the nights at home.*

You will need to negotiate each step with the survivor and reach an agreement. They can make each step as easy or difficult as they like. **Never prescribe tasks against the person's will**. It is very important that the person agrees with what you suggest. Once you reach an agreement on the course of action, explain how to conduct the exercise.

> As you begin your exercise, you may experience anxiety symptoms, such as sweating, shaking, rapid heartbeat, dizziness, or feeling faint. These symptoms are unpleasant but essentially harmless. You may feel a strong urge to leave the building. Try to control this urge by not giving in to it. Tell yourself "I am going to beat this fear once and for all." Do not be afraid of feeling anxious. Remember the vaccination example. You need such anxiety to build up your endurance against it. Always remember: This is a battle with fear. Either you will conquer your fear or it will conquer you.
>
> As you begin to tolerate anxiety better and better, you will notice an increase in your self-confidence. When this happens, challenge your fear by inviting it. This means doing things to increase your fear. For example, you may be standing near the door and therefore not feeling too anxious. You know that if you go further inside, you will be more anxious, thinking that it will not be easy to get out in case of an earthquake. Muster your courage and go into your home. If you know that going into the room where you experienced the earthquake will make you more anxious, go into that room to challenge your anxiety. If cracks in the wall plaster make you more anxious, go around looking for cracks and examining them. At every step of the way, ask yourself "What can I do now to invite my fear?" For example, if going up to the upper floors of the building makes you more anxious, do it. If thinking about your experiences during the earthquake makes you more anxious, think about them. Tell yourself "An earthquake might happen right now." Sometimes heavy vehicles passing by cause vibrations in buildings. If such vibrations scare you, go to a location where you can feel them better. These are just some examples of how you can challenge fear and you may be able to find many other ways of doing it. Once you have learned how to do this, you can consider the battle won. This is an early sign that shows you will be successful in this treatment.
>
> End the exercise only when you feel that you can leave the building at your own will and not because of your fear. This will mean that you have achieved total control over your fear and are no longer helpless against it. You can congratulate yourself for this achievement! You will be feeling great about yourself. The next time you go back, you are likely to be less anxious than you were the first time. This is because you have greater control over your anxiety. Each further step will seem easier to you as you make progress with your exercises.
>
> If your anxiety gets too intense, stay where you are and find somewhere to sit. Focus your mind on symptoms of anxiety. Tell yourself "I will not give in to this fear. I will not let it take control over me." Do NOT try to divert your attention elsewhere. Do not, for example, start reading something, talking to someone, or examining something. Otherwise, you would be defeating the purpose of the exercise. If at some point you give in to your fear and leave the building, do not worry. This does not mean failure yet. Have a short break and wait outside. Try to muster more courage and go back inside. If you fail again, you can always give it another try some other day. Keep trying and you will eventually succeed. Once you successfully complete the step, move on to the next step and then to the next one until you complete the whole exercise.

Once the person achieves this task and resettles at home, they may find it easier to deal with their fear of other buildings. A single exercise might be sufficient in some cases in helping them resume their normal life activities. Others, however, may need additional exercises with other buildings, such as homes of friends or relatives, schools, shopping places, banks, hospitals, government offices, cinemas, and so on. Note that it is important to ask the person not to distract their attention by occupying themselves with another activity. This is another form of avoidance, which may lead to failure in treatment.

When you are helping someone bear in mind the following points.

WARNING

- In the early days of the disaster do not encourage the person to enter buildings before the authorities have notified the public that it is safe to do so.
- Do not ask the person to enter buildings known to be damaged and uninhabitable.

Closing the session

In closing the session it is often useful to emphasize that treatment success depends entirely on the person's determination and efforts to get better.

Now that we have agreed on what you need to do, you need to understand clearly that success or failure in treatment depends entirely on you. You will have to take the responsibility for the outcome. If you make an effort to overcome your problems, your chances of recovery are very high. Almost all people who fail in treatment do so because they do not carry out their homework exercises. You may experience some setbacks along the way but you need not worry about them as long as you keep making an effort. I will guide you through this process and may even help you with some exercises you find too difficult. I will expect progress each time I see you. You also need to bear in mind that you do not have unlimited time in treatment. Most people begin to recover with this treatment within the first few weeks. This means I will be able to gage your chances of recovery quite early in treatment. If you are not making sufficient progress, this will most likely mean you are not making an effort, in which case there may not be any point in going on with treatment.

Involving close ones in treatment

Always consider involving a person's close ones in treatment. Inform them about the treatment and ask them to provide support and encouragement for the person throughout treatment. You can also ask them to monitor the person's progress with homework exercises, as this may make success in treatment more likely. In addition, ask the person to share each success with homework exercises with close ones, because this often motivates the person for further success. Furthermore, encourage the person to help other family members who may be suffering from similar traumatic stress problems by using what they learned during treatment (or by simply encouraging their close ones to utilize the self-help manual). This would benefit not only the family but would also help the person develop sense of control over their own problems.

Section 4: Monitoring progress

Monitoring progress means finding out whether the person you are helping has complied with your anti-avoidance instructions, conducted their homework exercises, and shown any improvement in their problems. It also involves helping them overcome any difficulty they might have in conducting their exercises. When the first treatment session is delivered properly, 80% of the earthquake survivors carry out their exercises without running into much difficulty. Others may need further help.

Session 2

Evaluating improvement in traumatic stress problems

Administer the *Traumatic Stress Symptom Checklist* and the *Fear and Avoidance Questionnaire* to assess improvement in the person's condition. Make sure no items are skipped, as otherwise the total scores may not reflect progress in a reliable fashion. Every time you administer them write down the total scores in the Progress Table below, so that you can see at a glance how the treatment is progressing.

they would most likely rate this activity as involving *'little difficulty'* or *'no difficulty.'* These ratings indicate **successful completion** of the exercise relating to that activity. With successful treatment, you will see at least 60% reduction in total score at some point. This means substantial reduction in the person's fears and avoidance behaviors.

A drop in the *Traumatic Stress Score* will give you an idea about the extent of improvement in traumatic stress and depressive symptoms. About 60% reduction in the total score means **substantial improvement** in traumatic stress, while 80% or more reduction means almost **complete recovery.**

Normally, 90% of the people are able to overcome their fear or distress in most situations in 4 weeks. A few people may, however, need as long as 10 weeks to get better. The first signs of improvement may appear any time between 1 and 4 weeks after start of treatment, usually after 2 weeks. The questionnaire scores 2–3 weeks after start of treatment will tell you whether the person is likely to get good results with this treatment. At that point, you should expect at least 40% reduction in the questionnaire scores. Less than 40% improvement may mean that treatment is not progressing as it should.

Progress Table

Questionnaires	Treatment weeks										
	0	1	2	3	4	5	6	7	8	9	10
Traumatic Stress Symptom Checklist											
Fear and Avoidance Questionnaire											

Note that **Week 0** refers to the very first assessment you conducted **before** starting the treatment. Each week compare the scores with previous ones to see how much progress is made. This would be easier if you calculate percentage of change in total scores. To do this, subtract a particular week's score from Week 0 score, divide the difference by the Week 0 score, and multiply the result by 100. For example, if the Traumatic Stress Score is 40 at Week 0 and 20 at week 3, this means 50% improvement in traumatic stress problems ($40 - 20 = 20 / 40 = 0.50 \times 100 = 50\%$).

The *Fear and Avoidance Questionnaire* will help you assess the person's success in overcoming distress or fears. If they have overcome their anxiety associated with a particular activity listed in this questionnaire,

You can also assess progress on the basis of the person's reports of various changes in their condition. They may feel more confident in themselves and less afraid of earthquakes. They may be less preoccupied with past trauma events and less distressed when they are reminded of them. They may also report improvement in other stress problems. They may, for example, sleep better, feel less irritable, and concentrate better on their work. Such changes are also likely to be noticed by their family and friends.

Once you have completed the assessment, share the results with the person. Seeing a drop in their scores may strengthen their resolve to make more progress. Bear in mind that it may take a few weeks before one sees a substantial reduction in scores. Thus, if the scores show no decline at this point, this does not necessarily mean lack of progress.

Evaluating progress with homework exercises

Next, ask the person whether they made any progress with their homework exercises. Find out what exactly they did to confront their fear or distress, how it went, and how they felt afterwards. How do they feel now about the progress they made? Did it have any positive impact on their daily functioning? Do they feel more confident in dealing with their fear or distress? Note that the most important sign of improvement in the first few weeks of treatment is increased self-confidence in confronting fear or distress and reduced avoidance of various situations. In such cases you can expect marked reduction in traumatic stress problems in subsequent weeks. Congratulate the person for any progress made and provide **strong praise** for each achievement. Encourage the person to celebrate such progress with close ones.

Dealing with problems that impede progress in treatment

If the person is reporting no progress, they are most likely to have encountered problems in conducting homework exercises. Let us see the most common reasons for this and how you can overcome them.

Confronted avoided situations, but felt too distressed and gave up

Find out if this is because the person did not plan homework exercises in a graduated fashion. This is the most common cause of failure in treatment. If so, work out a graduated exercise plan together with the person, breaking the task into easier steps, as described earlier. Provide strong support and encouragement (for example, "*I have total confidence in your ability to do this. Just give it a try and see for yourself.*") Note that the person does not have to complete the whole task in 1 week. If necessary, a single task may be executed step by step over the course of several weeks. You may also consider getting a close friend or a family member to accompany the person during a difficult exercise.

If the person has made several attempts and decided that they are unable to cope with distress even in a gradual and step by step fashion, you can recommend some mental exercises to help build up their tolerance of distress before they actually attempt a particular task. Below is a description of these exercises.

Set aside some time to go through in your mind all distressing events you experienced during the earthquake. Try to picture in your mind the events one by one as they happened, without omitting any detail, no matter how distressed you might get. When you are finished, start all over again. Repeat this exercise until you can easily tolerate the distress. With sufficient practice, you will notice an increase in your tolerance of distress and a decrease in the frequency of such thoughts. When you no longer feel the need to avoid these thoughts in your mind, this means you have succeeded in overcoming them.

If you do not find this strategy helpful enough, you may consider another. Write down your trauma experiences in detail as they happened from beginning to end without omitting any detail, as if you are writing your trauma story in a letter to a close friend. Read this letter over and over again, while also focusing on the events in your mind. Do this exercise over and over again until you see that you can easily tolerate the distress. You can also do this exercise in a different way, such as relating your trauma story to a close one over and over again. You can even audio-tape your story and listen to it repeatedly afterwards, if you have the means to do so.

Once you have done this, you may find it easier to tackle the distressing situations that you initially had difficulty confronting. It is important, however, that you test and strengthen further the beneficial effects of this exercise in real life situations that bring back trauma memories. Let us suppose, for example, that you have difficulty going to locations where there are destroyed buildings. Go to one such location to see how you feel. You may even choose the location where you actually experienced the traumatic events. You may find that you are better able to tolerate distress in that situation. Spend some time there and try to challenge your distress by going through your trauma story in your mind in the same way as you have done before until you have complete control over your distress. This exercise will prove to you that you can tolerate distress even when you are in situations that bring back most distressing memories of your trauma.

Confronted feared / distressing situations but felt no distress or fear

The person may not have properly challenged their fear or distress while they were in the situation. They may have done things to reduce their anxiety. For example, they may have made an attempt to enter a building but stayed close to the door, thinking that they can easily escape in case of an earthquake. Or, if their task involved taking a bath while alone at home, they may have had a close one waiting outside the bathroom door while taking a bath. Ask the person if they have done anything to make sure that they were 'safe' while in the feared situation. If they have, this might explain why they did not experience fear. In this case, ask them to repeat the exercise without resorting to such 'safety' measures. If they have avoided anxiety during the exercise by distracting their attention to something else, ask them to repeat the exercise without avoiding anxiety.

Paused or quit treatment after an aftershock happened

Survivors often experience an increase in their fear after an aftershock and find it more difficult not to avoid feared situations. This may also happen after hearing news of a major earthquake somewhere else in the country or even in another country. Tell the person that aftershocks are common after major earthquakes and other major earthquakes can happen any time in earthquake-prone countries. Remind the person of the reasons why they started this treatment in the first place. Ask them to take the increase in their fears as a good opportunity to challenge them. Tell them that stopping treatment at this point means accepting **defeat**.

Fears worsened after rumors about an impending earthquake

After a major earthquake rumors about further earthquakes expected to occur on a particular date are fairly common. People tend to believe such rumors because this makes them feel safe until the date of the expected earthquake. Remind the person that they heard such rumors many times before and none came true. Experts tell us that it is impossible to predict the exact date of an earthquake. Remind the person that, whenever they hear such rumors and notice an increase in your fear, they should consider this an opportunity to challenge it.

Closing the session

To summarize, the second session involves assessment of progress and finding solutions to problems encountered. In closing the session, discuss with the person their exercise plans for the next week and provide strong support and encouragement. If the person has failed in some tasks, tell them that there will always be setbacks in treatment and that they will eventually succeed, provided they keep making an effort.

Session 3

The third session involves much of the same procedures as the second one. Assess the person's problems using the questionnaires and check progress with homework exercises. Two weeks into treatment, you can expect some signs of improvement in traumatic stress problems in 90% of the cases. At this point you can make an assessment to see if the person can continue treatment without your help. This is most likely if the following are true:

- The person has not had much difficulty carrying out homework exercises or was able to overcome any difficulties encountered.
- There is at least 40% reduction in questionnaire scores. The person reports general improvement in traumatic stress problems (for example, less preoccupied with past trauma events, feels less distressed when reminded of them, feels less fearful about future earthquakes, sleeps better, less irritable, etc.).
- Changes in the person's problems are noticed by family and friends.
- The person feels confident about future homework exercises.

If these conditions are met, you can consider advising the person to continue with their exercises on their own and come back only if they experience problems. The latter is unlikely in most cases. You may also consider seeing them once more in 3 months simply to make sure that all went well for them.

Let us now see what you need to do with 1 out of 10 survivors, who will not meet these conditions. Such people are most likely to have failed with their homework exercises because of too much distress or fear. At this point you may consider conducting a session together with the person to guide them throughout the whole process. In planning for this session, find out which exercise, if completed successfully, is likely to have most impact on their self-confidence in overcoming fear or distress. For some people this might be feared situations, such as buildings. In others, it might be situations that bring back distressing memories of the trauma, such as the location where the most distressing event occurred. Let us assume that this exercise concerns visiting some relatives who live on the top floor of a five-floor building. Below is a description of how you can conduct the session. Note that the principles of treatment are the same, whether the exercise involves situations that evoke fear or distress associated with trauma memories.

The person's anxiety is likely to be most intense when you arrive at the location where you will conduct the session. Therefore, provide ample encouragement and praise for the person's courage and determination to confront their fear. If they are too anxious and feel a strong urge to leave, tell them they are free to leave whenever they want but this would only mean **surrendering** to their problem. Remind them that by resisting this urge they will learn to tolerate and gain control over their anxiety. If the person is too anxious, you can make the task easier by dividing it into more manageable bits. For example, ask the person to go only into the ground floor of the building and stay somewhere near the door in the first instance. As they gain more self-confidence, ask them to invite their fear by going further into the building. Whenever the person's anxiety increases, make sure that they do not mentally avoid fear by distracting their attention away from the situation, think about something else, or make believe that they are not there. Ask them to **challenge** their fear by thinking that an earthquake might happen any time. When the person feels more confident at some point, ask them if they can challenge their fear by going up to the next floor on their own. Your presence there might make the person feel safer and thus reduce their anxiety. If the person is prepared to do this, continue with the session, while you wait on the ground floor. Alternatively, you can go up to the next floor together and, when the person feels more comfortable, you can leave and wait at the next floor up. Repeat this process until you reach the top floor. If, at any stage, the survivor feels too anxious to take the next step, you could say the following:

In the beginning you thought even entering the building was too difficult for you. We are now here in the building, well away from the door. If an earthquake happens, there is no way we can leave the building quickly enough. Yet, you feel more in control now. If I asked you to go out now and come back in again to the same floor, would you be able to do that? [The answer is often yes]. Well, this is exactly what I meant earlier when I said that you would be feeling more and more confident in facing your fears if you stayed in the situation. Would you have ever imagined you would be capable of doing even this much? [The answer is often no.] Well, this is how it happens. Going up to the next floor might seem too difficult to you now but when you get there you will be telling me the same thing. This is how it will go all the way to the top floor. You can quit anytime you like but would you not have liked to pay your relatives a visit and surprise them now? We could all have a cup of coffee together and celebrate your victory!

Note that two aspects of this discourse are most important. First, it draws attention to the progress made thus far; the survivor is in the building, well away from the door, already feeling confident about repeating the same task. Such awareness of being able to tolerate and control anxiety is often a turning point in the session on which the person can build up further progress. Second, the therapist reinforces motivation for further progress by linking the latter to several potential rewards (e.g. the relatives being surprised about the visit, victory over fear, and everyone celebrating the victory with a cup of coffee). Such reward often reinforces motivation to continue with the session. In most cases the chances are that you will complete the session and celebrate victory with a cup of coffee at the top floor! In the rare case that you do not, do not worry about not having completed the session. Whatever progress achieved thus far is likely to have some impact on the person. If circumstances allow it, you can of course always plan for more sessions to complete the process. Otherwise, you can simply ask the person to continue with the exercise on their own and come back only if they feel in need of your help for continuing with treatment. The session might well have provided them with sufficient impetus to continue exercises on their own.

Being in a feared situation may bring back trauma memories in some cases, particularly those who experienced events, such as collapse of their house, being trapped under rubble, or witnessing the death of close ones, etc. Flooding of such distressing memories into mind may at times be quite overwhelming, both for the person and for you. The person may burst into tears and start to relate the trauma story to you. In such situations pause the session and allow some time for the survivor to relate the story. While providing emotional support, facilitate recall of distressing memories by asking brief prompting questions about the story. In relating their story, survivors often find a unique opportunity to express a wide range of emotions experienced during and after the traumatic events, such as fear, horror, helplessness, regrets, shame, guilt, and anger. In such a situation simply listen to the person, showing sympathy, understanding, and emotional support. Ask the person to relate the story several more times, each time mentally focusing on the most distressing details and retaining the trauma images in their mind for as long as they can. You will notice that the person is better able to tolerate distress each time they tell the story. At some point the person will be surprised to see that they no longer experience the same distress, even when they deliberately try to evoke it by thinking about the most distressing aspects of their trauma. They often describe this feeling with joyous expressions like "*huge weight lifted off my chest*" or "*I feel free like a bird now.*" This is often a turning point in treatment, not only because the person has now learned how to tolerate distressing memories, but also because the effects of this session is most likely to last in the long term.

In closing the session, have a discussion with the person to see how they feel about other exercises with which they had difficulty. Ask them if they feel prepared to tackle them on their own. At this point they are most likely to say yes. Define one or two more homework exercises and specify their location and timing **in agreement with the person**. Tell them that you expect to see them next time having conducted the exercises and that you are looking forward to their success story.

Session 4

The procedures in this session are the same as in the first two sessions. Administer the questionnaires, provide feedback about signs of improvement, review last week's homework exercises, and provide verbal praise for the person's achievements in the last week. You can expect progress with most survivors after you have conducted a session with them. At this point you will have to decide whether they need further sessions with you or whether they can continue on their own. Below are some guidelines to help you with this decision.

⇒ If 'substantial recovery' (defined as at least 60% reduction in questionnaire scores) has occurred, consider terminating the sessions. Advise the person to continue exercises on their own until 'complete recovery' (at least 80% reduction in questionnaire scores) occurs.

⇒ If the person has had success with the previous week's homework exercises but is not yet confident enough to continue treatment on their own, continue with further homework exercises and weekly monitoring sessions until substantial recovery occurs.

⇒ If the person needs your help with other difficult homework exercises, consider conducting one or two more sessions with them. Note, however, that the need for such sessions arises quite rarely.

⇒ Some people may need further support, particularly if their stress problems are complicated by depression. Recovery in such cases

may take a little longer than in others. Thus, if you feel that the person needs more time because of slow but definite progress, continue with weekly sessions until substantial recovery occurs.

Note that there are no exact criteria to help you decide when to terminate treatment. The above considerations are merely intended to provide you with some guidance in this respect. Such a decision may not be easy in some cases. Whenever you are uncertain, you may consider one or two more sessions.

We have limited the description of treatment to four sessions, because 90% of earthquake survivors recover after four sessions delivered in 4 to 6 weeks. How much time you can spend on one person will also depend on the post-disaster circumstances. If you are aiming to help as many people as possible, you will need to use your time rather sparingly and minimize the time you spend with each person. In other circumstances you may consider delivering as many sessions as required to achieve substantial improvement in the person.

Dealing with less common problems in treatment

In the previous section we reviewed some of the common problems that you may encounter in treatment and how you can deal with them. There are a few other problems that you may come across at some stage during treatment. These problems are rather uncommon (occurring in less than 10% of the cases), but you will need to know what to do if you encounter them.

Increase in traumatic stress symptoms

In some people confronting distressing or feared situations might lead to an increase in stress symptoms in the early phases of the treatment. For example, they may have more anxiety, sleeping difficulty, and nightmares. This is a fairly rare occurrence and, when it happens, it is no cause for concern. These symptoms subside as they continue with their exercises. Remember the vaccination example earlier in this section. This is like developing a slight fever after a vaccination. In such cases, simply reassure the person that these stress symptoms will disappear with treatment.

Worsening of depression during treatment

Depression is a common problem after earthquakes caused by disabling fear and related traumatic stress symptoms. Depressive symptoms often get better with treatment, as a person gains control over fear and other stress problems. However, they may also get worse for other reasons, such as financial difficulties, illness or loss in the family, marital problems, etc. You will notice the signs of depression in the person. They will look more anxious or distressed than usual, have a tendency to cry, express feelings of despair and hopelessness, and report worsening of other depressive symptoms (see Section 1). Any worsening in the person's depression will also be reflected in their *Traumatic Stress Score*. Check their last score to see if there is an increase. Remember that scores over 38 indicate probable depression. If the person has depression severe enough to impede treatment, their score is likely to be above 50. If there is worsening in depression, you will need answers to the following questions to make a decision on what to do in this situation:

- Is the person having thoughts of putting an end to their life and making plans to this effect, because they feel no longer able to cope with their problems?
- Are they no longer determined to go through this treatment thinking that there is no hope of getting better for them?
- Do depressive symptoms, such as loss of interest in things, feeling tired or lacking in energy, memory and concentration problems, or irritability, make it difficult for them to carry out homework exercises?

WARNING

If the answer to any of these questions is YES, then pause treatment and refer the person to a mental health specialist. They may need additional treatment for depression. Continue with treatment when the person has sufficiently recovered from depression.

In referring a depressed person to a mental healthcare specialist, it is useful to inform them about the following points.

- Although drugs (antidepressants) may be helpful in reducing depression, they are not likely to be a cure for traumatic stress problems. Such problems are most likely to come back after the person stops taking medication.
- The person should continue with the treatment in this booklet, when depressive symptoms no longer impede homework exercises. This might be possible after 6 to 8 weeks of drug treatment or perhaps even earlier.

- Antidepressants are often used for about 6 months in treating depression. There may not be a need for such long drug use, if the person can resume psychological treatment at an early stage. With successful psychological treatment, the person may be able to come off medication after 10 to 12 weeks of drug treatment. Advise the person to discuss this issue with their doctor.
- After restarting psychological treatment, the person needs to come off medication by gradually decreasing the dose under the guidance of their doctor. Make sure that the person conducts some of the homework exercises without medication so that they can see that their recovery is due to **their own efforts** and **not** to the tablets. They need to know that the limited effects of antidepressants on fear and related traumatic stress symptoms often disappear when they are discontinued.

Flashbacks during homework exercises

You learned what flashbacks are in Section 1. Although a flashback is an unpleasant experience, it is often harmless. Reassure the person that what they experience during a flashback is by no means a sign of 'going crazy' or losing their mind. Flashbacks rarely cause a problem in treatment, because they tend to disappear as a survivor makes progress in treatment. You can recommend the following actions to control this symptom when it occurs.

⇒ *Try to monitor your flashbacks and see what triggers the symptom. It could be a sight, sound, smell, word, thought, image, emotion, or anything that reminds you of your experience during the earthquake. Make a list of the situations that trigger them. When you encounter these situations, be aware that the symptom may appear.*

⇒ *When you realize that the symptom is about to appear, sit down and breathe deeply and regularly. Focus on what is happening around you. Try to watch carefully what people are doing, what they are saying. Or try to focus your attention on something. For example, look carefully at an object near you and study its shape, color and texture. Pick it up and feel what kind of emotion it produces. Focus all your attention on this object.*

⇒ *You could carry a small bottle of cologne with you. Pat some cologne on your face and hands and focus on the refreshing feeling. You could also carry a string of worry beads with you. As the symptom begins, hold the beads and start counting them in two's or three's. Focus on the prayer beads and be careful not to make a mistake when counting.*

⇒ *You may find other effective ways of focusing your attention elsewhere. These could be things like walking, telling yourself where you are, the date and time, or humming a tune.*

⇒ *Talk to your family about your situation and tell them about this symptom. If the symptom appears while you are with them, they can help 'bring you back to reality.' They could do this by touching you or telling you where you are.*

Summary of treatment procedures

Recall from Section 2 that in severe cases where a flashback causes **total loss of awareness of the surroundings**, a person might engage in harmful acts to self or others.

WARNING

After starting treatment if the person you are helping has had any flashbacks during which they lost total awareness of their surroundings or did something to endanger themselves or others around them, refer them to a mental health specialist before you continue with this treatment.

You are not likely to come across this problem if you have heeded our warning in Section 2 about referring such cases to a mental health specialist before treatment.

SESSION 1

1. Provide information on:
   (a) Traumatic stress and how it affects work, social, and family life.
   (b) How irrational fears differ from realistic fears.
   (c) Treatment aim → To overcome impact of trauma by learning to confront and tolerate fear or distress.
   (d) How treatment works → Increasing resilience against fear and distress.
2. Give anti-avoidance instructions → *"Do not avoid feared or distressing situations as you come across them in daily life."*
3. Give homework exercises in relation to particular feared or distressing situations and explain how to deal with distress or fear.
4. Emphasize importance of personal efforts in recovery.
5. Involve close ones in treatment.

SESSION 2

1. Administer questionnaires to assess improvement.
2. Review progress with homework exercises:
   (a) If progress made → Praise person's achievement.
   (b) If no progress → Identify problems and offer solutions.
3. Agree on next week's tasks and provide encouragement.

SESSION 3

1. Administer questionnaires to assess improvement.
2. Review progress with homework exercises:
   (a) If progress made → Praise person's achievement.
   (b) If sufficient improvement in traumatic stress problems observed → Discontinue monitoring sessions and advise person to continue with homework exercises and come back in 3 months for a final assessment.
   (c) If no progress → Help person conduct a difficult homework exercise to build up their self-confidence.
3. Agree on next week's tasks and provide encouragement.

SESSION 4

1. Administer questionnaires to assess improvement.
2. Review progress with homework exercises:
   (a) If progress made → Praise person's achievement.
   (b) If sufficient improvement in traumatic stress problems observed → Terminate treatment and advise person to continue with homework exercises and come back in 3 months for a final assessment.
3. If no progress → Help survivor conduct more homework exercises until substantial recovery occurs.

Section 5: Helping children

You can deliver the treatment to children individually or in groups. Group settings are particularly useful in delivering treatment to children of age 8 to 16. It is best to work with groups of about 10 children, although circumstances might require treatment delivery to larger groups (e.g. in schools) in the early aftermath of a disaster.

Traumatic Stress Symptom Checklist – Child Version

Below are some questions about the problems some people have after earthquakes. Answer these questions by putting X under the appropriate column.

	No	A little	Fairly	Very much
1. Do you keep thinking about what happened during the earthquake even when you do not want to?				
2. Do you suddenly feel like the same events are happening all over again and feel scared?				
3. Do you try to keep away from situations that remind you of the earthquake?				
4. Do you have frightening dreams?				
5. Have you lost interest in doing things you used to like?				
6. Do you have difficulty sleeping?				
7. Do you feel like other people do not understand what you have been through during the earthquake?				
8. Do you have difficulty remembering any events that happened during the earthquake?				
9. Do you find yourself unable to feel emotions like joy or sadness as you used to?				
10. Do you feel you will not live as long as you used to think?				
11. Do you get startled by sudden noises or movements?				
12. Do you feel on edge thinking there might be an earthquake anytime?				
13. Do you feel bad when something reminds you of the earthquake?				
14. Do you find yourself trying not to think about the earthquake?				
15. Do you have difficulty remembering things or concentrating on something?				
16. Do you have racing of the heart, sweating, trembling, dizziness, headaches, or stomach aches when something reminds you of the earthquake?				
17. Are you more snappy than usual?				
18. Are you afraid of doing certain things for fear of earthquakes (like going into safe buildings, taking a shower, staying at home alone, or sleeping in the dark)?				
19. Have you been feeling sad and tearful lately?				
20. Do you find yourself feeling guilty about something at times?				
21. Do you ever find yourself wishing you were dead?				
22. Do you have less appetite than usual?				
23. Do you get more easily tired than usual?				
24. Do you feel restless or fidgety?				
TOTAL SCORE				

Now work out the total score. Give 0 points for each X in the 'No' column, 1 point for each X in the 'A little' column, 2 for each X in the 'Fairly' column, and 3 for each X in the 'Very much' column. Add up the scores to obtain a total **Traumatic Stress Score** and write it underneath the questionnaire next to Total Score. Higher scores indicate more severe traumatic stress problems. Next, administer the *Fear and Avoidance Questionnaire* (see Section 2) to have an idea about the severity of the child's fear problems. You will use these questionnaires to assess progress each week.

Session 1

Start the session introducing the purpose of the meeting. Referring to the problems they marked on the questionnaires, get the children to talk about their fear problems for a while until they all understand that everyone has similar problems. Then, explain the treatment and tap their response to the idea of confronting feared situations (for example, sleeping alone or in the dark). Some children may readily agree with the treatment idea and display expressions of courage in challenging their fear. Encourage such children to express themselves fully, so that they serve as a model for others. Some of them might have overcome various fears (or phobias) in the past by challenging them; give such children a chance to tell their story. Praise their courageous behavior. Once they agree to do things to overcome their fear, ask them to write down what they want to do as homework exercises (for example, "*I will sleep alone at night; I will sleep with lights off; I will go to school and attend my classes; I will visit my friends in their home;*" etc.). Refrain from setting tasks against their will. In group settings children tend to compete with each other for approval and praise from the group leader. Use such tendency to boost their motivation for overcoming fear. For example, you may end the session with a comment such as "*let's see who will beat their fear first.*"

Subsequent monitoring sessions

In each subsequent weekly session, first administer the questionnaires, work out total scores, and write them down in the appropriate column in the Progress Table below. Next, ask the children whether they did their homework exercises. Find out what exactly they did, how it went, how they felt afterwards. How do they feel now about the progress they made? Do they feel more confident in dealing with their fear or distress? Provide ample praise for those who made progress in overcoming their fear. Encourage them to work on other homework exercises.

In children who show no progress, the most likely reason is failure to conduct homework exercises because of too much fear. In such cases give easier exercises or break homework exercises into easier steps. Also, inform the family about the treatment aims and ask close ones to provide strong support and encouragement for the child in conducting homework exercises. If necessary and feasible, you may also consider helping the child with one or two homework exercises in much the same way as described for adults in Section 4.

Conduct further weekly sessions until substantial improvement is achieved. As in adults, at least 60% reduction in the questionnaire scores is a sign of substantial improvement. Recovery after a few more sessions is as likely as in adults. In some cases where other family members have similar fear-related traumatic stress problems, consider treating the whole family together with the child. This is important, because it is difficult to help a child when their parents or siblings are suffering from fear and other related traumatic stress problems.

Progress Table

Questionnaires	Treatment weeks										
	0	1	2	3	4	5	6	7	8	9	10
Traumatic Stress Symptom Checklist											
Fear and Avoidance Questionnaire											

Section 6: Delivering treatment in a single session

After major disasters there may be situations where the person you want to help may not be able to attend weekly sessions for various reasons. Or you may not have the time to see the person more than once. In such situations you can consider delivering the treatment in one session. Research has shown that 80% of earthquake survivors benefit from what they learn in a single session. If you are working in a survivor shelter or camp where there are hundreds of people in need of urgent help, you may not have the time to help each person individually. In such situations, you can deliver the treatment session in groups.

Delivering treatment to individuals in a single session

When you want to deliver the treatment in one session, follow the steps below:

⇒ First, assess the person's condition, as described in Section 2.
⇒ Tell the person that you will be seeing them once to teach them how to overcome their fear and distress.
⇒ Deliver the first treatment session, as described in Section 3.
⇒ Provide a copy of the self-help manual and advise the person to read it and follow the instructions. (With illiterate survivors, you may consider giving it to a literate member of the family or a close friend to guide the person through the manual.)

This is all you need to do. If feasible, you may also consider helping the person with one homework exercise (as described in Section 4) to boost their self-confidence. Whenever possible, consider delivering the session to the whole family, as other family members may also be suffering from traumatic stress. You could do this during a home visit lasting about 2 hours.

Delivering treatment in groups

You can deliver treatment to groups of 20–30 survivors in about 1 to 2 hours. The treatment steps are the same as in individual treatment. First, distribute the *Traumatic Stress Symptom Checklist* and *Fear and Avoidance Questionnaire* and obtain the survivors' ratings before the session. Identify a few survivors with high scores on the questionnaires, as you will use their case to illustrate various points during the session.

Opening the session

In the first few minutes make a brief introduction regarding the purpose of the meeting.

> *Now that you have finished filling in the questionnaires we can begin the session. We are all here to discuss the problems we have been experiencing since the earthquake and how to go about dealing with them. First, let me give you some idea about the problems people in this group have been experiencing. Let us see what kind of problems have been marked in the questionnaire. I have here, for example, the ratings of Ms. X [a survivor with high scores on both questionnaires].* She is having problems with sleeping, memory, and concentration . . . *and she is unable to do many things in her daily life because of fear of earthquakes. Perhaps she could tell us more about her problems.*

Such an introduction will immediately focus the group's attention on a problem that survivors are often most keen to talk about: fear. Give Ms. X a chance to talk about her problems. She will most likely start relating her trauma story, for example, where they were during the earthquake, what they did to protect themselves, what they witnessed, etc. Allow some time for her story but do not let it go on for too long. There will be others waiting to tell their story. Always bear in mind that the purpose of the session is NOT to facilitate sharing of trauma stories. Do not allow long trauma stories and make an effort to keep the group's attention on the problems marked in the questionnaires. Allow more time for group members who provide demonstrative examples of the debilitating effects of fear. For example, if someone has had to quit work because of fear, give them a chance to talk about their problem. When someone mentions such a problem, conduct a small poll in the group to find out how many of them are experiencing similar problems. **Do not spend more than 15 minutes on this phase.** The purpose of this introduction is to define the problem for the group and draw their attention to distress or fear as the cause. This introduction will also make everyone aware that they are not alone in experiencing fear-related problems.

Explaining the treatment

A useful strategy in explaining treatment aims is to help survivors draw their own conclusions about the best way of dealing with fear, rather than didactically telling them what to do. For example:

*OK, you can now see how most people are affected by the earthquake. Most of you are distressed by memories of the earthquake and have fears of similar events happening to you in the future. Such anxiety is responsible for many of your stress problems [such as being alert all the time, sleeping problems, memory/concentration difficulty, irritability, helplessness, and depressed mood.] Because you avoid distressing/feared situations, you are unable to do many things that are important in your life. This makes you even more helpless and depressed. Fear is your worst **enemy** here, considering how it affects your life. Instead of fighting and defeating the enemy, you have so far chosen to surrender to it, letting it take control of your life. If avoiding distress/fear maintains your stress problems, what is the logical thing to do here to overcome these problems? [Most survivors say 'to overcome fears by not avoiding them']. Yes, confronting your anxiety is indeed the most effective way of dealing with your problem. You need to do this regularly until you learn to tolerate and control your anxiety. This means you will have to make an effort not to avoid situations or activities that make you anxious. You stand a good chance of recovery with this treatment.*

You will find in the group several people who have had past experience of dealing with various fears. There will be some who had a phobia (of certain animals, heights, or closed spaces, for example), who overcame the problem by confronting their fear. Others may have had a past trauma (e.g. a road traffic accident, physical assault, etc.), from which they recovered by using the same strategy. Ask the group who had such fears at some point in their lives and recovered using this method. When someone volunteers this information, allow the person to talk about their experience. If necessary, get another person to relate their story. In groups people usually relate such stories with a sense of victory and pride. They not only provide very useful real-life examples of recovery from fear for the group but also instill hope and courage in others. If anyone disagrees with this approach, you can deal with their arguments as described earlier for individual treatment in Section 3. Once you have done this, the path is clear for the next step.

Defining treatment goals and encouraging anti-avoidance

As in individual treatment, you will use the *Fear and Avoidance Questionnaire* to exemplify treatment goals. If possible, provide everyone with a copy of the questionnaire they filled in. Ask the group to mark the fears that cause most problems in their life and prioritize them in order of their importance. These will be their homework tasks. The rest of the session is much the same as in individual treatment. You will not have time to define homework exercises for each group member but do this with one or two survivors to demonstrate to the others how they should work out their homework exercises. When this is completed, ask the group if they have understood the treatment and if they have any questions.

Closing the session

In closing the session, distribute copies of the self-help manual, explain its purpose, and advise the group to read it and follow the instructions. You can end the session with the following statements:

Now that you know what to do about your problem, the choice is yours: you either do something to beat your fear or it will beat you. You need to understand clearly that success or failure in treatment depends entirely on you. If you make sufficient efforts to overcome your problems, your chances of recovery are very high. Almost all people who fail in treatment do so because they do not carry out their homework exercises. You may experience some setbacks along the way but you need not worry about them as long as you keep making an effort. I suggest you help each other with your exercises. Also, try helping your family, friends, and neighbors with what you have learned here.

In the group you are likely to come across some smart and articulate persons who understand the treatment very well, show strong motivation, and display remarkable enthusiasm and talent for helping others. You can ask such people to help others with their homework exercises.

Section 7: Helping people with prolonged grief

Grief is a natural reaction to loss, which often resolves within 6 to 12 months. In some people, however, it may persist beyond this period and last for many years. When this happens, grief is no longer considered as a natural reaction and it is termed **prolonged grief**. In this section you will see how you can help people with this condition. The person you are helping for prolonged grief might also have traumatic stress problems due to a personal experience of the disaster. Or they may have lost a close one during the earthquake but had no direct exposure to the disaster. The treatment in this section is applicable in both cases.

Assessment of grief problems

You will use two questionnaires to assess grief-related problems. The first one will help you determine the severity of grief reactions while the second one will help you identify the problem behaviors that need attention in treatment. These questionnaires are also often useful in helping the person understand the nature of their grief problems and why they may need help with them.

Assessing severity of grief symptoms

Ask the person to fill in the questionnaire as instructed. You will be using this questionnaire weekly during treatment, so either use a copy or ask the person to mark their responses on a separate sheet of paper.

Grief Assessment Scale

Below are statements that describe feelings and thoughts that some people have after the loss of a close one. Please indicate how frequently you have experienced these feelings and thoughts **IN THE LAST MONTH** by putting a cross (**X**) under the appropriate column.

	0 Never	0 Sometimes	1 Often	2 Always
I feel bitter for having lost him / her.				
I go to places that he / she used to go in the hope that I might find him / her there.				
I feel detached / estranged from others after his / her death.				
I feel that a future without him / her will always be empty and pointless.				
His / her death makes me feel like a part of me has died.				
I cry when I think about him / her.				
I cannot accept the fact that he / she is dead.				
I have lost trust in people because of his / her death.				
I feel lonely without him / her.				
I do things that remind me of him / her in day to day life (for example, keeping his / her pictures or belongings out in the open, thinking or talking about him / her, visiting his / her grave, etc.)				
I feel that life is empty or meaningless without him / her.				
I feel guilty when I enjoy myself.				
I acquired some of his / her harmful habits or behaviors (e.g. smoking or drinking).				
I yearn for him / her.				
I have physical complaints (e.g. headaches, pains, etc) that started after his / her death.				
I see him / her stand before me.				
I feel as if my feelings have died after his / her death.				
I feel I have no control over my life.				
I cannot stop thinking about him / her.				
I feel helpless without him / her.				
I have physical complaints that he / she used to have when he / she was alive.				
I cannot do things that remind me of him / her in day to day life (for example, looking at his / her pictures, visiting his / her grave, talking about him / her, etc.).				

Grief Assessment Scale (cont.)

	0 Never	0 Sometimes	1 Often	2 Always
I hear his/her voice.				
I cannot believe that he/she is dead.				
I blame myself for not having tried hard enough to save him/her.				
I feel angry with him/her because he/she left me.				
I have dreams of him/her.				
I feel envious of people who have not lost their loved ones.				
I feel angry for having lost him/her.				
I feel insecure because of his/her death.				
TOTAL SCORE				

Now work out the total score. Give 0 points for each X in the 'Never' or 'Sometimes' columns, 1 point for each X in the 'Often' column, and 2 points for each X in the 'Always' column. Add up the points to obtain a total *Grief Score* and write it underneath the questionnaire next to Total Score.

Identifying problem behaviors

People usually display two types of grieving behaviors. They may avoid particular situations or activities that bring back distressing memories of the loss. For example, they may avoid visits to the cemetery, talking about the lost one, looking at his/her pictures, or going to the location where s/he died. They may also repeatedly engage in activities to keep the memory of the lost one alive at all times. For example, they may feel like talking about the lost one all the time, make frequent visits to his/her grave, keep his/her pictures all around the house, not give away his/her clothes or other belongings, and keep his/her room exactly as it was before the event, etc. Such behaviors have a **ritualistic** quality, meaning that they are repetitive and excessive. One feels an **urge** to engage in them, which is often difficult to resist. Resisting them often causes distress. We will refer to them as '**ritualistic grief behaviors**' in this section.

Both types of grief behaviors help the person avoid loss-related distress. Such avoidance blocks the natural course of the grief process by making it difficult for the person to accept the reality of the loss. Acceptance of loss is essential for natural recovery from grief. The aim of treatment is to help the person change these behaviors so that natural recovery can take its course.

The questionnaire below will help you identify these grief behaviors. You will use this information later in defining the person's homework exercises. Ask the person to fill in the questionnaire below after reading the instructions carefully.

Behavior Checklist for Grief

After the loss of a close one some people feel the urge to do certain things to keep the memory of the lost one alive all the time. Others have difficulty with certain activities that bring back distressing memories of the lost one. Below are some statements that describe such activities. Please indicate how much they apply to you IN THE LAST WEEK by putting a cross (X) under the appropriate column. If you have lost more than one close person, you may consider each statement in relation to any of them.

	Not at all	Slightly	Fairly	Very much
I feel like seeing his/her belongings out in the open.				
I have difficulty looking at his/her pictures.				
I avoid going to the place where he/she died.				
I feel like seeing his/her pictures out in the open.				
I feel like going to the places where we used to go together.				
I have difficulty mentioning his/her name.				

Behavior Checklist for Grief (cont.)

	Not at all	Slightly	Fairly	Very much
I avoid meeting his / her friends.				
I have difficulty cooking / eating the meals that he / she used to like.				
I avoid visiting his / her grave.				
I have difficulty listening to the music he / she liked.				
I feel like talking about him / her.				
I have difficulty going to the places where we used to go together.				
I avoid talking about him / her.				
I have difficulty looking at his / her belongings.				
I feel like visiting his / her grave.				
Other:				
TOTAL SCORE				

Bear in mind that the person may have other forms of grief behaviors not covered by the questionnaire. You can obtain this information by questions such as

- "*Are there any other situations or activities that you avoid because they bring back distressing memories of your loved one?*" or
- "*Are there other things that you keep doing because they remind you of your loved one or because they keep his / her memory alive?*"

Make sure such information is added to the questionnaire under the 'Other' item. Now, work out the total score by giving 0 points for answers in the '*Not at all*' column, 1 point for answers in the '*Slightly*' column, 2 points for answers in the '*Fairly*' column, and 3 points for answers in the '*Very much*' column. Add up the points to obtain a total score and write it underneath the questionnaire next to Total Score.

How to decide whether the person needs treatment for grief

Consider the following in making this decision.

⇒ If the person's grief has continued with similar or increasing intensity beyond **12 months** and their *Grief Score* is **25 or more**, there is an 80% chance that they have prolonged grief that requires treatment. The higher the score, the greater the need for treatment.

⇒ Grief may cause intense distress and significant disruption in life activities. Consider how the

person's life has changed since their loss. Grief symptoms may have dramatically reduced the quality of their life. They may be neglecting their health, as well as home and work responsibilities. Because of the changes in their emotional state and the way they relate to other people, their relationships with their family and friends may have suffered. Because of their constant preoccupation with their loss, they may be underperforming at work. **If they feel you need help for these problems**, they can benefit from the treatment in this booklet, whatever their *Grief Score* might be.

Does normal grief need treatment?

As noted earlier, most people recover from grief and resume a relatively normal life within 6 to 12 months. If the person is still within this period, they most likely do not need any treatment. However, if they have unusually severe grief reactions and extensive avoidance behaviors and / or ritualistic grief behaviors (as would also be indicated by their high questionnaire scores) this might be a sign of their difficulty in accepting the reality of their loss. Such grief behaviors are considered normal in the very early stages of the loss and they usually become less frequent in subsequent weeks and months as the person resumes normal life activities. If they have not, this might be an early sign that recovery from grief might take longer than usual. In such cases you may consider using the treatment in this section to facilitate the natural course of grief. This might help prevent possible unresolved grief problems in the future.

Which one to treat first: traumatic stress or prolonged grief?

If the person you are helping has had a personal experience of trauma events during the earthquake or witnessed the events that led to loss of their close one, they may have traumatic stress problems in addition to prolonged grief. In such cases, consider treating both conditions at the same time. If, however, the person finds it too difficult to deal with both problems at the same time, you can take them one at a time, starting with the one that the person finds relatively easier to deal with and then turning to the other one. On the other hand, some people may have such intense grief that they may be unwilling to do anything about their other problems. In such cases consider helping them with grief first.

Treatment of prolonged grief

Treatment of grief is similar in principle to treatment of traumatic stress. The idea is to change certain behaviors that maintain grief reactions. You can achieve this by helping the person (a) not to avoid situations that bring back memories of their loss and (b) refrain from engaging in ritualistic behaviors. Let us now examine how you can do this.

Session 1

Step 1: Explaining the treatment

Explain to the person what prolonged grief is, how it affects one's life, why it needs treatment, and what treatment is about and how it works. Examine the following text carefully to see how you can best do this.

> I can see from your initial assessment results that you still have substantial grief-related problems. Most people recover from grief after 6–12 months to the extent that they can resume reasonably normal functioning. If you look carefully, you will see that this is the case with most people who lost their loved ones during the earthquake. People usually respond to sudden loss with initial shock and disbelief but then they accept the loss and go through a period of grief. They eventually recover from grief and return to a reasonably normal life. Some people, however, find it difficult to accept the reality of their loss and develop behaviors that may block natural grief process. Such behaviors are usually of two types. Some people avoid particular situations or activities that bring back distressing

> memories of the loss. For example, they may avoid visits to the cemetery, talking about the lost one, looking at his / her pictures, or going to the location where s/he died. Others may repeatedly engage in certain activities to keep the memory of the lost one alive at all times. For example, they may feel like talking about the lost one all the time, make frequent visits to his / her grave, keep his / her pictures all around the house, avoid giving away his / her clothes or other belongings, and keep his / her room exactly as it was before the event.

> This treatment will help you change these behaviors so that you can complete your grief. You can do this by not avoiding situations that bring back memories of your loss and by doing things that will help you come to terms with the reality of your loss. You may experience distress in the process but you will learn to tolerate and control it. This will help you get over your grief once and for all. Just think how this problem has taken control over your life. You will need to decide whether you want to live with this problem or do something about it. If you choose the latter option, you will need to conduct exercises to overcome your distress caused by the activities listed in this questionnaire [Behavior Checklist for Grief]. I will help you with this process. You are free to carry out your exercises at your own pace, tackling them gradually or one step at a time, if you like. Most people recover within 2 months, so you will need to complete your exercises within this time. We will then choose one final homework task to mark the end of your mourning and also of your treatment.

A potential problem in engaging the client in the idea of treatment deserves mention here. Some people regard their grief process as normal, no matter how prolonged and disabling their grief might be. They may have such intense grief (usually associated with child loss) that they may simply not care about their own problems. Such people may be reluctant to accept treatment for their grief problems. In such cases, try to negotiate a deal with the person, asking them to give the treatment a chance by conducting one or two homework exercises and then decide whether or not they want to continue with treatment. Once they do this, most people find the early impact of treatment sufficiently rewarding to continue with treatment.

Step 2: Defining homework exercises

Once the person agrees to treatment, the next step is to define and prescribe homework exercises that will facilitate the grief process. Use the *Behavior Checklist for Grief* for this purpose. As a general rule, the items marked as 'fairly' or 'very much' need attention in treatment. The homework exercises that correspond to each *Behavior Checklist for Grief* item are as follows:

⇒ Remove lost one's belongings from sight (store them away).
⇒ Look at his / her pictures.
⇒ Go to the place where he / she died.
⇒ Remove his / her pictures from sight (or stop looking at them).
⇒ Do not go to the places where you used to go together with him / her.
⇒ Do not avoid mentioning his / her name during conversations.
⇒ Meet with his / her friends.
⇒ Cook / eat the meals that he / she used to like.
⇒ Visit his / her grave.
⇒ Listen to the music that he / she liked.
⇒ Do not talk about him / her.
⇒ Go to the places where you used to go together with him / her.
⇒ Talk about him / her.
⇒ Look at his / her belongings.
⇒ Do not visit his / her grave.

Note that the idea is to encourage the person to experience and tolerate distress by getting them to reverse the behavior that serves to reduce their distress. Thus, if the person avoids talking about the lost one, for example, their exercise involves talking about the lost one. If they frequently feel an urge to talk about the lost one and feel distressed when they do not do this, then their exercise involves **not** talking about the lost one. In either case the exercise facilitates grief by affording an opportunity to confront the reality of the loss and experience grief. Make a list of homework exercises that apply to the person. Remember to include exercises that correspond to grief behaviors indicated under the 'Others' item in the *Behavior Checklist for Grief.*

Once the list of tasks is drawn up, the next step is to explain to the person how to go about executing these homework exercises. Examine carefully the following account.

*You can start working on your tasks in any order you like. If you like, you can start with the easier ones and, when you feel you can tolerate distress better, move on to more difficult ones. Look at your task list and decide which ones are the easiest and which ones are more difficult to achieve. You can also break a difficult task into **easier steps**. For example, if you are keeping your lost one's pictures or belongings out in the open so that you can see them all the time, you*

can begin your task by removing these items one by one, instead of all of them at once. Or you can remove them in a particular order, starting with the 'easier-to-remove' items first. Similarly, you can give away his / her belongings one by one, starting with the easiest items first. If you feel you cannot stop cemetery visits at once, you can reduce their frequency gradually. You may experience a certain amount of distress during your exercises. This is natural and not undesirable. Remember always that this will help you go through your grief in a natural fashion. In the process you may experience anger, blame, or guilt. Some of these exercises may make you feel like giving up on your lost one or betraying his / her memory. This is normal and most grieving people have such feelings. You will recover from them as your treatment progresses.

The aim of treatment is not to deprive you of all memory of your lost one forever. It is normal to keep some pictures of the lost one in the living room or make cemetery visits from time to time, as most people do. These tasks are simply designed to help you come to terms with your loss. When the treatment is over and you are no longer distressed by the thought of removing them from your sight, you can put back some of the pictures in your living room.

Bear in mind that there is a time frame for this treatment. It is designed for a maximum of 10 weeks, as most people are able to complete their homework exercises within this period. Plan your treatment accordingly. Consider the number of homework tasks you have. If you have 10, for example, this means you can complete all tasks in 10 weeks by working on one task each week. You can, however, work on as many tasks as you want each week and complete the treatment even earlier. This is entirely up to you.

Note that the way a person should confront distress related to their loss is essentially the same as that described for fear in Section 3. If you are using this booklet to help someone only with grief problems, it is advisable that you read Section 3 to gain a better understanding of the treatment. Treatment procedures in dealing with avoidance behaviors are essentially the same, whether avoidance is caused by fear of earthquakes or distress associated with a loss. Once the person fully understands the treatment aims and agrees with the homework tasks, you can close the session by clarifying the homework tasks for the following week. Make sure that you set these tasks **in agreement with the person**. Also, do not forget to make a task easier by breaking it into more manageable steps, if the person is not prepared to do it all at once.

Prescribing additional homework tasks for traumatic stress

If the person you are helping has traumatic stress problems caused by the earthquake and is willing to tackle both problems at the same time, prescribe additional homework exercises, as described in Section 3. Some of these exercises may relate to both earthquake trauma and the loss of a loved one. For example, for people who were trapped under the rubble of their house and who witnessed the death of a close one, a visit to the site where the event occurred would provide an opportunity to overcome distress caused by both trauma memories and the loss of a close one. Such an exercise would be helpful in overcoming both problems.

Involving close ones in treatment

It is often helpful to get family members or close friends involved in treatment so that they understand the treatment aims and help the person through the process. When not fully informed about the treatment procedures, family members may not provide the support that the person needs in conducting their homework exercises and may even object to certain tasks, such as removing the belongings of the deceased from sight or giving them away, for example. Furthermore, bear in mind that other family members may have prolonged grief problems too, in which case treatment would need to be directed at the whole family.

Monitoring progress

You will need to monitor progress weekly to ensure that the person conducts homework exercises as required. As monitoring sessions involve more or less the same procedures, we will describe a typical session here.

Evaluating progress in treatment

Administer the *Behavior Checklist for Grief* every week and *Grief Assessment Scale* every 4 weeks in treatment.

Every time you do this, write down the total scores in the Progress Table below, so that you can see the changes at a glance. Make sure that the person does not skip any items. Otherwise, the total scores will not reflect progress in a reliable fashion. You need to administer these questionnaires once **before** you start treatment so that you can see how the person's problems change during treatment. This is called Week 0 assessment (column labelled 0 in the Progress Table). Each week compare the scores with the previous ones to see how much progress is made. It would help in your assessment if you calculate percentage improvement in scores. To do this, subtract the last week's score from Week 0 score, divide the difference by the Week 0 score, and multiply the result by 100. For example, if the *Grief Assessment Scale* score at Week 0 is 40 and week 4 score is 20, this means there is 50% improvement in grief symptoms ($40 - 20 = 20 / 40 = 0.50 \times 100 = 50\%$).

Both questionnaires measure the severity of grief problems. You can use the *Behavior Checklist for Grief* in assessing progress in homework exercises. Recall that the person's homework tasks were based on the items rated as '*fairly*' or '*very much.*' After start of treatment a rating of '*not at all*' or '*slightly*' on any item means that the person has successfully completed the task relating to that behavior. A reduction of 60% or more in the total scores of these two questionnaires indicates **substantial improvement** in grief problems. A reduction of 80% or more reflects **almost complete recovery**.

Evaluating progress with homework exercises

Next, ask the person whether they conducted the previous week's homework exercises. Find out exactly what they did, how it went, and how they felt afterwards. How do they feel about the progress they made? Did it have any positive impact on their daily functioning? Congratulate the person for any progress made and provide strong praise for each achievement.

Progress Table

Questionnaires	Treatment weeks										
	0	1	2	3	4	5	6	7	8	9	10
Grief Assessment Scale											
Behavior Checklist for Grief											

In closing the session, discuss with the person their homework exercises for the next week and provide strong support and encouragement.

Dealing with problems that impede progress

If the person has attempted a particular exercise and failed, this is most likely because they found it too distressing. There are several ways to help a person who has failed to conduct certain homework exercises. You can make their tasks easier, provide additional exercises to make them easier, or provide direct assistance with their tasks. These are reviewed below.

Making homework tasks easier

The most common cause of failure with a homework task is not planning it in a gradual or step by step fashion. If this is the case with the person you are helping, together work out a gradual exercise plan, breaking the task into more manageable steps, as described earlier. Provide strong support and encouragement (for example, "*I have total confidence in your ability to do this. Just give it a try and see for yourself.*") Note that the person does not have to complete the whole task in 1 week. If necessary, a single task may be executed step by step over the course of several weeks. You may also consider getting a close friend or a family member to help the person with the exercises.

Giving additional homework exercises to overcome distress

Some people may have witnessed the painful death of close ones during the earthquake. Certain homework exercises (for example, cemetery visits or going to the site where the close one died) may thus be too distressing because they evoke memories of these events. If the person has attempted such an exercise and decided that they cannot do it even in a gradual fashion, you can recommend some mental exercises to help build up their tolerance of distress before they actually attempt a particular task.

Set aside some time to go through in your mind all distressing events you experienced during the earthquake. Try to picture in your mind the events one by one as they happened, without omitting any detail, no matter how distressed you might get. When you are finished, start all over again. Repeat this exercise as many times as necessary until you feel you can easily tolerate the distress evoked by these memories. With sufficient practice, you will notice an increase in your tolerance of distress and a decrease in the frequency of such thoughts. *You will also see that you are no longer able to evoke intensely distressing thoughts in your mind, no matter how hard you try.*

If you do not find this strategy helpful enough, you may consider another. Write down your trauma experiences in detail as they happened from beginning to end without omitting any detail, as if you are writing your trauma story in a letter to a close friend. Read this letter over and over again, while also focusing on the events in your mind. Do this exercise over and over again until you see that you can easily tolerate the distress. You can also do this exercise in a different way, such as relating your trauma story to a close one over and over again. You can even audiotape your story and listen to it repeatedly afterwards, if you have the means to do so.

Once you have done this, you may find it easier to tackle the situations that bring back these memories. Try making a cemetery visit or going to the site where you experienced the trauma events and see how you feel. You may find that you are better able to tolerate distress in that situation. Spend some time there and try to challenge your distress by going through your trauma story in your mind in the same way as you have done before until you have complete control over your distress. This exercise will prove to you that you can tolerate distress even when faced with most distressing reminders of your trauma.

Providing direct assistance with homework exercises

If the person is unable to conduct the above exercises for some reason, you may consider helping them with these exercises. Simply get them to relate their trauma story to you over and over again until they can easily tolerate the distress. If you have the means, audiotape the session and ask the person to listen to it over and over again at home. This process will help the person overcome the distress caused by trauma memories.

You may also consider conducting this exercise at the location where the person's close one died. This is often a difficult task for most people, particularly if they witnessed the death of their loved one. During the session the person may break into tears and start talking about the trauma experience. This may be an emotionally taxing experience for both the person and yourself, so be prepared for it. Try to maintain a certain emotional distance from the person's trauma story, so that you can keep the session under control. Encourage the person to relive the experience by getting them to talk about the lost one and the events that led to his / her death. Get them to focus on the most distressing images and try to keep them in their mind as long as they can. Ask them to relate the story over and over again until they can do this without much distress. This process often leads to a sense of relief in the person, which they often express as '*great burden lifted off my chest.*' As a final test, ask the person to recall the most distressing aspect of their trauma experience. If they cannot evoke the same degree of distress they had in the beginning, this means the session has been successful.

Making home visits to assist with homework exercises

After loss of a close one, some people may keep the deceased person's room exactly as it was before the event, as if she / he was still living there. The lost one's pictures may be spread around, clothes still hanging in the same wardrobe, and other personal belongings in the same place as they were before the event. Some people may have difficulty removing them from sight, even in a gradual fashion. In such cases you may consider making a home visit to help the person store away some of the personal belongings or pictures of the deceased or give away some of his / her clothes. A home visit may also help you understand better the relative significance of such items for the person and devise a program by which they can 'let go' of these items in a more gradual and effective fashion.

Resuming normal life activities

As the person begins to make progress with their tasks, they will notice an increased sense of well being within the first few weeks of treatment. At this point encourage them to make an effort to resume their normal life activities. For example, ask them to take better care of themselves and their appearance, attend social gatherings, meet with friends, or do other things that they previously enjoyed doing. Resuming these activities may help the person regain interest in them. If engaging in these activities makes them feel guilty, tell them that these feelings will reduce as they continue with such activities.

Terminating treatment: Closure of grief process

When the person makes substantial recovery from grief problems (at least 60% reduction in grief symptoms), it is time to consider 'closure' for grief. To help you decide

on the timing of closure, consider also the following changes in the person's condition.

- They are more able to tolerate the distress they experience when something reminds them of their loss or when thoughts about it enter their mind.
- They are less preoccupied with thoughts or memories of their loss.
- They are more acceptant of the reality of their loss.
- Avoidance or ritualistic mourning behaviors have decreased to an extent that they no longer disrupt daily functioning.
- They experience an increase in their sense of well being.
- They are better able to function in daily life.
- They are beginning to resume normal life activities.
- Their family and friends notice the change in them.

When most of the above is true, it is time for closure. This point is often reached in about 2 months. The task at hand at this point is to designate an event that best represents closure of the grieving process. To identify this event, ask the person the following question: "*What is it that you can do as the one last thing that will mean finally accepting the loss of your loved one and separating from him or her?* This could be a small family gathering or a religious or other ceremony at the cemetery, a final visit to the location where the loved one died, giving away his / her belongings (or a particular item among them), or any other activity that carries a special meaning for the person. The important point here is that this final task is perceived by the person as the most appropriate one to mark the end of the mourning process.

Once the closure event takes place, you may see the person one last time to advise them to continue practicing what they have learned in treatment with any remaining grief problems. Bear in mind that 60% to 80% recovery means good treatment outcome but there may still be a few problems that the person may have to tackle in the long term. Once this point is reached, however, the rest is plain sailing. You can congratulate yourself for your achievement as a therapist!

When can you expect improvement in treatment?

This depends entirely on how much effort the person makes in conducting their homework exercises. The harder they work on them, the faster they improve. Normally, 80% of the people make significant progress with their tasks in 4 weeks and begin to notice a distinct improvement in their condition. Some people may need as long as 10 weeks or more to get better. At least 40% reduction in grief scores at week 4 is usually a good sign, indicating that the person is making good progress in treatment.

Summary of treatment procedures for prolonged grief treatment

1. Assess severity of grief symptoms (Grief Assessment Scale).

2. Identify avoidance and ritualistic grief behaviors (Behavior Checklist for Grief).

3. Establish need for treatment: At least one of the following is present:
   (a) Grief Assessment Scale score is 25 or higher.
   (b) Grief symptoms cause significant functional impairment.
   (c) Person perceives need for help (or requests help).

4. Explain treatment aims → To facilitate grief process by not avoiding distressing reminders of lost one and not engaging in ritualistic grief behaviors.

5. Set homework exercises targeting avoidance and ritualistic grief behaviors (and traumatic stress, if necessary).

6. Set time frame for treatment (up to 10 weeks).

7. Involve close ones in treatment.

8. Monitor progress by weekly sessions:
   (a) Administer questionnaires to assess improvement.
   (b) Evaluate progress with homework exercises:
       (i) If progress made → Praise person's achievement.
       (ii) Agree on next week's tasks and provide encouragement.
       (iii) If no progress made → Identify problem and offer solutions:
       • Make exercises easier by breaking them into more manageable steps.
       • Give mental exercises to overcome distress.
       • Provide direct assistance with homework exercises.
       • Make home visits to assist with homework exercises.

9. Set final homework task for closure of grief.

10. Terminate treatment.

Appendix C: Recovering from earthquake trauma
A self-help manual

Metin Başoğlu and Ebru Şalcıoğlu

Trauma Studies, Department of Psychological Medicine, Institute of Psychiatry, King's College London & Istanbul Center for Behavior Research and Therapy

About the Authors

Professor Metin Başoğlu and Associate Professor Ebru Şalcıoğlu are currently the directors of the Istanbul Centre for Behavior Research and Therapy (ICBRT / DABATEM) in Istanbul. They are also affiliated with the Institute of Psychiatry, King's College London, where Prof. Başoğlu is head of Trauma Studies. Prof. Başoğlu has published extensively on the phenomenology and behavioral treatment of anxiety disorders, including post-traumatic stress disorder. He is internationally recognized for his extensive research with war, torture, and earthquake trauma and their treatment. After the 1999 earthquakes in Turkey the authors developed brief behavioral treatments for earthquake survivors and a self-help booklet designed to help people recover from the traumatic effects of earthquakes. This work appeared in a book entitled *A Mental Healthcare Model for Mass Trauma Survivors: Control-Focused Behavioral Treatment of Earthquake, War, and Torture Trauma*, which is published by Cambridge University Press. More information about the authors' work can be found at http://www.dabatem.org.

Introduction

Many people experience various traumatic stress problems after major earthquakes. Although some recover from the traumatic effects of the earthquake after a while, others may continue to experience problems for many years. The aim of this booklet is to show how you can get over these problems by yourself and protect yourself from long-term traumatic effects of earthquakes. The self-help treatment described in this booklet has been based on *Control-Focused Behavioral Treatment*, which is designed to help people recover from traumatic stress by increasing their resilience against anxiety or distress. This treatment has been developed through work with more than 6000 survivors of the 1999 earthquakes in Turkey. It has been tested and demonstrated to be highly effective in scientific studies (Başoğlu et al., 2003a; Başoğlu et al., 2003b; Başoğlu et al., 2005; Başoğlu et al., 2007). The first version of this booklet has been piloted with more than 1000 earthquake survivors and tested in a study, which showed that more than 80% of survivors who utilize this manual recover from traumatic stress and depression (Başoğlu et al., 2009).

This booklet may have been given to you by a mental healthcare provider who may be planning to see you from time to time to check up on your progress. He or she may have conducted an initial assessment of your psychological status and deemed self-help to be suitable in your case. In that case you can simply utilize the booklet on your own and keep in contact with your therapist as advised. If, however, you are intending to use this booklet on your own without the supervision of a mental healthcare provider, you will have to pay close attention to the WARNINGS you come across in the booklet. These warnings will let you know whether or not this treatment is suitable for you. They will also let you know when to seek alternative help from a mental healthcare provider for some problems you might encounter in treatment. Note that if this treatment is not suitable for you or if you failed to administer the treatment effectively by yourself, this does NOT mean that your problem is untreatable. You might well benefit from the same treatment under the supervision of a qualified therapist.

References

Başoğlu, M., Livanou, M., Şalcıoğlu, E., et al. (2003a). A brief behavioural treatment of chronic post-traumatic stress disorder in earthquake survivors: Results from an open clinical trial. *Psychological Medicine*, **33**, 647–654.

Başoğlu, M., Livanou, M., Şalcıoğlu, E. (2003b). A single session with an earthquake simulator for traumatic stress in earthquake survivors. *American Journal of Psychiatry*, **160**, 788–790.

Başoğlu, M., Şalcıoğlu, E., Livanou, M., et al. (2005). Single-session behavioral treatment of earthquake-related posttraumatic stress disorder: A randomized waiting list controlled trial. *Journal of Traumatic Stress*, **18**, 1–11.

Başoğlu, M., Şalcıoğlu, E., Livanou, M. (2007). A randomized controlled study of single-session behavioural treatment of earthquake-related post-traumatic stress disorder using an earthquake simulator. *Psychological Medicine*, **37**, 203–213.

Başoğlu, M., Şalcıoğlu, E., Livanou, M. (2009). Single-case experimental studies of a self-help manual for traumatic stress in earthquake survivors. *Journal of Behavior Therapy and Experimental Psychiatry*, **40**, 50–58.

Part 1: Assessing your psychological status

Exposure to earthquakes is an intensely frightening experience that may lead to severe and disabling **traumatic stress** problems. Although some people recover from these problems in a few months, others may continue to have problems for years or even a lifetime, if left untreated. Traumatic stress may severely impair work, social, and family functioning and lead to other problems, such as depression and drug or alcohol dependence. This section will help you assess your psychological status after your earthquake experiences, possible need for treatment, and whether the treatment in this booklet is suitable for your problems. Reading this section you will also understand what kind of psychological problems people commonly have after earthquakes.

Assessing traumatic stress problems

Below is a questionnaire that includes statements concerning various traumatic stress problems that people have after earthquakes. Please read each statement and indicate how much you were bothered by the problem in the LAST WEEK by putting a cross (X) under the appropriate column. Make sure you do not skip any statement. You will be using this questionnaire weekly during treatment, so either make a copy of it or mark your responses on a separate sheet of paper.

Traumatic Stress Symptom Checklist

	0 Not at all bothered	1 Slightly	2 Fairly	3 Very much bothered
I cannot help thinking about certain memories / images related to the earthquake.				
Sometimes all of a sudden past events pass before my eyes like a movie and I feel as if I am re-living the events.				
I frequently have nightmares.				
I cannot do certain things easily for fear of an earthquake (e.g. entering undamaged houses, taking a shower, being alone or sleeping in the dark).				
I have lost interest in things.				
I feel distant and estranged from people.				
I feel as if my feelings are dead.				
I have difficulty sleeping.				
I lose my temper more easily.				
I have difficulty remembering things or concentrating on what I am doing.				
I am on edge all the time for fear of an earthquake.				
I get startled when there is a sudden noise or movement.				
I feel upset when something reminds me of my experiences during the earthquake.				
I try to get rid of thoughts and feelings about my experiences during the earthquake.				
I have difficulty remembering certain parts of my experiences during the earthquake.				
Making long-term plans seems meaningless to me because the earthquake made me realize I may die anytime.				
I have physical symptoms such as palpitations, sweating, dizziness, and tension in my body when something reminds me of my experiences during the earthquake.				
I feel guilty.				

Traumatic Stress Symptom Checklist (cont.)

	0 Not at all bothered	1 Slightly	2 Fairly	3 Very much bothered
I feel depressed.				
I cannot enjoy life as I used to.				
I feel hopeless about the future.				
I have thoughts of killing myself from time to time.				
I have less energy for my daily activities.				
TOTAL SCORE				

Now you need to work out your total score on this questionnaire. You have scored 0 points for each X in the '*Not at all bothered*' column, 1 point for each X in the '*Slightly*' column, 2 points for each X in the '*Fairly*' column, and 3 points for each X in the '*Very much bothered*' column. Add up your points for all statements to obtain your total STRESS SCORE and write it underneath the questionnaire next to TOTAL SCORE. Now let us see what the total *Stress Score* is likely to mean.

STRESS SCORE 34 OR MORE: There is an 80% chance that you have traumatic stress problems requiring treatment.

STRESS SCORE 38 OR MORE: There is an 80% chance that you also have mild to moderate depression.

STRESS SCORE MORE THAN 50: There is an 80% chance that you have fairly severe traumatic stress and depression.

What is depression?

As depression occurs fairly commonly in people after major earthquakes, you should know more about this condition. Depression is a condition that may occur in response to traumatic or stressful life events, such as those you have experienced during and after the earthquake. These include repeated exposures to earthquakes, loss of close ones, property, or occupation, and financial difficulties. A depressed person feels intense anguish, unhappiness, or distress. They no longer enjoy life as they used to. They lose interest in a lot of activities they enjoyed before. They feel helpless, pessimistic, and hopeless about the future. They have sleep problems and feel too tired to go about their everyday business. They may have decreased or increased appetite. Accordingly, they may lose or gain weight. During the day they often feel worried and

cannot stop thinking about their problems. They may become forgetful or find it difficult to concentrate on what they are doing. There may also be physical symptoms like sweating, dizziness, numbing of the extremities or other parts of the body, palpitations, feeling faint, shortness of breath, or localized pains. A loss of sexual desire can also be experienced. They may sometimes wish to die as a means of relief. In more severe cases they may contemplate suicide, or even take this as far as a suicide attempt. A loss of self-confidence is common, as is a sense of uselessness and worthlessness. The person may feel guilty because they have trouble carrying out their everyday responsibilities. Remember that simply feeling sad or low does not mean you are depressed. You need to have many of the symptoms described above to be considered as having depression.

How to decide whether you need treatment

As noted above, if your *Stress Score* is 34 or more, there is an 80% chance that you need treatment for your problems. The higher your score, the more severe your problem and the more you are likely to need help. If your score is higher than 50, you most probably feel a strong need for help. Remember, however, that this score is only a rough guide in estimating your need for treatment. You may have a score of 15 or lower and still feel the need for help. **Therefore, if you are distressed enough by your problems to feel the need for help, this means that you do need help, regardless of your *Stress Score*.** For example, you may be experiencing intense fear because of continuing aftershocks but only a few of the traumatic stress problems in the above questionnaire. If this is true for you, then consider the treatment in this booklet, as this treatment includes useful information about how you should deal with fear of earthquakes. This information might be useful in **protecting** you from traumatic effects of future earthquakes.

On the other hand, if your score is higher than 34 but you do not think that you need treatment, consider carefully how your stress problems affect your life. Because of your **fear or distress** you may be having difficulty leading your life normally. You may be having difficulty doing many things in your everyday life because of distress or fear. Your problems might have affected your work and social and family life. If this is true for you, just give yourself a chance by initiating the treatment and see how you feel.

Assessing grief

(Skip this section if you have not lost a loved one)

Grief is a natural reaction to loss, which often resolves within 6 to 12 months. In some people, however, it may persist beyond this period and last for many years.

When this happens, grief is no longer considered as a natural reaction and it is termed **prolonged grief**. In this section you will see what prolonged grief involves and why it requires treatment. If you have lost a loved one recently your grief does not require treatment but you may nevertheless find the information in this section useful. Knowing how to handle normal grief might facilitate it and reduce the chances of unresolved or prolonged grief in the future.

How to assess grief

Below is a questionnaire that will help you to assess the severity of your grief. It will also help you understand what grief symptoms involve. Read the instructions and fill in the questionnaire as requested. You will be using this questionnaire again during treatment, so either make a copy of it or mark your responses on a separate sheet of paper.

Grief Assessment Scale

Below are statements that describe feelings and thoughts that some people have after the loss of a close one. Please indicate how frequently you have experienced these feelings and thoughts **IN THE LAST MONTH** by putting a cross (**X**) under the appropriate column.

	0 Never	0 Sometimes	1 Often	2 Always
I feel bitter for having lost him / her.				
I go to places that he / she used to go in the hope that I might find him / her there.				
I feel detached / estranged from others after his / her death.				
I feel that a future without him / her will always be empty and pointless.				
His / her death makes me feel like a part of me has died.				
I cry when I think about him / her.				
I cannot accept the fact that he / she is dead.				
I have lost trust in people because of his / her death.				
I feel lonely without him / her.				
I do things that remind me of him / her in day to day life (for example, keeping his / her pictures or belongings out in the open, thinking or talking about him / her, visiting his / her grave, etc.).				
I feel that life is empty or meaningless without him / her.				
I feel guilty when I enjoy myself.				
I acquired some of his / her harmful habits or behaviors (e.g. smoking or drinking).				
I yearn for him / her.				
I have physical complaints (e.g. headaches, pains, etc.) that started after his / her death.				
I see him / her stand before me.				
I feel as if my feelings have died after his / her death.				

Grief Assessment Scale (cont.)

	0 Never	0 Sometimes	1 Often	2 Always
I feel I have no control over my life.				
I cannot stop thinking about him / her.				
I feel helpless without him / her.				
I have physical complaints that he / she used to have when he / she was alive.				
I cannot do things that remind me of him / her in day to day life (for example, looking at his / her pictures, visiting his / her grave, talking about him / her, etc.).				
I hear his / her voice.				
I cannot believe that he / she is dead.				
I blame myself for not having tried hard enough to save him / her.				
I feel angry with him / her because he / she left me.				
I have dreams of him / her.				
I feel envious of people who have not lost their loved ones.				
I feel angry for having lost him / her.				
I feel insecure because of his / her death.				
TOTAL SCORE				

Now work out your total score on this questionnaire. You gained 0 points for each X in the '*Never*' or '*Sometimes*' columns, 1 point for each X in the '*Often*' column, and 2 points for each X in the '*Always*' column. Add up your points for all items to obtain your total GRIEF SCORE and write it underneath the questionnaire next to TOTAL SCORE.

How to decide whether you need treatment for grief

Consider the following in deciding whether or not you need treatment for grief:

- If your grief has continued with similar or increasing intensity beyond **12 months** and your total *Grief Score* is **25 or more**, there is an 80% chance that you have prolonged grief that requires treatment.
- Grief may cause intense distress and significant disruption in life activities. Consider how your life has changed since your loss. Grief symptoms may have dramatically reduced the quality of your life. You may be neglecting your health, as well as home and work responsibilities. Because of the changes in your emotional state and the way you relate to other people, your relationships with your family and friends may have suffered. Because of your constant preoccupation with your loss, you may be

underperforming at work. **If you feel you need help for these problems,** you can benefit from the treatment in this booklet, whatever your *Grief Score* might be.

> Treatment of grief is NOT about forgetting or completely abandoning your lost one. The treatment will simply help you recover from disabling grief symptoms so that you can lead a reasonably normal life. Even if you regard your grief as normal and think that you do not need treatment, consider giving the treatment a chance and see how you feel soon after you started it. You can then decide whether or not to continue with it.

Do I need treatment for normal grief?

As noted earlier, most people recover from grief and resume a relatively normal life within 6 to 12 months. If you are still within this period, then you probably do not need any treatment. However, consider the following questions:

1. Are you **frequently** *doing things that remind you of your loss in day to day life (for example, keeping your lost one's pictures or belongings out in the open, constantly thinking or talking about him / her, making frequent visits to his / her grave, etc.)?*

2. *Do you frequently avoid doing things that remind you of your loss in day to day life (for example, looking at your lost one's pictures, visiting his/her grave, talking about him/her, etc.).*

If your answer to either question (or both) is YES, you might be experiencing some difficulties in coping with your loss. Such behaviors might be an early sign that your recovery from grief might take longer than usual. You may therefore benefit from reading Part 5, where you will find information on what you can do to facilitate your grief and avoid this possible problem.

Is this treatment suitable for you?

Before starting the treatment, you need to rule out possible problems in carrying out the treatment on your own. Let us first see if you have any psychiatric conditions that need attention before you start the treatment. Please answer the questions below and pay close attention to the warnings.

Warnings

⇒ *Have you recently had thoughts of ending your life and made any plans to this effect?*
If YES, contact a mental health professional before going any further. You may have severe depression requiring drug treatment first. However, bear in mind that drugs may help with depression but not with other fear-related traumatic stress problems. Therefore, make sure that you start the treatment in this booklet after you recover from depression. Consult with your doctor about the best time to start psychological treatment.

⇒ *Since the earthquake have you ever had any flashbacks lasting more than 10–15 minutes, during which you lost total awareness of your surroundings or did something to endanger yourself or others around you?* (See the description in the footnote[1] below to understand better what a flashback is.)
If YES, contact a mental healthcare provider. Your condition may require treatment by a therapist. Once your flashbacks disappear or are brought under control, you may consider the treatment in this booklet.

⇒ *Do you currently have a psychiatric condition for which you were admitted to a psychiatric hospital and received drug treatment in the past?*
If YES, contact your doctor first. Once your psychiatric problem is brought under control, you may consider the treatment in this booklet.

⇒ *Do you have any physical conditions (such as serious heart problems or high blood pressure requiring treatment or pregnancy) that might be affected by heightened anxiety?*
If YES, consult with a doctor first and find out if your condition is likely to be affected by a treatment that may involve heightened anxiety as a result of entering feared or distressing situations. If it is, you may need to receive this treatment under the supervision of a therapist.

⇒ *Do you currently consume substantial amounts of alcohol or other sedatives on a regular basis?*
If YES, contact a mental healthcare provider. If you were using alcohol or drugs before the earthquake, you will need help for this problem first. If you started using these substances after the earthquake, you can receive the treatment in this booklet under the direction of a therapist as you begin to reduce your intake of these substances. The treatment may be helpful in coming off these substances.

---

[1] A flashback is a sudden feeling *as if you are re-living* the traumatic events of the earthquake. It usually lasts for a few seconds or minutes but in exceptional cases for as long as 10–15 minutes. When it happens, you may feel like *you are watching a filmstrip of your traumatic experiences.* You may see what you saw during a previous experience, hear the sounds that you heard, feel the objects you touched, or smell the smells you smelled all over again. You may also experience the fear and terror you experienced before with the same intensity. And because you think you are in the same situation all over again, you may rush outside, begin screaming, cry for help or think that your family is in danger and try to rescue them. For the duration of the flashback you may not be aware of what is going on around you. If someone speaks to you, for example, you may not be able to hear them. And once the flashback is over, you may not remember what has happened.

Part 2: How does treatment work?

To understand how treatment works it would help to know first the causes of your problem. In Part 1 we established that your main problem is **traumatic stress**. Let us briefly examine what causes traumatic stress.

Fear of earthquakes

An earthquake is an intensely frightening experience for most people. Aftershocks intensify people's fear and after a while make them feel totally **helpless**. This is because earthquakes occur **unpredictably** and there is no way of avoiding them. Fear is a natural reaction that helps people to protect themselves in the face of real danger. It is therefore normal to be afraid of earthquakes. However, it is important to distinguish **irrational** from **rational** fears. Taking realistic safety measures against earthquakes, such as strengthening one's house and learning how to protect oneself during an earthquake, reflects normal fear. However, after a major earthquake some people fear earthquakes so much that they are unable to stay alone at home, sleep in the dark, take a bath as usual, or get undressed when going to bed. Some cannot sleep in the room where they experienced the earthquake. Many people stay in shelters under difficult conditions for a long time even when their house is undamaged and inhabitable. Some people can stay at home during the day but not at night. Such fears are not rational, given that they do not afford realistic protection from earthquakes. Beyond a few precautionary measures, there is not much one can do to avoid earthquakes and therefore one has to resume normal life as soon as it is possible to do so after a major earthquake.

Remember also that people are faced with many other dangers in life. We can be run over by a car when we go out on the street. Yet we do not live in daily fear of having a car accident. A flowerpot could fall on our head and kill us as we are walking along the road. Because we do not notice these risks in our everyday lives, we are not afraid of them. But, whether we are afraid or not, the dangers still exist for us. We build these risks into our lives, because otherwise it would be impossible to carry on living normally.

Distress associated with trauma memories

In addition to earthquake tremors, some people may have experienced other traumatic events, such as collapse of their house, being trapped under rubble, witnessing the death of their loved ones or others, or witnessing disturbing scenes during rescue efforts. Distressing memories of such events may frequently enter their mind against their will, despite their efforts to keep them away. Certain events, activities, or objects may also remind them of these distressing events and make them feel upset. For example, they may be distressed when they visit the site where the event happened, go to a hospital, or hear ambulance sirens, etc. Particular sights, sounds, smells, thoughts, emotions, and even bodily sensations may remind them of their traumatic experiences. Because such trauma reminders are very common in daily life, they spend much of their time in considerable distress.

What is avoidance behavior?

After an earthquake people often tend to keep away from certain situations where they think they may be caught up helpless in an earthquake. They do not enter particular buildings, even when they are not damaged by the earthquake. This is called **avoidance behavior**. People also tend to avoid various situations that bring back distressing memories of their earthquake experience. Some people avoid so many different situations or activities that they are unable to conduct their daily activities in the usual way. Such fear and avoidance often make them feel even more **helpless** and many eventually get **depressed**. To get a better idea of how your fear and avoidance might be affecting your life, fill in the questionnaire below. Read the instructions carefully to understand how you should fill it in. (You will be using this questionnaire weekly, so either make a copy of it or mark your responses on a separate sheet of paper.) If you have avoidance behaviors that are not included in this questionnaire, make sure that you add them to the list under *Other Feared Activities*.

Fear and Avoidance Questionnaire

Below is a list of activities that may cause anxiety, fear, or distress in people who have experienced an earthquake. Please indicate by putting X under the appropriate column how much difficulty you have in carrying out these activities because of associated anxiety, fear, or distress.

None = *Not difficult at all / I can do it easily.*
Slightly = *Slightly difficult / Sometimes cannot do it.*
Fairly = *Fairly difficult / Cannot do it most of the time.*
Extremely = *Extremely difficult / Cannot do it at all.*

	0 None	1 Slightly	2 Fairly	3 Extremely
Going into safe buildings by day				
Going into safe buildings at night				
Staying in safe buildings at night				
Staying alone in safe buildings by day				
Staying alone in safe buildings at night				
Sleeping alone in safe buildings at night				
Sleeping alone in a room at night				
Sleeping before the time that the earthquake occurred				
Sleeping at home with no one else awake				
Being in the dark				
Sleeping in the dark				
Taking a bath in a safe house with other people there				
Taking a bath in a safe house alone				
Taking as long in the bathroom as before				
Getting undressed (into pyjamas / nightdress) before going to bed				
Closing or locking the doors when sleeping in a safe house at night				
Watching news about the earthquake on television				
Reading news about the earthquake in the newspapers				
Joining in conversations about the earthquake				
Talking about earthquake experiences				
Being in confined spaces				
Going anywhere high up				
Using an elevator				
Going to the upper floors of safe buildings				
Going to the lower floors of safe buildings				
Going shopping				
Going out alone				
Travelling alone on public transport				
Going past collapsed buildings				
Going close to collapsed buildings				
Looking at damaged buildings				
Looking at pictures of acquaintances that died in the earthquake				

Fear and Avoidance Questionnaire (cont.)

	0 None	1 Slightly	2 Fairly	3 Extremely
Visiting the graves of acquaintances that died in the earthquake				
Looking at things that make you think there could be an earthquake (e.g. the sky, the sea, animals, etc.)				
Thinking about things that happened during or after the earthquake				
Other feared activities (please indicate below):				
TOTAL SCORE				

Now work out your total score on this questionnaire. For each item give yourself 0 points for '*None*,' 1 point for '*Slightly*,' 2 points for '*Fairly*,' and 3 points for '*Extremely*' responses. Add up your points for all items to obtain your total **Fear and Avoidance Score** and write it underneath the questionnaire next to Total Score. People who have experienced a devastating earthquake in the epicenter region avoid an average of 10 activities in this questionnaire and obtain an average score of 32. These figures will give you some idea about how you compare with other earthquake survivors in this respect.

Take a look at activities you marked as '*Fairly difficult*' or '*Extremely difficult*' and examine how realistic these fears are. Consider how consistent you are in avoiding certain situations and not others. For example, if you are avoiding being in a building at night but not during the day, does this really make you any safer, given that earthquakes may happen any time of the day? Consider also the price you pay in avoiding these situations. Ask yourself "*How much do my fears interfere with my work, social, and family life?*" For example:

- You may be living in difficult or even dangerous conditions in a shelter, because you are afraid of going into buildings, even when they are undamaged.
- Because of your fear of buildings, you may not be able to go to work or undertake any important function in life that requires entering particular buildings, such as schools, shops, government offices, etc.
- If you cannot go shopping, this problem may make it hard for you to carry out your responsibilities at home.

- If you cannot stay at home alone or take a bath without anyone present at home, this may create problems within the family.
- Your social life may suffer, because you may be unable to visit friends or relatives in their home or join them in various leisure activities, such as going to the cinema, restaurants, parties, weddings, or other social gatherings.
- Think about how much effort you make every day to avoid memories and reminders of your earthquake experience. You may have stopped reading newspapers, listening to TV news, or seeing friends who remind you of the earthquake.

If you think these avoidances significantly interfere with your life, this is another indication that you need treatment (regardless of your traumatic stress score).

How does fear contribute to traumatic stress problems?

The stress problems you have indicated in the *Traumatic Stress Symptom Checklist* are directly related to your fear / distress and avoidance. For example, because you are in fear and trying to avoid earthquakes, you are constantly vigilant, watching out for signs of an impending earthquake. Consequently, you are easily startled by sudden noises or movements, lose your sleep, feel irritable, and have problems with your memory and concentration. Because you are desperately trying to achieve the essentially impossible task of avoiding earthquakes, you may be feeling helpless and depressed. In turn, depression makes your life even more difficult, because this means you have lost all hope in effectively dealing with your problems. Furthermore, fear and depression interfere with important responsibilities in your life, make it more difficult for you to cope with everyday problems, and thereby cause additional stress for you.

What does treatment involve?

The main principle of treatment is to break this vicious cycle by learning how to **TOLERATE** and **CONTROL** fear or distress caused by the trauma. This can be achieved by confronting situations and thoughts that evoke fear or distress, rather than avoiding them. For example, if you are afraid of staying alone at home, you will need to make an effort to stay alone at home so that you can overcome your fear. If you are trying to keep distressing thoughts away from your mind, you will need to try and focus on these thoughts until you no longer feel the urge to avoid them. You will see how you can do this in Part 3.

Why make an effort not to avoid fear or distress?

You have experienced unfortunate events, which made a psychological impact on you. The fact is that there is no way of turning the clock back and undoing the things that happened. The only way you can recover from the impact of these events is to look forward and see what you can do about your problem. **Building up your RESILIENCE by CONFRONTING and CHALLENGING your fear or distress is the best strategy in overcoming your problem**. You cannot do this if you keep avoiding fear or distress. To use an analogy, confronting fear or distress is like getting vaccinated against a virus. When a small dose of the virus is in your system, your body can build up its defense against the virus. This is also called **immunization**. People can be immunized against traumatic stress by confronting fear or distress. Confronting fear or distress is also like practicing weight-lifting. The more you do it, the stronger you get.

Your problem is not the unfortunate events that you have experienced or what you think might happen if you do not try to prevent them from happening again. Many other people experience similar events during earthquakes but recover after a while. Your problem is that you are unable to **confront**, **challenge**, **tolerate**, and **control** your distress or fear. Distress or fear is your worst **ENEMY** and you **SURRENDER** to this enemy by letting it take control of your life and make you more and more **helpless** as time goes by. Avoiding

feared situations may provide instant relief from anxiety but this only perpetuates the problem because, no matter how hard you try, it is impossible to avoid earthquakes. Moreover, you pay a high price by desperately trying to avoid them. Remember that **it is impossible to live a normal life without taking any risks**. A more realistic approach is to take reasonable safety precautions as much as possible and continue with your normal life. This treatment is about making you more resilient against stress so that you can lead a normal life.

DISTRESS – FEAR – AVOIDANCE
is your worst enemy.

At this point you are facing a critical choice in your life:
either you **BEAT** your fear
and **TAKE CONTROL** over your life
or
SURRENDER and live a life in distress, fear,
and helplessness.

How do people cope with fear?

The treatment might make more sense to you if you consider examples of how people cope with fear. After major earthquakes, such as the one you experienced, many people eventually realize that they have to confront and overcome their fear of buildings for the simple reason that they cannot live in shelters forever. Accordingly, they begin to enter buildings, staying there for a short period each time, and gradually increase the time they spend in a building as their confidence grows. If you have a look around, you may see such people around among your friends or neighbors.

Some people have phobic fears of animals (dogs, cats, spiders, snakes, etc.) or particular situations, such as enclosed spaces, heights, crowded places, etc. Just ask the people you know if they had such fears in the past and what they did to overcome them. Some of them will tell you that they beat their fears by gradually confronting the feared objects or situation in much the same way as described in this booklet. You may have had a similar experience yourself in the past, in which case you should have no difficulty in understanding what this treatment is about.

Part 3: Beating fear and distress

In Part 2 you learned that avoidance of feared or distressing situations is the main problem that makes you helpless and lose control over your life. If you are in the very early days or weeks of the disaster your main goal in treatment is **not to lose control over your life by starting not to avoid feared or distressing situations**. In this section you will see how you can fight your fear or distress caused by ongoing aftershocks. If it has been some months since the earthquake and you have already lost control over your life because of intense fear and avoidance, your main goal in treatment is **to regain control over your life by not avoiding fear and distress**. This means making an effort to do the things you used to do before the earthquake so that you can function reasonably well in all important areas of your life. Let us now see how you can achieve this.

Identifying avoidance behaviors

In Part 2 you filled in the *Fear and Avoidance Questionnaire*. Have a look at the activities you marked as *'Fairly difficult'* or *'Extremely difficult.'* Make a list of these activities. Remember that if you avoid other situations or activities not included in the questionnaire, you were supposed to include them under *'Other feared activities.'* Make sure you include them also in your list. This list will guide you in your daily exercises to overcome fear and distress.

Many of the avoidance behaviors you listed concern situations that you come across every day in your life. After the earthquake you may have organized your life in such as way that you do not have to come across situations that you find frightening or distressing. For example, because you can no longer do the shopping yourself, you may have delegated this chore to someone else in the household. You may be taking a bath only when someone else is present in the house. You may have also given up certain outdoor or social activities. You may be used to your 'new' life and these changes may now seem normal to you. Remember that a life in fear is not normal and your normal life was the one you lived **free of fear** before the earthquake. Let us now see what you can do to resume a normal life.

Beating your fear of buildings

Taking refuge in shelters is a normal safety precaution in the early days of a devastating earthquake and does not necessarily reflect a psychological problem. If you are reading this booklet in the very early days of an earthquake, you need to consider the fact that aftershocks are common after major earthquakes and they can cause further damage and casualties. You would, therefore, need to be very careful in choosing the right timing for any action you might take to overcome your fear of buildings, particularly in the early days of the disaster. Bear in mind the following points before you make any attempt to enter buildings.

WARNING

- **In the early days of the disaster do not enter buildings before the authorities have told the public that it is safe to do so.**

- **Do not enter buildings known to be damaged and uninhabitable.**

Let us suppose that your house is undamaged and you have been living in a shelter for some time. Even though the authorities said that it is now safe to go back home, you cannot do this because of fear. Here is what you can do. If you are not feeling confident enough to move back to your house in one go, **you can do it gradually in easier steps**. For example, you can proceed as follows:

STEP 1: Go near the building and stand near the door.
STEP 2: Go into the building, have a look around, and then leave.
STEP 3: Go into your home, have a cup of coffee, and then leave.
STEP 4: Go back home, tidy up the place, and then leave.
STEP 5: Spend the whole day at home and leave in the evening.
STEP 6: Spend the day and the evening at home and leave late at night.
STEP 7: Start spending the nights at home.

You may make each step as easy or difficult for yourself as you like, depending on how you feel about it. As you attempt each step, you may experience a certain amount of anxiety. Anxiety symptoms may include sweating, shaking, rapid heartbeat, dizziness, feeling faint, numbing of the extremities, and feeling short of breath. These symptoms are unpleasant but essentially harmless. When you experience these symptoms, you may feel a strong **urge** to leave the building. Try to control this urge by not giving into it. Tell yourself "I am going to beat this fear once and for all." Do not be afraid of feeling anxious or fearful. Remember the analogy about vaccination against a virus. Your anxiety is the virus that you need to build up your endurance or strength against it. Always remember:

> This is a battle with fear.
> Either you will conquer your fear
> or
> it will conquer you.

As you begin to tolerate anxiety better, you will notice an increase in your self-confidence. As your self-confidence grows, **challenge your fear by inviting it**. This means doing things to increase your fear. For example, you may be standing near the door and thus not feeling too anxious. You know that if you go further inside, you will be more anxious, thinking that it will not be easy to get out in case of an earthquake. Muster your courage and go into your flat. You may think that going into the room where you experienced the earthquake will increase your fear. Make a point of going into that room to challenge your fear. The cracks on the wall plaster might make you more anxious. Instead of turning your eyes away from them, go around looking for cracks and examining them. At every step of the way, think as follows: "*What can I do now to invite my fear?*" For example, if going up to the upper floors of the building makes you more anxious, do it. If thinking about your experiences during the earthquake makes you more anxious, think about them. Tell yourself "*An earthquake might happen right now.*" Sometimes heavy vehicles passing by cause vibrations in buildings. If such vibrations scare you, go and stand at a location where they are most strongly felt. These are just some examples of how you can challenge fear and you may be able to find many other ways of doing it.

> Once you have learned how to challenge your fear successfully, you can consider the battle won. This is an early sign that shows you will be successful in this treatment.

At each step terminate the exercise only when you feel that you can leave the building **at your own will and not because of your fear**. This will mean that you have achieved total control over your fear and are no longer helpless against it. **You can congratulate yourself for this achievement!** You will be feeling great about yourself. The next time you go back, you are likely to be less anxious than you were the first time. This is because your sense of control over the situation has increased. Each further step will seem easier to you as you progress through treatment. Therefore, do things to invite your fear while you are there. Remember that the point of this exercise is to learn to tolerate and control distress or fear. You will need to experience anxiety to achieve this.

In situations where your anxiety or fear gets too intense, stay where you are and find somewhere to sit. Focus your mind on symptoms of anxiety. Tell yourself "*I will not give in to this fear. I will not let it take control over me.*" **Do NOT try to divert your attention elsewhere**. Do not, for example, start reading something, talking to someone or examining something. Otherwise, you would not be able to learn how to tolerate your fear.

> Your first successfully completed exercise will prove to you that you can control your anxiety or fear. If you think that this task was relatively easy, remember that you will be just as successful in completing more difficult ones using the same strategy.

What happens when you fail to control your anxiety at some point? For example, you gave in to your fear and left the building. In such a situation, do not worry. This does not mean failure yet. Have a short break and wait outside. Try to muster more courage and go back inside. If you fail again, you can always give it another try some other day. Keep trying and you will eventually succeed. Once you successfully complete the step, move on to the next step and then to the next one until you complete the whole exercise.

You can conduct similar exercises for your fear of other buildings. If you are avoiding visits to homes of friends or relatives, make a point of visiting them. Again, if you cannot do this all at once, **break it into easier steps**. If you have difficulty going shopping, make a point of going shopping, instead of letting someone else do it for you. If necessary, beat your fear step by step, challenging your fear at every step. For example:

STEP 1: Go near the shop and stand near the door.
STEP 2: Go into the shop, have a look around, and then leave.

STEP 3: Go into the shop, buy one item, and then leave.
STEP 4: Go into the shop, buy all the items you need, and leave.
STEP 5: Repeat the same steps with other places where you have more difficulty shopping.

Your daily life may require entering various other buildings in the region, such as schools, business places, banks, hospitals, government offices, cinemas, and so on. Every time you need to go to one such place, take this as an opportunity to beat your fear. (Once again, it is worth noting that you should make sure that the building is NOT one that is known to be damaged in the earthquake.)

Beating your fear of earthquakes at home

There are things that you can do to overcome your fear of earthquakes in your daily life at home. It is reasonable to take some safety precautions in your house, such as making sure that objects on the wall, cupboards, or other furniture will not fall over during an earthquake and injure someone. There may be other such realistic safety measures that you may have been advised to take by the authorities in your country. It is natural and advisable to take such precautions. You may, however, be doing many other things in the hope that they will make you safer. You may be *feeling* safer with such actions but they do not realistically *make* you any safer. **Such actions are just signs of your anxiety or a state of excessive alertness and they achieve nothing more than fuelling your fear.** You will need to **challenge** your fear of earthquakes by changing these behaviors. Below are some examples of what you can do:

⇒ Take a bath as usual, making sure that you do not cut short your time in the bathroom for fear of earthquakes. If you have stopped taking a bath when you are alone at home, make an effort and do it.
⇒ At night get undressed before going to bed, turn the light off, close the bedroom door, and do not keep the TV or radio on until you sleep.
⇒ Do not avoid sleeping in the dark or when you are alone at home.
⇒ Do not keep someone in the family awake at night in case an earthquake happens.
⇒ If you are afraid of sleeping alone in the house, make a point of sleeping alone whenever you need to.

⇒ If you have stopped sleeping in the room where you experienced the earthquake, make a point of sleeping in that room.
⇒ Do not seek the company of someone in the house because it makes you feel safer. Make sure you can stay in the house all by yourself. Do not go out of your way to visit friends, relatives, or neighbours when you are in fear. Take every opportunity to overcome your fear of being alone in the house.
⇒ Stop trying to avoid earthquakes by watching out for signs of an impending earthquake. For example, do not repeatedly check the ceiling lights or keep a glass of water on the table to detect signs of any movement. Do not keep listening to sounds of dogs or birds or keep watching the sky or the sea for any signs of an impending earthquake. Stop watching TV or listening to the radio all the time in the hope that you may hear something about future earthquakes. Do not keep checking with your friends to see if they have heard any rumors about an earthquake in the near future.
⇒ If you have developed a fear of various other situations that you did not have before the earthquake, make a point of not avoiding them. For example, confront and overcome any fear of confined spaces, heights, lifts, going out alone, swimming, or travelling in public transport.

There may be many other things that you can do to overcome your fears. Just ask yourself "*What is it that I do in the belief that it will protect me in case of an earthquake?*" Make a list of them. Then examine each action carefully to see if it realistically makes you any safer. Bear in mind in your evaluation that feeling safe and *actually being safe* are entirely different things. Remember also that it is impossible to avoid earthquakes by being alert all the time or trying to detect early signs. The best you can do is to take some realistic precautions and learn to live with the reality of earthquakes.

Beating distress caused by trauma reminders

You may be avoiding various situations because they remind you of your distressing earthquake experiences. These reminders may bring back memories of the earthquake, collapse of the building, being trapped under rubble, your close ones or other people trapped under rubble, sights of devastation, severely injured or dead people, mutilated bodies, etc. Some of the avoidance behaviors you marked in the *Fear and Avoidance Questionnaire* may relate to distressing reminders of these experiences. Every time you come across these reminders, take it as an opportunity to build up your resilience against distress by not avoiding them. Below are some examples of what you can do to achieve this.

⇒ Do not avoid sights of devastation or destroyed buildings. If you need to pass by such locations in your everyday life, make sure that you do not take a different route. Look closely at these sights, examine them, and do not try to avoid any memories of the earthquake that may come to your mind. If necessary, make a point of going to these locations **just to prove to yourself that you can overcome your distress**. Spend as much time there as necessary until you feel completely in control over your distress.

⇒ Do not avoid talking about things you experienced during the earthquake with friends, acquaintances, or others.

⇒ Take every opportunity to participate in conversations or discussions about earthquakes.

⇒ Do not avoid earthquake-related news in the media. On the contrary, challenge your distress and listen to such news on TV or radio or read them in the newspapers.

⇒ Do not avoid any other reminders of the earthquake. If necessary, make a point of looking at pictures of acquaintances that died in the earthquake, seeing particular people or visiting particular locations in the region that bring back your memories, and attending community meetings, ceremonies for the dead, anniversaries of the disaster, and so on.

⇒ Whenever something reminds you of your earthquake experiences, do not try to avoid memories, thoughts, or images about your experiences by pushing them away from your mind. Do not try to divert your attention from these thoughts or prevent them from entering your mind by occupying yourself with other activities, such as keeping the radio on, reading something, or doing housework. Instead, **focus your attention on these thoughts and go through the earthquake events as they happened over and over again until you no longer feel the need to avoid them in your mind**. You will see that when you do not try to avoid such thoughts, they will come to your mind less often.

What to do in case of difficulty with confronting distress

When you stop avoiding trauma reminders you will inevitably experience a certain degree of distress. It is important that you make an effort to confront such distress and see if you can overcome it. If you have made several attempts and decided that you are unable to cope with your distress even in a gradual and step by step fashion, do not worry. There are some exercises that you can do to build up your tolerance of distress before you actually confront particular situations. For example, set aside some time to go through in your mind all distressing events you experienced. Try to picture in your mind the events one by one as they happened, without omitting any detail, no matter how distressed you might get. Focus on the most distressing images and try to keep them in your mind as long as you can. When you are finished, start all over again. **Repeat this exercise as many times as necessary until you feel you can easily tolerate the distress evoked by these memories**. With sufficient practice, you will notice an increase in your tolerance of distress and a decrease in the frequency of such thoughts. You will also see that you are no longer able to evoke intensely distressing thoughts in your mind, no matter how hard you try.

If you do not find this strategy helpful enough, you may consider another. Write down your traumatic experiences in detail as they happened from beginning to the end without omitting any detail, as if you are writing your trauma story in a letter to a close friend. Read this letter over and over again, while also focusing on the events in your mind. Do this exercise over and over again until you see that you can easily tolerate the distress. You can also do this exercise is a different way, such as relating your trauma story to a close one over and over again. You can even audiotape your story and listen to it repeatedly afterwards, if you have the means to do so.

Once you have done this, you may find it easier to tackle the distressing situations that you initially had difficulty confronting. **It is important, however, that you test and strengthen further the beneficial effects of this exercise in real life situations that bring back trauma memories**. Let us suppose, for example, that you have difficulty going to locations where there are destroyed buildings. Go to one such location to see how you feel. You may even choose the location where you actually experienced the traumatic events. You may find that you are better able to tolerate distress in that situation. Spend some time there and try to challenge your distress by going through your trauma story in your mind in the same way as you have done before until you have complete control over your distress. **This exercise will prove to you that you can tolerate distress even when you directly confront reminders of your trauma.**

Remember that 90% of people with your problems are able to overcome distress by confronting distressing situations in real life and therefore do not need to use the methods described here. You are therefore most likely to be one of them if you make an effort.

However, IF you are considering quitting treatment, because:

1. You feel discouraged at this point, thinking that you will never be able to overcome your distress in real life situations,

OR

2. You feel discouraged after making several failed attempts to confront real life situations and think that you will not be able to overcome your distress,

GIVE THE TREATMENT A CHANCE BY USING THESE METHODS FIRST.

Involve your close ones in your treatment

Involving your close ones in your treatment has several important advantages. First of all, they should know what your treatment is about so that they can support and encourage you throughout your treatment. Second, you may also need their cooperation in conducting some exercises. For example, if you have a fear of staying alone at home in the evenings, there may be times when you may want to ask them to leave you alone in the house. Third, if they know about what you are setting out to achieve, you can share your success with them each time you make significant progress. Fourth, you can ask them to monitor your progress.

When you know that someone is watching your progress, you are more likely to succeed in your treatment. Finally, your family or friends may have the same stress problems and you may be able to help them by setting an example with your success in treatment. Therefore, try to get them to read this booklet and encourage them to use it in overcoming their own problems. You can monitor and support each other during treatment.

When is the best time to start treatment after an earthquake?

The answer is **as soon as possible**. Treatment in the early days of the disaster means simply not avoiding feared or distressing situations after having taken the necessary safety precautions. For example, if your home is undamaged and still inhabitable, you can make sure that you go back home (instead of staying in shelters) when the authorities tell you that it is safe to do so. If you are already at home you can carry out the exercises described earlier to overcome your fear or distress. You can do this even if you have lost your home and are living in difficult circumstances in a shelter. You do not need extra time or much prior planning to conduct most of the exercises. Simply be aware of any tendency in yourself to avoid particular situations and make an effort not to avoid them as you encounter them in the daily course of your life. Such awareness will help you to stamp out the problem before it emerges.

Evaluating progress in treatment

If your circumstances allow it, we highly recommend that you take time to fill in the *Traumatic Stress Symptom Checklist* and *Fear and Avoidance Questionnaire* every week, so that you can monitor your progress regularly in treatment. Even if you cannot fill in these questionnaires every week, try and use them once every few weeks to see how your progress is going. Every time you use the questionnaires write down the total scores in the **Progress Table** below. This way you can see at a glance how your treatment is progressing.

Progress Table

Questionnaires	Treatment weeks										
	0	1	2	3	4	5	6	7	8	9	10
Traumatic Stress Symptom Checklist											
Fear and Avoidance Questionnaire											

Before you start treatment fill in both questionnaires to determine the severity of your stress problems. This is called **Week 0 assessment**. Write down the total scores under the column marked 0 in the Progress Table. Fill in the same questionnaires every week and insert your total scores under the appropriate column in the Progress Table. Make sure you do not skip any items in the questionnaires. Otherwise, your total scores will not reflect your progress in a reliable fashion.

At each week compare your scores with your Week 0 scores to see how much progress you have made. If you like, you can calculate percentage improvement in total scores by subtracting a week's score from Week 0 score, dividing the difference by the Week 0 score, and multiplying the result by 100. Let us take the *Traumatic Stress Symptom Checklist*, for example. If your Week 0 total score is 40 and week 3 score is 20, this means a 50% improvement in your traumatic stress problems $(40 - 20 = 20 / 40 = 0.50 \times 100 = 50\%)$.

If you carry out the treatment as you should, you are most likely to experience certain changes in your condition after 2 to 4 weeks. Having done the things that you were unable to do before, you may feel more confident in yourself and less afraid of earthquakes. You may notice that you are less preoccupied with past trauma events and less distressed when you are reminded of them. You may also feel a general improvement in your stress problems. You may, for example, sleep better, feel less irritable, and concentrate better on your work. Such changes are also likely to be noticed by your family and friends. However, there are different grades of improvement and you can best assess them by examining your questionnaire scores. Let us now see how you can do this.

Your score on the *Fear and Avoidance Questionnaire* will help you assess your success in overcoming your distress or fears. This is most important, because recovery from all other problems depends on improvement in your trauma-related distress or fears. Recall that your aim in treatment is to do things you marked as '*fairly*' or '*extremely*' difficult in this questionnaire. If you have managed to do these things successfully, you would be rating them as involving '*slight*' or '*no difficulty.*' These ratings indicate **successful completion** of each exercise. With successful treatment, you will also see at least 60% reduction in the total scores of this questionnaire at some point.

Reduction in your total score *Stress Score* will give you an idea about the extent of improvement in your traumatic stress and depressive symptoms. At least 60% reduction in the total score means good treatment outcome; 80% reduction means an excellent outcome.

When to expect improvement in treatment

This depends entirely on how much effort you make in treatment. Normally, 80% of the people are able to overcome their fear or distress in most situations in 4 weeks and begin to notice a distinct improvement in their condition after 2 to 4 weeks. Some people may, however, need as long as 10 weeks to get better. Your questionnaire scores 4 weeks after you started treatment will tell you whether or not you are likely to get good results with this treatment. At that point, you should expect at least 40% reduction in your scores. Less than 40% improvement may mean that you have encountered some problems in treatment. In that case, you should refer to Part 5 to see how you can overcome these problems.

Part 4: Treating prolonged grief

(*You may skip this section if you have not lost a loved one during the earthquake.*)

Treatment of grief is similar in principle to treatment of traumatic stress problems. The idea is to change certain behaviors that maintain grief reactions. People usually display two types of grieving behaviors. They may avoid particular situations or activities that bring back distressing memories of the loss. For example, they may avoid visits to the cemetery, talking about the lost one, looking at his / her pictures, or going to the location where s / he died. This is because they find it difficult to tolerate the distress caused by any reminder of their loss. This is similar to avoiding reminders of other earthquake-related traumatic events that evoke fear or distress.

A person may also engage in activities or '**ritualistic behaviors**' to keep the memory of the lost one alive at all times. For example, they may feel like talking about the lost one all the time, make frequent visits to his / her grave, keep his / her pictures all around the house, feel unable to give away his / her clothes or other belongings,

and keep his / her room exactly as it was before the event, etc. Such behaviors have a **ritualistic** quality, meaning that they are regular and excessive. One feels an **urge** to engage in them, which is often difficult to resist. Moreover, not engaging in them often causes anxiety.

Both avoidant and ritualistic mourning behaviors are aimed at **avoidance of distress** and, as such, block the natural course of the grief process by making it difficult for the person to accept the reality of the loss. **Acceptance of the loss is essential for natural recovery from grief.** The aim of treatment is to help you change these behaviors so that natural recovery can take its course. You can achieve this by (a) not avoiding situations that bring back memories of your loss and (b) not engaging in ritualistic behaviors. Let us now examine what you need to do to facilitate your recovery from grief.

Step 1: Identify problem behaviors

The first step is to identify problem behaviors that block recovery. Fill in the questionnaire below after reading the instructions carefully.

Behavior Checklist for Grief (BCG)

After the loss of a close one some people feel the urge to do certain things to keep the memory of the lost one alive all the time. Others have difficulty with certain activities that bring back distressing memories of the lost one. Below are some statements that describe such activities. Please indicate how much they apply to you IN THE LAST WEEK by putting a cross (X) under the appropriate column. If you have lost more than one close person, you may consider each statement in relation to any of them.

	Not at all	Slightly	Fairly	Very much
I feel like seeing his / her belongings out in the open.				
I have difficulty looking at his / her pictures.				
I avoid going to the place where he / she died.				
I feel like seeing his / her pictures out in the open.				
I feel like going to the places where we used to go together.				
I have difficulty mentioning his / her name.				
I avoid meeting his / her friends.				
I have difficulty cooking / eating the meals that he / she used to like.				
I avoid visiting his / her grave.				
I have difficulty listening to the music he / she liked.				
I feel like talking about him / her.				
I have difficulty going to the places where we used to go together.				
I avoid talking about him / her.				
I have difficulty looking at his / her belongings.				
I feel like visiting his / her grave.				
Other:				

If you can think of other behaviors similar to the ones listed in the questionnaire, make sure you add them to the list. Next, work out your total score by giving yourself 0 points for answers in the 'Not at all' column, 1 point for answers in the 'Slightly' column, 2 points for answers in the 'Fairly' column, and 3 points for answers in the 'Very much' column.

Step 2: Define your tasks in treatment

You will need a structure in dealing with your problems. Accordingly, you will need to set yourself some **TASKS** to work on during treatment. Take a look at the behaviors you marked as 'Fairly' or 'Very much' in the above questionnaire. Make a list of them. Your aim in treatment is to change these behaviors by (a) **not avoiding the activities that cause distress** and (b) **refraining from repeatedly doing things that maintain your grief**. If you have difficulty in engaging in various activities that remind you of your lost one, your tasks may include the following:

- Looking at his / her pictures.
- Looking at his / her belongings.
- Cooking / eating the meals that he / she used to like.
- Going to the place where he / she died.
- Meeting with his / her friends.
- Talking about him / her.
- Visiting his / her grave.
- Listening to the music he / she liked.
- Going to the places where you used to go together.
- Going to the site where he / she died.

If you have difficulty in refraining from engaging in ritualistic activities, then your tasks may include the following:

- Removing his / her pictures from sight or stop looking at them.
- Removing his / her belongings from sight or stop looking at them.
- Giving away his / her belongings.
- Not going to the place where he / she died.
- Not going to the places where you used to go together.
- Not talking about him / her.
- Not visiting his / her grave.
- Not carrying with you things that belonged to him / her (for example, a picture, key ring, scarf, watch, ring, bracelet, etc.).

Note that these two groups of tasks involve different activities but they share one thing in common: they both involve confronting distress associated with your loss. Depending on the nature of your problem, you may have to select more tasks from one group than the other.

Step 3: Work on your tasks

Once again, the purpose in conducting your tasks is to learn to tolerate the distress caused by your loss so that you can complete the normal grief process. The way you should confront distress related to your loss is essentially the same as described for fear in Part 3. If you are using this booklet only for your grief problems, we suggest that you read Part 3 to gain a better understanding of treatment needs to be conducted. Treatment procedures in dealing with avoidance behaviors are essentially the same, whether avoidance is caused by fear of earthquake or distress associated with a loss.

You can start working on your tasks in any order you like. **If you like, you can start with the easier ones and, when you feel you can tolerate distress better, move on to more difficult ones**. Look at the task lists above and decide which ones are the easiest and which ones are more difficult to achieve. You can also break a difficult task into **easier steps**. For example, if you are keeping your lost one's pictures or belongings out in the open so that you can see them all the time, you can begin your task by removing these items one by one, instead of all of them at once. Or you can remove them in a particular order, starting with the 'easier-to-remove' items first. Similarly, you can give away his / her belongings one by one, starting with the easiest items first. If you feel you cannot stop cemetery visits at once, you can reduce their frequency gradually. You may experience a certain amount of distress in achieving each task but this is natural and not undesirable. Remember always that this will help you to learn to tolerate the distress caused by your loss so that you can complete your grief in a natural fashion.

The distress you experience in executing these tasks may include feelings of anger, blame, or guilt. Executing these tasks may also make you feel guilty because they may come across to you as giving up on your lost one or as 'betraying' his / her memory. This is natural and most grieving people have such thoughts and feelings. You will recover from such emotions as your treatment progresses and you will most likely feel different about the issues that bring about these emotions.

Note also that the aim of treatment is not to deprive you of all reminders of your lost one forever. It is normal to keep some pictures of the lost one in the living room or make cemetery visits from time to time, as most people do. These tasks are simply designed to help you come to terms with your loss. When the treatment is over and you are no longer distressed by the thought of removing them from your sight, you can put back some of the pictures in your living room. You should make sure, however, that you do not revert back to the same excessive or avoidant mourning behaviors you had before the treatment.

Step 4: Resume your normal life activities

As you begin to make progress with your tasks, you will notice an increased sense of well being within the first few weeks of treatment. At this point it is important that you make an effort to resume your normal life activities. For example, you can begin to take better care of yourself and your appearance, attend social gatherings, meet with friends, or do other things that you previously enjoyed doing. If you stopped doing these things because you lost interest in them, making an active effort to start doing them may help you regain your interest in these activities. If you have been avoiding such activities because they make you feel guilty, you should still make an active effort not to avoid them. You will see that feelings of guilt will reduce as you resume your normal life activities.

Setting a time frame for treatment

It is important that you set yourself a time frame to complete your grieving process. This treatment is designed for 10 weeks, because most people are able to complete this process within about 3 months. So bear this time frame in mind and plan your treatment accordingly. Take a look at how many tasks are defined for you. If you have 10 tasks, for example, this means you can complete all tasks in 10 weeks by working on one task each week. You can, however, work on as many tasks as you want each week and complete the treatment even earlier. This is entirely up to you.

Defining a closure point for grief

When you reach the end of treatment within 3 months, this will also mean the termination of your grief process. Completion of your last task could define the **CLOSURE** point of your grief. This could be the most difficult task or one with the most significant symbolic meaning for you. Ask yourself "*What is it that I can do as one last thing that will mean finally accepting the loss of my loved one and separating from him or her*? This could be a small family gathering or ceremony at the cemetery, a final visit to the location where your loved one died, giving away his / her belongings (or a particular item among them), or any other activity that carries a special meaning for you. What is important here is that you see this final task as the most appropriate one to mark the end of your grieving process. The timing of this event is important. It could be earlier or perhaps a bit later than 3 months. **When you feel you have come to terms with the reality of your loss, gained sufficient control over problem mourning behaviors, and resumed your normal life activities, you are ready for closure.** Once again, closure does not mean forgetting about your loved one or separating from his / her memory forever. It simply means your grief is now completed in the way that it should have naturally resolved in the first place.

Treating traumatic stress together with grief

If you have traumatic stress problems in addition to prolonged grief, you may conduct tasks relating to both problems during the same period. In some cases a particular task may concern both problems. For example, visiting the site where you experienced the earthquake and where your loved one died would constitute a task relating to both problems. If you find it too difficult to work on both problems at the same time, you can tackle them in turn. Start with the one you find relatively easier to deal with and then turn to the other one.

Evaluate your progress in treatment

You can monitor your progress by filling in the *Behavior Checklist for Grief* every week and *Grief Assessment Scale* (see Part 1) every 4 weeks in treatment. Every time you do this, write down the total scores in the PROGRESS TABLE below, so that you can see the changes in your scores at a glance. Make sure you do not skip any items or questions. Otherwise, your total scores will not reflect your progress in a reliable fashion.

Progress table

Questionnaires	Treatment weeks										
	0	1	2	3	4	5	6	7	8	9	10
Grief Assessment Scale											
Behavior Checklist for Grief											

You need to assess your grief problems once before you start treatment so that you can see how your symptoms change during treatment. This is called **Week 0 assessment** (column labelled 0 in the Progress Table). It is important that you fill in the *Behavior Checklist for Grief* every week because it will show you which tasks you have successfully completed and help you to set new tasks for each week.

If you are carrying out the treatment as you should, you are likely to experience the following changes in your condition after about 4 weeks:

- You are more able to tolerate the distress you experience when something reminds you of your loss or when thoughts about it enter your mind.
- You are less preoccupied with thoughts or memories of your loss.
- You are beginning to accept the reality of your loss.
- There has been some reduction in your grief symptoms, resulting in an increase in your sense of well being.
- You are better able to function in your daily life.
- Your family and friends notice the change in you.

Let us now see how you can assess your progress based on your questionnaire scores. You can compare your scores at week 4 and week 10 with your Week 0 scores to see how much progress you have made. If you like, you can calculate percentage improvement in scores by subtracting a week's score from Week 0 score, dividing the difference by the Week 0 score, and multiplying the result by 100. For example, if your *Grief Assessment Scale* score at Week 0 is 40 and week 4 score is 20, this means there is 50% improvement in your grief score ($40 - 20 = 20 / 40 = 0.50 \times 100 = 50\%$).

The *Behavior Checklist for Grief* reflects the severity of your grief. Recall that your tasks were based on the items you rated as '*fairly*' or '*very much.*' After you start treatment a rating of '*not at all*' or '*slightly*' on any item means that you have successfully completed a particular task. A reduction of 60% or more in the total questionnaire score indicates successful treatment outcome.

The *Grief Assessment Scale* is another measure of the severity of your grief. It is different from the *Behavior Checklist for Grief* in that it measures a wider range of grief symptoms, including thoughts and emotions concerning the loss. A reduction of 60% or more in the total score of this scale indicates successful treatment.

When can you expect improvement in treatment?

This depends entirely on how much effort you make in conducting your tasks. The harder you work on them, the faster you improve. Normally, 80% of the people make significant progress with their tasks in 4 weeks and begin to notice a distinct improvement in their condition. Some people may need as long as 10 weeks to get better. Therefore, allow yourself 4 to 10 weeks to complete your tasks and recover. Your scores at week 4 will be a good indicator of your progress. At that point, you should see about 40% reduction in your questionnaire scores. Less improvement might mean that you have encountered some problems in treatment. In that case, you should refer to Part 5 to see how you can overcome these problems.

Part 5: Dealing with problems in treatment

In this section you will see how you can deal with some problems that you might encounter during treatment. It is worth noting that most people complete their treatment without running into these problems. Nevertheless, these problems are reviewed here so that you know what to do in case you experience them.

Dealing with worsening depression during treatment

Depression is a common problem after earthquakes caused by disabling fear and related traumatic stress symptoms. Depressive symptoms often get better with treatment, as a person gains control over fear and other stress problems. However, they may also get worse for other reasons, such as financial difficulties, illness or loss in the family, marital problems, etc. Any worsening in your depression will also be reflected in your *Stress Score*. Check your last score on this questionnaire to see if there is an increase. Remember that scores over 38 on this questionnaire indicate probable depression. If you have depression severe enough to impede treatment, your score is likely to be above 50. If this is the case with you, answer the following questions to decide on what to do:

WARNING

1. Are you having thoughts of putting an end to your life and making plans to this effect, because you feel you can no longer cope with your problems?

2. Are you no longer determined to go through this treatment thinking that there is no hope of getting better for you?

3. Are problems like loss of interest in everything, feeling tired or lacking in energy, memory and concentration problems, or irritability making it difficult to continue with treatment?

If your answer to any of these questions is YES, then you should see a mental healthcare provider before you continue with this treatment. You may need additional treatment for your depression. When you no longer have these problems you may continue with this treatment.

No matter how hopeless things might seem, remember that it is your depression that makes you feel this way and that it is possible to treat depression using medication. It might also be helpful to bear in mind some useful information about drug treatment:

⇒ Medication (antidepressants) is not likely to be a cure for your fear-related stress problems. While you may experience some improvement in these problems with drug treatment, your problems are most likely to come back after you stop taking medication.

⇒ We strongly recommend that you start the treatment in this booklet while you are still taking medication. This could be at the earliest stage when you sufficiently recover from depression (meaning you no longer have the symptoms indicated in the above warning box). Discuss this issue with your doctor so that he or she can let you know when you can start this treatment again. This might be possible after 6 to 8 weeks of drug treatment.

⇒ Antidepressants are often used for about 6 months in treating depression. In your case there may not be a need for such long use, if you can start psychological treatment at an early stage. Discuss this issue with your doctor so that he or she can plan for your withdrawal from medication at an earlier stage. For example, if you started psychological treatment after 6 to 8 weeks of drug treatment, 4 weeks of psychological treatment might allow you to start coming off medication after about 10 to 12 weeks of drug treatment. This would be possible, however, only if you complete all your exercises within 4 weeks and overcome your fears.

⇒ We recommend that you come off medication, gradually decreasing the dose under the guidance of your doctor. Make sure that you have completed all your exercises before you are completely free of medication.

⇒ Always bear in mind that any improvement in your distress- or fear-related stress symptoms while you are on medication is most likely to be due to **your own efforts** and not to the tablets you are taking. Antidepressants reduce depression symptoms but have only a limited effect on fear-related problems, which often disappears when they are discontinued.

Dealing with increased stress symptoms

In some people confronting a distressing or feared situation might lead to an increase in stress symptoms in the early phases of the treatment. For example, you may have experienced an increase in your general level of anxiety, your sleeping pattern may be disrupted, you may have nightmares, or you may become more irritable. This is a fairly rare occurrence and, when it happens, it is no cause for concern. Bear in mind that this is only temporary and the stress symptoms will subside as you continue with your treatment. Remember the vaccination example we gave in Part 2. This is like developing a slight fever after a vaccination. This is a sign that the treatment is working.

Having said this, however, you should also bear in mind that increased anxiety or distress might make a previously existing problem of **irritability** or **fits of uncontrollable anger** worse. If you have this problem and noticed a worsening in this condition make sure that you heed the following warning:

WARNING

If at any stage of the treatment you feel a tendency to harm yourself or others due to irritability or fits of uncontrollable anger, give the treatment a break and contact a mental healthcare provider. You may need treatment under supervision.

Dealing with panics during treatment

Panic is severe anxiety or fear that lasts a very short time. It is usually accompanied by sweating, shaking, shortness of breath, feeling faint, numbing in parts of the body, hot and cold flushes, racing of the heart and sometimes chest pains, and fear of dying, losing one's mind, or control. Although distressing, these symptoms are harmless and last only a short while. Panics occur rarely in treatment but in case you encounter this problem, it is worth knowing what it involves. In a situation like this, sit down somewhere and wait for the panic to subside. Sometimes, people experiencing panic breathe very rapidly, and this can have an aggravating effect. Breathing regularly and deeply may make the panic subside quickly. What is important here is for you to recognize the symptoms and know that there is nothing to worry about. Once the panic is over, you can continue with your treatment.

Dealing with flashbacks during treatment

You learned what flashbacks are in Part 1. Like panics, this symptom occurs fairly rarely during treatment.

Although a flashback is an unpleasant experience, it is often harmless and likely to disappear as you make progress in treatment. What you experience during a flashback is by no means a sign of losing your mind. You can do the following to control this symptom:

⇒ Try to monitor your flashbacks and work out what triggers the symptom. It could be a sight, sound, smell, word, thought, image, emotion, or anything that reminds you of your experience during the earthquake. Make a list of the situations that trigger them. When you encounter these situations, be aware that the symptom may appear.

⇒ When you realize that the symptom is about to appear, sit down and breathe deeply and regularly. Focus on what is happening around you. Try to watch carefully what people are doing, what they are saying. Or try to focus your attention on something. For example, look carefully at an object near you and study its shape, color and texture. Pick it up and feel what kind of emotion it produces. Focus all your attention on this object.

⇒ You could carry a small bottle of cologne with you. If you do, pat some cologne on your face and hands and focus on feeling refreshed. You could also carry a string of worry beads with you. As the symptom begins, hold the beads and start counting them in two's or three's. Focus on the prayer beads and be careful not to make a mistake when counting.

⇒ You may find other effective ways of focusing your attention elsewhere. These could be things like walking, telling yourself where you are, the date and time, or humming a tune.

⇒ Talk to your family about your situation and tell them about this symptom. If the symptom appears while you are with them, they can help 'bring you back to reality.' They could do this by touching you or telling you where you are.

In severe cases where a flashback causes total loss of awareness of the surroundings, a person might engage in harmful acts to self or others, but you are not likely to be one of them if you have heeded our warning in Part 1 about not undertaking this treatment before you see a therapist. Nevertheless, bear in mind the following:

Dealing with other problems that impede progress in treatment

In Part 3 we noted that the extent of your progress after 4 weeks of treatment will give you a good idea about how you are doing in treatment. If you experienced none of the problems reviewed so far but still had little or no improvement in your condition, you may have encountered some other problems. Most probably you were not able to work on your tasks the way you should. Let us see the most common reasons for this and how you can overcome them.

You attempted to confront a feared situation, but felt too anxious and gave up.

You may have started with too difficult situations. Break your task into easier steps (as described in Part 3) and start with the easiest step. Alternatively, select an easier situation where you can control your fear better and start again.

You started working on your grief problems, felt too distressed, and gave up.

You may have started with too difficult situations. Break your task into easier steps and start with the easiest step. Alternatively, select an easier situation where you can tolerate your distress better and start again. If this does not work, read '*What to do in case of difficulty with confronting distress*' in Part 3.

You confronted feared or distressing situations but experienced no distress or fear.

You may not have properly challenged your fear or distress while you were in the situation. You may have done things that made you feel safe. For example, you may have made an attempt to enter a building but stayed close to the door, thinking that you can easily escape in case of an earthquake. Or you may have had a close one waiting outside the bathroom door while you were taking a bath and his / her presence might have made you feel safer. **Think carefully: have you done anything to make sure that you feel safe while you were in the feared situation?** If yes, this might be the reason why you did not experience fear. In this case, repeat the exercise without resorting to such 'safety' measures. Alternatively, you may have avoided your anxiety or distress while conducting your task by distracting your attention to something else. Repeat the exercise, this time not avoiding your anxiety or distress. Focus your attention on things around or thoughts that make you anxious or distressed.

An aftershock happened after you started the treatment, your fears got worse, and you paused or quit treatment.

Aftershocks are common after major earthquakes. They may happen anytime and there is no way of controlling or avoiding them. Take this as a good opportunity to challenge your fears. Resume treatment, telling yourself that you will lead a normal life despite the aftershocks. Bear in mind that stopping treatment at this point means accepting **defeat**.

You heard rumors about an earthquake expected to occur on a particular date and gave up treatment.

Such rumors are common after an earthquake. You probably heard such rumors many times before and none came true. People tend to believe such rumors because the thought that an earthquake will happen on a particular date makes them feel safe until that date. In this way they think they can avoid the possible consequences of an earthquake. In actual fact, experts tell us that it is impossible to predict an earthquake. Instead of trying to avoid earthquakes, you should try to gain control over your fear. Whenever you hear such rumors and notice an increase in your fear, consider this an opportunity to beat your fear. If you can challenge your fear in such situations, you will have greater confidence in yourself.

Index

Printed in the United States
By Bookmasters